HEPATOCELLULAR CARCINOMA

HEPATOCELLULAR CARCINOMA

Diagnosis, investigation and management

Edited by

Anthony S.-Y. Leong

Professor of Anatomical Pathology
University of Newcastle
New South Wales, Australia
Medical Director, Hunter Area Pathology Services
New South Wales, Australia

Choong-Tsek Liew

Associate Professor, Department of Anatomical and Cellular Pathology
The Chinese University of Hong Kong
Shatin, Hong Kong

Joseph W.Y. Lau

Chairman and Professor, Department of Surgery
The Chinese University of Hong Kong
Shatin, Hong Kong

Philip J. Johnson

Chairman and Professor, Department of Clinical Oncology
The Chinese University of Hong Kong
Shatin, Hong Kong

A member of the Hodder Headline Group
LONDON • SYDNEY • AUCKLAND
Distributed in the US and Canada by
Oxford University Press, Inc., New York

First published in Great Britain in 1999 by
Arnold, a member of the Hodder Headline Group,
338 Euston Road, London NW1 3BH

http://www.arnoldpublishers.com

Distributed in the US and Canada by
Oxford University Press Inc.,
198 Madison Avenue, New York, NY10016
Oxford is a registered trademark of Oxford University Press

Whilst the advice and information in this book are believed to be true and
accurate at the date of going to press, neither the authors nor the publisher
can accept any legal responsibility or liability for any errors or omissions
that may be made. In particular (but without limiting the generality of the
preceding disclaimer) every effort has been made to check drug dosages;
however, it is still possible that errors have been missed. Furthermore,
dosage schedules are constantly being revised and new side-effects
recognized. For these reasons the reader is strongly urged to consult the
drug companies' printed instructions before administering any of the drugs
recommended in this book.

British Library Cataloguing in Publication Data
A catalogue record for this book is available from the British Library

Library of Congress Cataloging-in-Publication Data
A catalog record for this book is available from the Library of Congress

ISBN 0 340 74096 5

1 2 3 4 5 6 7 8 9 10

Typeset in 10 on 12 pt Palatino by Genesis Typesetting, Rochester, Kent
Printed and bound in Great Britain by The Bath Press, Bath, Avon

What do you think about this book? Or any other Arnold title?
Please send your comments to feedback.arnold@hodder.co.uk

CONTENTS

Color plates appear between pages 48 and 49.

Contributors   xi

Foreword   xiii

Preface   xv

1   Epidemiology, risk factors, etiology, premalignant lesions and carcinogenesis   1
     A.S.-Y. Leong

     1.1   Introduction   1
     1.2   Epidemiology   1
     1.3   Risk factors and etiology   3
     1.4   Cirrhosis   7
     1.5   Hepatitis B virus (HBV)   7
     1.6   Hepatitis C virus (HCV)   8
     1.7   Chemical and plant carcinogens   8
     1.8   Radiation and thorotrast   9
     1.9   Precancerous changes   9
     1.10 Carcinogenesis   12
          References   13

2   Presentation and approach to diagnosis   19
     P.J. Johnson

     2.1   Introduction   19
     2.2   The common modes of presentation   19
     2.3   Rarer modes of presentation   21
     2.4   Clinical features of specific subtypes   22
     2.5   HCC in the non-cirrhotic liver   23
     2.6   Should we be screening for HCC?   23
     2.7   Approach to diagnosis   25
     2.8   The initial assessment   26
     2.9   Further investigations   26
     2.10 Approach to the diagnosis of recurrent disease after surgical resection or
          transplantation   27
     2.11 Conclusions   28
          References   28

3   Tumor markers   31
    S.K.W. Ho and P.J. Johnson

    3.1   Introduction   31
    3.2   α-fetoprotein (AFP)   31
    3.3   Serum ferritin   36
    3.4   γ-glutamyltranspeptidase (γ-GTP) isoenzyme   37
    3.5   Alkaline phosphatase (ALP)   37
    3.6   Des-γ-carboxy prothrombin (DCP)   37
    3.7   α-1-antitrypsin (AAT)   38
    3.8   Aldolase A   38
    3.9   5′-nucleotide phosphodiesterase V (5′-NPD)   38
    3.10 Tissue polypeptide antigen (TPA)   38
    3.11 α-L-fucosidase   39
    3.12 Conclusions   39
          References   39

4   Diagnostic imaging   43
    S.C.-H. Yu, M.S.Y. Chan and J.W.Y. Lau

    4.1   Overview   43
    4.2   Radiography   45
    4.3   Ultrasonography   46
    4.4   Computed tomography   51
    4.5   Magnetic resonance imaging   56
    4.6   Hepatic angiography   60
    4.7   Nuclear imaging   65
    4.8   Image-guided percutaneous biopsy   66
    4.9   Diagnostic algorithm   67
          References   69

5   Fine needle aspiration cytology diagnosis of primary liver cancer   75
    A.R. Chang

    5.1   Introduction   75
    5.2   Cooperation of pathologist and radiologist   76
    5.3   Complications   76
    5.4   FNA appearance of cells found in the normal liver   77
    5.5   Findings in hepatocellular carcinoma   78
    5.6   Ancillary studies   85
    5.7   Concluding remarks   86
          References   86

6   Pathology of hepatocellular carcinoma   89
    C.-T. Liew and A.S.-Y. Leong

    6.1   Introduction   89
    6.2   Morphology   89

6.3 Natural history and spread   101
6.4 Combined hepatocellular carcinoma and cholangiocarcinoma   102
6.5 Liver carcinoma in children   102
     References   104

7 Needle biopsy diagnosis of hepatocellular carcinoma   107
   A.S.-Y. Leong and C.-T. Liew

7.1 Introduction   107
7.2 Problems associated with needle biopsies   107
7.3 Differential diagnoses   108
7.4 Malignant tumors   121
7.5 Special stains   123
7.6 Conclusions   124
     References   126

8 Molecular aspects   131
   J Y-H Chan, K.-W. Lo, H.-M. Li and C.-T. Liew

8.1 Introduction   131
8.2 Molecular analysis of hepadnaviruses infection and HCC   131
8.3 Interactions between chemical carcinogens, HBV and cellular genes   135
8.4 Alterations of proto-oncogenes, tumor suppressor genes and genes
     associated with proliferation and inflammation   136
8.5 Genomic instability and chromosomal alterations in HCC   137
8.6 Gene transfer and gene therapy in HCC   142
     References   142

9 Surgical management (including liver transplantation)   147
   J.W.Y. Lau and C.K. Leow

9.1 Surgical anatomy of the liver   147
9.2 Classification of hepatectomies   149
9.3 Preoperative investigations   151
9.4 Assessing the risk to the patient   152
9.5 Postoperative follow-up   155
9.6 Liver resection   155
9.7 Postoperative complications   160
9.8 Prognosis   162
9.9 Adjuvant therapy   164
9.10 Palliative resection   165
9.11 Liver transplantation for irresectable HCC   165
9.12 Conclusions   167
     References   167

10   Non-surgical management   173
     T.W.T. Leung

     10.1   Introduction   173
     10.2   Systemic chemotherapy   173
     10.3   Immunotherapy   175
     10.4   Regional intra-arterial treatment   176
     10.5   Radiotherapy   179
     10.6   Direct intralesional treatment   185
     10.7   Hepatic arterial embolization   186
            References   186

11   Management of specific tumor complications   193
     C.K. Leow and J.W.Y. Lau

     11.1   Spontaneous rupture   193
     11.2   Obstructive jaundice   195
     11.3   Variceal hemorrhage   197
     11.4   Paraneoplastic syndromes   197
     11.5   Conclusion   200
            References   200

12   Palliative care   205
     A.T.C. Chan and P.J. Johnson

     12.1   Introduction   205
     12.2   Clinical evaluation   205
     12.3   Specific measures   208
     12.4   Hospice care   210
            References   210

13   Hepatocellular carcinoma in other regions of the world   213

     Africa   213
     A.C. Paterson and K. Cooper

            References   215

     Europe   219
     P.J. Johnson

     13.1   Introduction   219
     13.2   Epidemiology   219
     13.3   Diagnosis, clinical features and presentation   221
     13.4   Treatment   222
     13.5   Prognosis   223
     13.6   Fibrolamellar hepatocellular carcinoma   223
            References   223

Japan   225
M. *Kage and M. Kojiro*

13.7   Incidence of hepatocellular carcinoma (HCC)   225
13.8   Etiologic factors in HCC in Japan   225
13.9   Clinical aspects   225
13.10 Pathomorphologic features   226
13.11 Pathomorphologic characteristics of early HCC   226
13.12 Histologic features of the non-cancerous liver tissue   229
       References   229

Korea   231
C. *Park and Y.-N. Park*

13.13 Introduction   231
13.14 Pathology   232
13.15 Genetic alterations   232
       References   233

Taiwan: Progress in the past decade (1988–1997)   235
J.-H. *Kao and D.-S. Chen*

13.16 Introduction   235
13.17 Etiology   235
13.18 Carcinogenesis   237
13.19 Diagnosis   239
13.20 Therapy   240
13.21 Childhood HCC   243
13.22 Prevention   243
       References   244

USA: with emphasis on fibrolamellar carcinoma (FLHCC)   251
J.R. *Craig*

13.23 Incidence   251
13.24 Etiology of HCC   251
13.25 Fibrolamellar HCC – an uncommon but distinctive HCC variant in the USA   252
       References   254

14 Future prospects   257
    P.J. *Johnson*

14.1   Introduction   257
14.2   Prospects for effective treatment   257
14.3   Prospects for prevention   265
14.4   Conclusions and predictions   267
       References   267

Index   271

CONTRIBUTORS

A.T.C. CHAN
Associate Professor
Department of Clinical Oncology
The Chinese University of Hong Kong
The Prince of Wales Hospital
Shatin, Hong Kong

J.Y.-H. CHAN
Associate Professor
Department of Clinical Oncology
The Sir Y.K. Pao Centre for Cancer
The Chinese University of Hong Kong
The Prince of Wales Hospital
Shatin, Hong Kong

M.S.Y. CHAN
Consultant Radiologist
Department of Diagnostic Radiology
The Prince of Wales Hospital
Shatin, Hong Kong

A.R. CHANG
Associate Professor
Department of Anatomical and Cellular
  Pathology
The Chinese University of Hong Kong
The Prince of Wales Hospital
Shatin, Hong Kong

D.-S. CHEN
Professor of Medicine
Director, Hepatitis Research Centre
National Taiwan University Hospital
Taipei, Taiwan

K. COOPER
Professor and Head
Department of Anatomical Pathology
School of Pathology
South African Institute for Medical Research
  and University of the Witwatersrand
Johannesburg, South Africa

J.R. CRAIG
Medical Director Oncology Services
Director of Laboratories
St Jude Medical Center
Fullerton, California 92834
USA

S.K.W. HO
Scientific Officer
Department of Clinical Oncology
The Prince of Wales Hospital
Shatin, Hong Kong

P.J. JOHNSON
Chairman and Professor
Department of Clinical Oncology
The Chinese University of Hong Kong
The Prince of Wales Hospital
Shatin, Hong Kong
Director
The Sir Y.K. Pao Centre for Cancer
The Prince of Wales Hospital
Shatin, Hong Kong

M. KAGE
Associate Professor
First Department of Pathology
Kurume University School of Medicine
67 Asahi-Machi, Kurume-Shi
Fukuoka-Ken, 830 Japan

J.-H. KAO
Associate Professor
Department of Internal Medicine and
    Graduate Institute of Clinical Medicine
National Taiwan University College of
    Medicine and National Taiwan University
    Hospital
Taipei 10016, Taiwan

M. KOJIRO
Chairman and Professor
First Department of Pathology
Kurume University School of Medicine
67 Asahi-Machi, Kurume-Shi
Fukuoka-Ken, 830 Japan

J.W.Y. LAU
Chairman and Professor
Department of Surgery
The Chinese University of Hong Kong
The Prince of Wales Hospital
Shatin, Hong Kong

A.S.-Y. LEONG
Professor of Anatomical Pathology
University of Newcastle
New South Wales, Australia
Medical Director
Hunter Area Pathology Services
New South Wales, Australia

C.K. LEOW
Head and Associate Professor
Division of Hepatobiliary and Pancreatic
    Surgery
Department of Surgery
The National University of Singapore
National University Hospital
Singapore 119074

T.W.T. LEUNG
Associate Professor
Department of Clinical Oncology
The Chinese University of Hong Kong
The Prince of Wales Hospital
Shatin, Hong Kong

H.-M. LI
Research Associate
Department of Anatomic and Cellular
    Pathology
The Chinese University of Hong Kong
The Prince of Wales Hospital
Shatin, Hong Kong

C.-T. LIEW
Associate Professor
Department of Anatomical and Cellular
    Pathology
The Chinese University of Hong Kong
The Prince of Wales Hospital
Shatin, Hong Kong

K.W. LO
Scientific Officer
Department of Anatomical and Cellular
    Pathology
The Chinese University of Hong Kong
The Prince of Wales Hospital
Shatin, Hong Kong

A.C. PATERSON
Professor and Deputy Head
Department of Anatomical Pathology
School of Pathology
South African Institute for Medical Research
    and University of the Witwatersrand
Johannesburg, South Africa

C. PARK
Professor
Department of Pathology
Yonsei University College of Medicine
Seoul, Korea

Y.-N. PARK
Department of Pathology
Yonsei University College of Medicine
Seoul, Korea

S.C.-H. YU
Senior Medical Officer
Department of Diagnostic Radiology and
    Organ Imaging
The Prince of Wales Hospital
Shatin, Hong Kong

FOREWORD

When I returned from the UK to take up the Foundation Chair in Surgery at the Chinese University of Hong Kong, I was appalled at the devastation caused by hepatocellular carcinoma. The disease runs a galloping course among young men in the prime of life. The average survival from diagnosis to death is only 10 weeks. Despite my best efforts at surgical extirpation the results were, to say the least, disappointing. Indeed, some of my close friends and dear colleagues have succumbed to this terrible disease. It became obvious to me that a multidisciplinary approach was essential to combat the problem. Accordingly a Hepatoma Clinic was established at the Prince of Wales Hospital where hepatologists, oncologists, radiologists and surgeons saw patients with hepatocellular cancer together. In addition, we gathered a dedicated group of pathologists, cytologists, physicists, virologists and molecular biologists to attack the problem on the laboratory front.

I stepped down from the surgical front line with more than a tinge of regret, but as I reflect on my sojourn in the surgical arena in Hong Kong I am gratified to note that some in-roads have been made in the fight against hepatocellular carcinoma. Although the war against liver cancer is far from won, there has been significant successes on several fronts. Earlier diagnosis is now possible with the screening of high-risk populations. More accurate serological markers have been identified. Advances in surgery, anesthesia and intensive care have made liver resection, even in the cirrhotic patient, a routine operation with negligible mortality. In in-operable cases, new modalities such as internal irradiation and targeted chemotherapy offer a glimmer of hope. Eradication of hepatocellular carcinoma associated with hepatitis B may be within reach in a few decades with the introduction of mass immunization, but the emergence of tumors associated with other forms of viral hepatitis will create new challenges.

We were fortunate at the Prince of Wales Hospital that a talented group of individuals with different backgrounds and training could work as a harmonious and productive team. It has been my privilege to be part of that team. I am delighted that the same team has chronicled the advances made in the war against hepatocellular cancer over the past decade. I hope this book will serve as a stimulation and encouragement to them and to others in the field.

A.K.C. Li
MA, MD, BChir (Cantab), FRCS (England),
FRCS (Edinburgh), FRACS, FACS,
Hon.FPCS, Hon.FRCS (Glasgow),
Hon.FRSM
Professor of Surgery and Vice-Chancellor
Chinese University of Hong Kong

PREFACE

Hepatocellular carcinoma is a relatively uncommon disease in Western countries but its worldwide incidence is very large with a concentration in regions such as the Far East, including China, Japan, Taiwan, Hong Kong and South-East Asia, Southern Africa, and Southern and Eastern Europe. The magnitude of the problem is highlighted by the comparative incidence of hepatocellular carcinoma of 150 and 28.1 per 100 000 population in Taiwan and Singapore respectively, and that of 1–3 per 100 000 population incidence in Australia, North America and Western Europe. In countries such as Taiwan, Singapore, Japan and Hong Kong, hepatocellular carcinoma ranks among the top five leading causes of cancer death and therefore, it represents a major health problem.

Surgical resection presently remains the only form of curative therapy available, with many refinements being made in surgical management. However, recent years have witnessed a tremendous advancement in our knowledge of the etiology and pathogenesis of hepatocellular carcinoma, and major strides have been made with diagnostic and investigative procedures to allow the earlier identification of these tumors. Such achievements, largely the result of advanced imaging technology and other improved diagnostic procedures, are well reflected in the introduction of the concept of small hepatocellular carcinomas whose definition over the years has continued to change in terms of size, starting with a size < 5 cm, to the current definition of <2 cm according to the Liver Cancer Study Group of Japan.

Advances have also been made in chemotherapy and other non-surgical management regimes, such as transcatheter arterial chemoembolization (TACE), and greater attention has been paid to the often neglected area of palliative and terminal care of patients with this form of cancer. The knowledge gained of the etiology and pathogenesis of this aggressive neoplasm has been directed to screening and prevention. In-roads have been made at the molecular level, in particular the interaction of established etiological agents and various cancer-related genes such as the tumor suppresser gene *p53*. Together with the recognition of the hepatitis C virus as a leading cause of cirrhosis and hepatocellular carcinoma in some countries such as Japan, such advances have provided greater insights into hepatocarcinogenesis.

It is clear that the management of hepatocellular carcinoma can be successful only with a multidisciplinary approach and this book represents the extensive experience of such a team at the Chinese University of Hong Kong at the Prince of Wales Hospital. The group presents their cumulative local experience and provides a comprehensive update of the state-of-the-art in diagnosis, investigation and management of hepatocellular carcinoma. We are fortunate also to have contributions from other international experts in the field who provide reviews on the situation in their own countries.

The text is organized in a logical and systematic manner, allowing ready reference to both the specialist and generalist in all clinical and laboratory disciplines who deal with patients with hepatocellular carcinoma.

A.S.-Y. Leong
C.-T. Liew
J.W.Y. Lau
P.J. Johnson
Shatin, Hong Kong
1998

EPIDEMIOLOGY, RISK FACTORS, ETIOLOGY, PREMALIGNANT LESIONS AND CARCINOGENESIS

1

A.S.-Y. Leong

1.1 INTRODUCTION

This book is concerned with primary liver cancer (hepatoma, hepatocellular carcinoma) and the many related advances made during the recent years. Progress has largely been in our understanding of carcinogenesis as well as the development of more rapid and sensitive laboratory and radiological diagnostic procedures. This advancement has been the result of technological achievements. Newer molecular techniques have also allowed the development of hepatitis B virus (HBV) vaccines, putting into practice much of the groundwork laid in the preceding decade. The identification of the hepatitis C virus as a major causative agent of cirrhosis in some countries such as Japan, and the slow but progressive understanding of its natural history have provided many new insights into its impact on liver disease and cancer worldwide.

1.2 EPIDEMIOLOGY

The remarkable geographical distribution of hepatocellular carcinoma (HCC) was found to have no association with race or genetic factors but to be more closely related to environmental agents, particularly the prevalence of chronic HBV infection.

In many of the countries with a high incidence of HCC cancer statistics are far from complete, so that much of the data concerning this form of cancer must represent underestimates (Okuda *et al.* 1993). This notwithstanding, liver cancer is one of the most common internal malignancies worldwide, with an occurrence of at least 1 million new cases annually. It is the seventh most common malignant tumor in males and the ninth in females. The outcome of HCC is uniformly poor in most countries, with the overwhelming majority of patients dying in a few weeks, at best, months; the death toll from this disease is considerable (Omata, 1987; Rustgi, 1987; Munoz and Bosch, 1988; Simonetti *et al.*, 1991).

The strikingly uneven geographic distribution of liver cancer worldwide is reflected in Fig. 1.1 which shows countries grouped into those with high, intermediate and low incidence rates. A fourth group with poorly documented cancer statistics is also shown. The highest incidence is encountered in the countries of South-East Asia including Taiwan, Korea, Thailand, Hong Kong, Singapore, Malaysia and China, especially in the southeast, and those of tropical Africa. The incidence in Cambodia, Vietnam and Burma is suspected of being equally high, but the countries lack proper documentation to ascertain this fact. The incidence of HCC worldwide

Hepatocellular Carcinoma: Diagnosis, investigation and management. Edited by Anthony S.-Y. Leong, Choong-Tsek Liew, Joseph W.Y. Lau and Philip J. Johnson. Published in 1999 by Arnold, London. ISBN 0 340 74096 5.

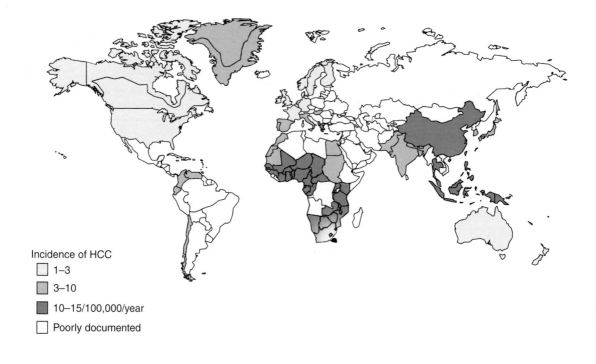

Incidence of HCC
- 1–3
- 3–10
- 10–15/100,000/year
- Poorly documented

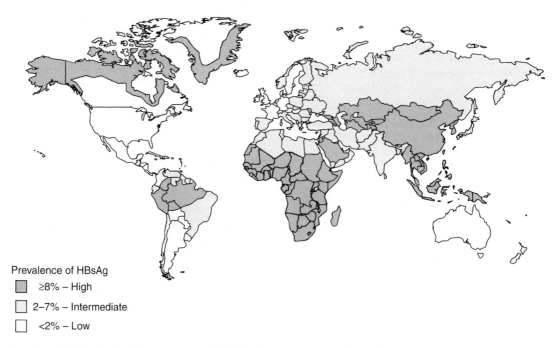

Prevalence of HBsAg
- ≥8% – High
- 2–7% – Intermediate
- <2% – Low

Fig. 1.1 Worldwide incidence of chronic HBV infection compared with the distribution of hepatocellular carcinoma. (Courtesy of Dr J.S.L. Tam, Hong Kong.)

parallels the incidence of HBV infection as shown in Fig. 1.1. In Asia, the incidence of HCC is about 10–20 per 100 000 population compared with that of 1–3 per 100 000 population in Australia, North America and Europe (Wu, 1983). There is also a variation in prevalence among the Asian countries, with Taiwan having an incidence of 150 per 100 000 (Rustgi, 1987), while that of Singapore is 28 per 100 000 population (Oon *et al.*, 1989). In some countries of high incidence such as Mozambique, liver cancer is the commonest of all cancers. The lowest rates of HCC are found in Western countries, South America and the Indian subcontinent, with intermediate rates in Japan, the Middle East and the Mediterranean countries (Munoz and Linsell, 1982; Rustgi, 1987; Munoz and Bosch, 1988; Bosch and Munoz, 1989; Lau and Lai, 1990; Simonetti *et al.*, 1991).

In general, with successive generations, the incidence of HCC in migrant populations slowly equates to that of the local population. For example, Indians who have settled in Hong Kong and Singapore have acquired incidence rates close to those of the rest of the population and approximately double those of their home country. The tumor incidence has decreased slowly among the Japanese and Korean migrants who have settled in California and Hawaii although the Chinese seem to be at high risk, whether they live in Hong Kong, Singapore, Shanghai, or elsewhere. In contrast, whites seemingly have a low incidence, even when they live in areas of high prevalence of HCC such as South-East Asia or Africa. This has been attributed to the continuance of the lifestyle and environment of their home countries. Much of the variation in incidence rates among migrant populations is paralleled by the HBV carrier rates in these populations (Rustgi, 1987; Lau and Lai, 1990; Simonetti et al., 1991; Tong and Hwang, 1994).

While HCC is rare in Western countries, the magnitude of the problem is reflected by the uniformly dismal outlook. In the USA, of an estimated 11 600 new cases per year of liver and biliary tract carcinoma, the annual death rate was 9300 (Lefkowitch, 1981). In Birmingham, UK, primary liver tumors comprised <0.5% of all cancers but the 5-year survival for HCC was nil and only slightly better for bile duct carcinoma (Waterhouse, 1974). This improved only marginally by 1982, but the results for patients <45 years of age were better, with 5-year survivals of 12 and 14% respectively for males and females (Toms, 1982).

In Africa and South-East Asia, an estimated 1 million deaths annually occur from hepatocellular carcinoma alone (Rustgi, 1987). In Hong Kong, the mortality rate for primary liver tumors (both HCC and intrahepatic bile duct carcinoma) was 19.5 per 100 000 population in 1991, second only to lung carcinoma (Director of Hospital Services Hong Kong, 1992).

1.3 RISK FACTORS AND ETIOLOGY

The marked differences in incidence rates of HCC worldwide has spawned tremendous interest in epidemiological factors and related etiologic agents. Besides variations in tumor incidence in migrant populations and geographic regions, lesser variations have been observed in racially homogenous countries such as Greece, Spain and Italy. These have been explained by differences in HBV carriage, alcohol consumption and smoking, or variable levels of exposure to hepatotoxins. For example, Switzerland, a highly developed and industrialized country, has a higher than average liver cancer rate compared with other European nations, raising the possibility of exposure to hepatotoxic chemicals. In China, high mortality rates from HCC have been reported from coastal and riverside areas with stagnant and polluted water supplies. In a massive survey of 840 million people in China from 1972 to 1977, it was found that the main endemic areas for liver cancer were along the south-east coast, particularly the deltas, valleys and islands. In these areas, the standardized mortality rate was >60 per

100 000 per year compared with <10% of this figure in low-incidence areas of the country (Yu, 1985). In Mozambique, a nine-fold difference between the coastal and inland region has been reported. Movement from a rural to an urban environment has apparently also been associated with increased risk in countries like Norway and Poland, whereas the reverse seems to be true in South Africa (Rustgi, 1987; Munoz and Bosch, 1988; Bosch and Munoz, 1989; Simonetti *et al.*, 1991). The effects of environmental changes have been attributed to differences in levels of exposure to hepatotoxins and improving living standards.

Improved living standards can produce paradoxical effects. While it may reduce the incidence of liver cancer in some communities, studies on time trends show a steady but indisputable increase in liver cancer rates. In the National Registry of Autopsies which records almost 90% of all autopsies performed in Japan, the rate of HCC has gradually increased from 1.91% among 19 356 autopsies in 1958–59 to 7.66% in 1986–87 (Okuda *et al.*, 1993). Similar increasing trends were demonstrated in Los Angeles where the rate rose from 0.15% in 1918–53 to 1.48% in 1964–83 (Craig *et al.*, 1989). There appears to be a general increase in the incidence of liver cancer throughout the world. According to one cancer registry study, there was an increase in incidence rate among males in 24 of 37 countries and among females in 26 of 37 countries (Saracci and Repetto, 1980). In Florence, Italy, an eight-fold increase was reported; in Shanghai, between 1959 and 1976, cancer mortality increased about 2-fold (Yu, 1985) and in Mexico a 2-fold increase was recorded over a 25-year period (Cortes-Espinosa *et al.*, 1997).

It is very unlikely that liver cancer has a single causative agent. More probably, like other carcinomas, this tumor is the result of a complex interaction between multiple etiologic factors and through a multistep mechanism.

1.3.1 AGE AND GENDER

Generally, the incidence of HCC increases with age in all populations, tending to fall a little in the elderly. There is a tendency for the age peak to be inversely related to the frequency of the tumor in various regions, i.e. in high incidence areas, the peak is in the youngest, whereas in areas of low incidence, liver cancer occurs most frequently in the elderly. For example, in Mozambique where 50% of patients with the tumor are <30 years old, the incidence of liver cancer among males aged 25–34 years is >500-fold that of the same age group in Western countries compared with only a 15-fold difference in the elderly. Similar age differences are observed among South-East Asian migrants and whites in California, and blacks and whites with liver cancer in South Africa.

Liver cancer occurs in adolescence and childhood and has been reported in patients as young as 2 years of age in Hong Kong (Fan and Wong, 1996). This is not unexpected in high incidence areas where the tumor is associated with the acquisition of chronic HBV infection early in life (Moore *et al.*, 1997). Congenital abnormalities and inborn errors of metabolism may account for some cases of childhood liver cancer, especially in Western countries (Bianchi, 1993). Other liver tumors include hepatoblastoma and fibrolamellar carcinomas, the latter having a recognized predilection for the young (Weinberg and Finegold, 1983).

With practically no exceptions, HCC is four-to-eight times more common in males than females in low and high prevalence regions respectively. Findings in experimental animals suggest that sex hormones and/or hormone receptors may play a role in the development of liver cancer. Experimental tumors in rats and mice can be more easily induced in males than females and orchidectomy reduces the carcinogenic effects of chemicals in male rats to the level found in females. The implantation of stilbestrol or estradiol pellets produces a similar but less marked effect (Newberne and Butler, 1978; Grasso, 1987). Androgen receptors have been demonstrated in hepatocellular carcinoma, leading to the suggestion that this tumor is androgen-dependent; however, it is controversial whether androgen receptors exist in the normal liver (Nagasue *et al.*, 1985). Liver adenomas associated with androgen or anabolic steroids (Kosaka *et al.*, 1996) may regress after withdrawal of the drug (See, *et al.*, 1992), a phenomenon also seen in tumors induced by oral contraceptive steroids.

Cytosolic and nuclear assays show elevation of androgen receptors in most liver cancers, with variable but generally normal or lower levels of estrogen receptors (Nagasue *et al.*, 1990; Eagon *et al.*, 1991). The use of several therapeutic compounds that interfere with hormone action and receptors have produced variable and disappointing results (Carr and van Thiel, 1990; d'Arville and Johnson, 1990). It is highly unlikely that sex steroids are carcinogenic on their own and they are more likely to act in combination with other factors as promotors of abnormal growth. The significantly higher frequency of liver cancer in males may be the cumulative result of other associated factors such as the increased incidence of cirrhosis in males and their greater propensity to smoke and consume alcohol. The rate of DNA synthesis in cirrhotic livers, a factor related to the risk of carcinoma in such livers, is higher in men than in women (Tarao *et al.*, 1993).

1.3.2 GENETICS AND CONGENITAL ABNORMALITIES

A genetic predisposition to cirrhosis and liver cancer has been shown in inbred stains of mice, but this has not been demonstrated in man. There have been reported family clusters with this tumor. Some 100 cases of liver carcinoma have been reported in children in seven families for up to three generations (Leuschner *et al.*, 1988; Cheah *et al.*, 1990):

however, these were invariably associated with chronic HBV infection as shown in 95 cases. Analysis of major histocompatibility complex antigens among patients and controls in both South Africa and China has not revealed a link with HBV infection or liver cancer.

There are rare examples of liver carcinoma occurring in association with conditions which have a genetic, congenital or metabolic origin. HCC has been documented rarely in familial polyposis coli (Laferia *et al.*, 1988), ataxia telangiectasia (Weinstein *et al.*, 1985), a type of familial cholestatic cirrhosis, biliary atresia, congenital hepatic fibrosis, neurofibromatosis, *situs inversus* and the fetal alcohol syndrome (Weinberg and Finegold, 1983; McGoldrick *et al.*, 1986).

Among the inborn errors of metabolism, the chronic form of hereditary tyrosinemia carries the highest risk of malignancy with one report describing 16 of 43 patients developing liver cancer (Weinberg *et al.*, 1976). These patients show a progression from micro- to macronodular cirrhosis, dysplasia and eventually HCC. Hepatectomy and liver transplantation before 2 years of age is now the recommended treatment (Dehner *et al.*, 1989). Type I glycogen storage disease may be associated with adenomas but carcinoma has rarely been reported (Bianchi, 1993). Hepatic porphyria of both intermittent and cutanea tarda types have a 61-fold increased risk for HCC (Kauppinen and Mustajoki, 1988).

HCC was the cause of death in 22% of patients with genetic hemochromatosis, representing a 219-fold risk over the general population (Purtilo and Gottlieb, 1973; Niederau *et al.*, 1985; Gangaidzo and Gordeuk, 1995). The disease commonly affects males and results in cirrhosis with its attendant risk of cancer. Although it has been suggested that iron may have a carcinogenic action through the production of free radicals (Okada, 1996), this has not been substantiated. Wilson's disease, another autosomal recessive disorder, also tends to affect males and it produces cirrhosis through accumulation of copper in the liver (Chu and Hung, 1993). A few cases of liver carcinoma have been reported in this disorder, all accompanied by cirrhosis. Rarely, liver cancer has complicated biliary cirrhosis, another condition in which excess copper accumulates in the liver.

α_1-Antitrypsin (α_1AT) deficiency is associated with jaundice and cirrhosis in early childhood, and with pulmonary emphysema and cirrhosis in adult life. α_1AT is an inhibitor of serine proteinases, which include trypsin, chymotrypsin and leukocyte elastase. The enzyme is synthesized in the liver and released into the blood. In α_1AT deficiency, the enzyme continues to be produced in the liver but is not secreted, accumulating as PAS-positive, diastase-resistant globules in the hepatocytes. There are up to 75 allelic variants of the Pi (protease inhibitor) genes, which control this enzyme. PiZ is the variant associated with low levels of serum α_1AT and it occurs as a homozygous and the more common heterozygous form. The mechanisms behind the association between α_1AT deficiency and HCC are still unknown. The α_1AT globules can be observed in the cells of both liver adenomas and carcinomas of patients who do not have the PiZ gene and who show no evidence of α_1AT deficiency. Such cases suggest that the failure to release the enzyme may have a promoting effect on the tumor by allowing proteases to destroy contact inhibition between transformed liver cells (Crystal, 1990). However, other exogenous factors may be operative, as the association with HCC appears to be statistically significant only for males (Eriksson *et al.*, 1986).

Membranous obstruction of the hepatic portion of the inferior vena cava, a type of Budd–Chiari syndrome, has been associated with HCC. While this condition is uncommon in the West, it is seen in Japan, India and among the blacks of South Africa. The lesion may be congenital, such as due to malformation of the Eustachian valve, or acquired due to mechanical injury, infection or thrombosis.

In one study from Japan, 29 of 71 cases (41%) developed HCC, and in South Africa 20% of all cases with HCC showed the lesion at autopsy and 47.5% of patients with radiologically demonstrable caval obstructions subsequently developed carcinoma (Simpson, 1982). While the mechanism causing carcinoma is not known, the passive congestion which results may act as a stimulus to liver cell regeneration.

1.3.3   OTHER FACTORS

While malnutrition is common in many of the geographic areas with a high incidence of liver cancer, the association is more likely due to HBV infection and exposure to hepatotoxins that are also prevalent in these areas. Indeed, existing information indicates that over-nourishment is more likely to promote neoplastic growth as shown by the association of a high intake of animal fat and cholesterol, and obesity, with breast, endometrial, colonic and pancreatic cancer (Willett and MacMahon, 1984). Prolonged parenteral nutrition in infancy may be complicated by cholestasis, liver fibrosis and cirrhosis, with rare cases of liver cancer occurring in such infants (Patterson *et al.*, 1985).

There is no evidence to link parasitic infections with HCC although the relationship between cholangiocarcinoma and liver flukes is well recognized (Ishii *et al.*, 1994). It is possible that certain types of medication may expedite hepatocarcinogenesis, as suggested by anecdotal case reports that have incriminated azathioprine, methotrexate, danazol, tamoxifen and cytoproterone acetate. There are also very rare cases of carcinoma developing in various forms of chronic liver disease including autoimmune chronic hepatitis (Jakovibits, 1981), and primary biliary cirrhosis (Melia, 1985).

Chronic alcohol abuse often complicates HCC, particularly in low-incidence areas where HBV infection is uncommon. While alcohol has been incriminated in the causation of carcinomas in the larynx, mouth and esophagus, it has never been shown to have a carcinogenic effect in hepatocytes. It is likely that its role is that of co-carcinogen with other agents such as HBV, HCV, hepatotoxins and tobacco (Saunders and Latt, 1993; Nalpas *et al.*, 1995; Schiff 1997). In addition, it is a cirrhosis-causing agent. Alcohol may also have a role through its induction of the microsomal cytochrome P450 system, which is responsible for the metabolic activation and inactivation of diverse chemical carcinogens including aflatoxins. The cytochrome P450 system is also highly inducible by smoking, which is a significant risk factor for HCC. Smoking also has a synergistic effect with alcohol and chronic HBV infection (Austin *et al.*, 1986; Trichopoulos *et al.*, 1987; Naccarato and Farinati, 1991).

1.4 CIRRHOSIS

A rare strain of rat was established in Japan in which severe hepatic necrosis occurred spontaneously. The rats that survived this episode invariably developed HCC after a period of chronic liver disease. Almost any form of chronic liver disease that leads to cirrhosis may be complicated by HCC. Cirrhosis is the most common association of HCC. It is the underlying disease in 80–90% of patients with primary liver cancer in most countries, non-alcoholic posthepatitic cirrhosis being most common. Cirrhosis, whatever the cause, is a precancerous condition.

It has been shown that cirrhotic livers with large nodules and thin stromas are more commonly associated with HCC than livers with small nodules and thick stroma (Shikata, 1976). It is suggested that those with large nodules have greater regenerative activities, with increased DNA synthesis in hepatocytes and more rearrangements of DNA sequences. Similarly, a higher incidence of carcinoma was noted among patients with alcoholic cirrhosis who had abstained and whose micronodular cirrhosis had turned macronodular. With abstinence, there is a surge of regenerative activity that transforms small nodules to large ones. Clinically, patients with alcoholic cirrhosis seldom develop carcinoma while they are still imbibing.

The actual role of cirrhosis in the pathogenesis of HCC remains speculative. Cirrhosis is clearly not a prerequisite for carcinoma and the latter is not an inevitable consequence. The two share a common cause, although some causes of cirrhosis (e.g. chronic HBV infection) are associated with a higher risk of carcinoma than others (e.g. alcohol).

1.5 HEPATITIS B VIRUS (HBV)

An etiologic association between HBV infection and HCC has been clearly established although the relationship is complex and may involve the role of age and sex, and risk factors such as alcohol, aflatoxins and smoking. HBV carrier rates parallel the incidence of carcinoma (Fig. 1.1). More than 250 million people worldwide are chronically infected with HBV and have a 200-fold increased risk of developing HCC. Variations in tumor incidence within a region generally relate to differences in carrier rates of the virus. When pockets of high incidence of HCC occur in areas of otherwise low incidence, they are usually confined to migrants with high carrier rates of HBV. The risk of becoming a carrier and the subsequent development of carcinoma is associated with the acquisition of the infection at birth or early in childhood, attributed to the immaturity of the immune system in this group. This risk falls to about 40% in those infected in childhood, whereas those infected as adults have a 10% risk of the carrier state (Melnick, 1983; Beasley and Hwang, 1984). Familiar clustering of HCC, when observed, is commonly due to HBV-related disease due to vertical transmission of the virus.

Between 1975 and 1986, prospective studies were conducted on 22 707 men in Taiwan of whom 15.2% were HBsAg-positive, 9.9% were anti-HBc-positive, 68.6% were anti-HBs-positive and 5.6% were negative for all three HBV markers. At the end of the study period, 152 of 161 cases of HCC developed in HBsAg carriers and nine in those positive for anti-HBc, seven of whom were also positive for anti-HBs. There were no cancers of HCC among the men who were negative for all three markers for HBV infection.

The relationship of other hepatitis viruses to liver cancer is less clear. There is an obligatory symbiosis between hepatitis D virus (HDV) and HBV making evaluation of its role in hepatocarcinogenesis difficult; however, there is evidence to indicate that HDV infection places an additional burden on the already damaged liver, thus contributing to the risk of carcinoma. In the case of hepatitis A and hepatitis E, infection does not lead to chronic liver disease and has no carcinogenic potential.

While HBV antigens can readily be demonstrated by immunostaining in the non-tumorous hepatocytes of carriers and patients with cirrhosis and HCC, they are less commonly found in tumor cells. Nonetheless, a human hepatoma cell line has been shown to produce HBsAg and transplanted tumor in nude mice has resulted in the production of all three major antigens of HBV as well as the DNA polymerase (Matsui *et al.*, 1986). HBV cannot be visualized in tumor cells in a replicative form but it can be demonstrated, once integrated, by molecular techniques. Integration of HBV DNA precedes the development of HCC. It occurs in the majority of tumors from both HBsAg-positive and -negative patients, but more frequently after replication of the virus has declined or ceased and the patient has become seronegative. When HBV DNA was used as a genetic marker, identical patterns of integration were found in multifocal hepatomas, and in primary tumors and their metastases. These findings indicated origin from a single clone of cells in which HBV integration had occurred before malignant transformation (Blum *et al.*, 1987; Govindarajan *et al.*, 1988).

1.6   HEPATITIS C VIRUS (HCV)

In some countries like Japan, HCV has emerged as a very common cause of chronic liver disease. Previously known as non-A, non-B hepatitis virus, antibodies to HCV have been found in as high as 76% of patients with HCC in Japan, Italy and Spain (Simonetti, 1989) and in 36% in the USA. The natural history of HCV is such that the disease appears deceptively benign in the early stages but ends up with cirrhosis and HCC (Colombo, 1996; Sharara *et al.*, 1996). The HCV carrier rate among Japanese blood donors is 1.2% and is lower in Western countries. At present, it is not known if HCV is integrated into the host chromosome. It may have an interaction with HBV or may act by simply causing cirrhosis but currently there is no evidence that it is oncogenic. HCV is proving important as a cause of chronic liver disease, cirrhosis and HCC as HBV in some countries (Yu and Chen, 1994; National Institutes of Health, 1997; Tibbs 1997).

1.7   CHEMICAL AND PLANT CARCINOGENS

Improvement in living standards is accompanied by the use of a wide variety of chemicals, in items such as foodstuffs, cleaning reagents, cosmetics and pharmaceuticals, as well as in farming, plastics, chemical, rubber, textiles and other industries. Many of these are toxic to the liver and have carcinogenic and mutagenic potential in the experimental situation. A number of pesticides, such as DDT, which was once widely used, were found to be carcinogenic. Other chemicals like nitrites, hydrocarbons, solvents, orgnochlorine pesticides, primary metals and polychlorinated biphenyls have also been implicated (Forman, 1991). In China, farmers in a newly reclaimed coastal region in the county of Qidong had difficulty in getting water from the ground and drank ditch water suspected of being contaminated with pesticides used in farming. A crude death rate from HCC of 62–101 per 100 000 population was observed among those who drank stagnant ditch water compared with 0–11.9 deaths per 100 000 among well water drinkers. When the government instituted the sinking of many more wells in the county, there was a 20–30% reduction in the frequency of liver cancer (Su, 1979).

While a vast array of naturally occurring substances which can be found in drinking water, foodstuffs, native and herbal remedies have been suspected carcinogens, most have not been proven to be so. Among these substances are the pyrrolizidine alkaloids found in species of *Senecio*, *Crotalaria* and *Heliotropium* plants, comfrey, which is used as a green vegetable, tea and animal fodder, and cycads which contain the glycoside cycasins have been shown to be hepatotoxic and can produce liver tumors in many animals. Other substances like tannic acid in tea and coffee, and safrole in oils used for medicines and flavoring are carcinogenic in rodents.

Aflatoxins in large doses produce severe liver injury. The fungi *Aspergillus flavus* and *A. parasiticus* produce two groups of aflatoxins, designated B_1, B_2, G_1 and G_2 because of their blue or yellow-green autofluorescence. Aflatoxin B_1 is the most hepatoxic although to be carcinogenic it appears that chronic exposure to the mycotoxin is necessary. Chronic feeding of aflatoxin B_1 induces liver cancer in many animal species, and in the monkey it produces not only HCC but also cholangiocarcinoma, pancreatic cancer, hemangioma and osteosarcoma. The fungi grow readily on grains, peanuts and food products in the humid tropical and subtropical regions, *A. flavus* being the most common cause of food spoilage in the tropics. Such regions also tend to have a high level of HBV infection so that epidemiologic analysis is made difficult.

In experimental animals, a carcinogenic effect has been demonstrated for other mycotoxins like sterigmatocystin, produced by *Aspergillus*, and luteoskyrin and cyclochlorotine, metabolites of *Penicillium islandicum* found in spoilt rice and grain, but some of these have not been shown to be a risk in man. The intake of aflatoxin B_1 by people of ten villages in China was shown to correlate with HCC mortality rates and at least six epidemiological studies have shown that people who drink pond-ditch water contaminated with the blue-green algal toxin microcystin experience higher HCC mortality rates, the toxin causing hepatic hemorrhage and necrosis (Yu, 1995). The ability to measure aflatoxin bound to serum albumin has shown that exposure can occur throughout the life span of the individual, including the perinatal period, in high incidence areas (Wild *et al.*, 1993).

1.8 RADIATION AND THOROTRAST

There was no evidence of increased liver cancer among victims of the Hiroshima and Nagasaki atomic bombing although there is good evidence that internal α and β radiation is carcinogenic. Thorotrast, colloidal thorium dioxide, which was used as an angiographic agent in 1930s, emits high levels of α, β and γ radiation with a long physical and biologic half-life. It accumulates in macrophages of the reticuloendothelial system, particularly the liver, and produces hepatic fibrosis, angiosarcoma, cholangiocarcinoma and HCC. In Western countries angiosarcoma was the more common tumor associated with Thorotrast, but in Japan, both cholangiocarcinoma and HCC were more common. It took a longer interval for HCC to develop compared to the other two tumors, requiring at least 10 years after deposition of Thorotrast in the liver (Okuda *et al.*, 1993).

1.9 PRECANCEROUS CHANGES

In contrast with other human carcinomas, the concept of premalignant lesions of the liver and cellular alterations preceding fully developed HCC has been controversial. Recent advances in imaging techniques, such as high-resolution ultrasonography, allow the detection, biopsy and resection of nodular lesions

<1 cm diameter, and liver transplantation occasionally provides explanted liver tissues with premalignant or early malignant lesions for more exacting morphological and molecular analysis.

The diagnostic criteria for early HCC include nuclear crowding, increased cytoplasmic basophilia and microacinar formation (Kondo *et al.*, 1987). These criteria have been successfully employed for evaluating ultrasound-guided needle biopsies of nodular hepatic lesions (Kondo *et al.*, 1989). Tumor size is another important criterion as a study involving 58 resected small nodular lesions revealed every lesion >1.5 cm in diameter to be an early carcinoma. However, the sizes of benign and early malignant lesions may overlap and adenomas can be >2 cm in diameter. The liver cell populations that precede the development of overt metastasizing HCC are morphologically characterized by hyperplastic expansive collections of hepatocytes which may have clear, basophilic or acidophilic cytoplasm or may show pleomorphism and megalocytosis. The gradual loss of adult liver enzymes and the appearance of fetal enzymes accompany these features. Such changes are recognized as dysplastic nodules (adenomatous hyperplasia) and liver cell dysplasia.

1.9.1 DYSPLASTIC NODULE (DN)

Dysplastic nodules and other premalignant states are discussed in further detail in Chapter 8.

The dysplastic nodule (DN) has also been known as adenomatous hyperplasia, hepatocellular pseudotumor, macroregenerative nodule, adenomatous regeneration, adenomatous hyperplastic nodule and borderline nodule. It is defined as a nodule that is usually, but not always, found in the setting of cirrhosis and it is distinct from the surrounding parenchyma in terms of size, color, texture and by bulging beyond the cut surface of the liver (Thiese, 1995). These nodules grow to a large size and appear tumor-like, and reported examples of DN have ranged from 1 to 15 cm, most measuring 2–3 cm. Such nodules are readily detected by modern imaging techniques and usually occur in individuals being screened for HCC. They may occur in the presence of established HCC and are often larger and more numerous in this situation. The term 'dysplastic nodule' does not refer to a nodule made up of dysplastic hepatocytes of small or large cell type, in fact, they often consist of normal-appearing hepatocytes with only foci of cellular atypia within the nodules. They are not encapsulated but are often partially or completely surrounded by a rim of fibrous tissue in the manner of ordinary cirrhotic nodules. The nodules have a bulging cut surface and show compression of the surrounding liver parenchyma. Unlike focal nodular hyperplasia, they do not show a central scar and do not contain necrotic or hemorrhagic areas as in HCC. Microscopically, these nodules are composed of normal-appearing hepatocytes arranged in plates of one or two cells-thick with areas of fatty change. While there may be some suggestion of a disordered growth pattern, there is no evidence of nuclear atypia. The nodules are devoid of portal tracts. Rarely, these nodules have been described in the absence of preceding chronic liver injury, especially following long-term steroid intake.

Dysplastic nodules have been divided into low- and high-grade categories. Low-grade lesions are defined by the absence of cellular or architectural atypia although areas of large cell dysplasia may be present making distinction from ordinary regenerative nodules difficult. It has been suggested that an increased number of arteries without corresponding bile ducts (so-called 'unpaired arteries') is evidence of a dysplastic nodule (Thiese, 1997). High-grade dysplastic nodules show focal or diffuse cytologic or architectural atypia in the form of diffuse small cell dysplasia or microacinar formation. The areas of atypia appear as subnodules or nodule-in-nodule, pushing against the surrounding hepatocytes within the dysplastic nodule. These subnodules have been shown to proliferate more rapidly than the surrounding nodule and may be difficult to distinguish from well-differentiated HCC. They may also display iron resistance in an otherwise siderotic nodule, increased copper, fatty change, Mallory's hyaline, clear cell change or thickened trabeculae.

One clinicopathological study showed that about 50% of patients with biopsy-proven DNs developed carcinoma over 6–50 months (Takayama *et al.*, 1990). Cases have been described in which carcinomas were clearly embedded within adenomatous lesions (Ohno *et al.*, 1990), and in one report, a HBV-related carcinoma within an adenomatous lesion was shown to have an identical clonal HBV integration pattern as the surrounding hepatocytes, indicating a common origin (Esumi *et al.*, 1986). There is also evidence that these nodules are monoclonal in nature.

Nodular regenerative hyperplasia (NRH) is a condition in which the entire liver is interspersed with foci of hyperplastic hepatocytes consisting of plates of more than one cell thick in the periportal areas. In some instances these regenerative nodules progress to multiple adenomatous lesions of up to several centimeters in diameter. It is suspected that NRH may be a premalignant condition (Stromeyer and Ishak, 1981) and indeed progression of NRH to carcinoma has been reported (Sogaard, 1981).

1.9.2 LIVER CELL DYSPLASIA

Liver cell dysplasia refers to the presence of large hepatocytes with bizarre, hyperchromatic and occasionally multiple nuclei (large cell dysplasia – LCD). These cells occur in groups and may sometimes occupy entire cirrhotic nodules. The nature of these cells is controversial, with one contention that dysplastic hepatocytes represent a premalignant change. While there has been support for the premalignant concept from subsequent studies, reports from South Africa and Japan have refuted this concept, suggesting that liver cell dysplasia may be a regenerative or hyperplastic phenomenon rather than premalignant (Gerber, 1986; Anthony, 1987). More recent support for the premalignant concept comes from ploidy studies which indicate that morphologically dysplastic hepatocytes are associated with DNA aneuploidy (Roncalli *et al.*, 1989; Thomas *et al.*, 1992), although conflicting results have also been reported (Henmi *et al.*, 1985).

Another form of liver dysplasia was described in which the cells have small nuclei and relatively less than normal, often basophilic cytoplasm, yielding an increased nuclear-to-cytoplasmic ratio. This has come to be known as small cell dysplasia (SCD) (Watanabe *et al.*, 1983). These cells also show nuclear pleorphism and sometimes multinucleation. SCD was readily identified in studies from Asia and has been associated with HCC, but this association is less so among North American and European populations.

A recent study of various atypical features including LCD, SCD, cytoplasmic basophilia, small microacinar structures, peripheral distribution of nuclei, nuclear irregularities and thickened liver plates found that when used separately, none was useful in discriminating between cirrhosis without tumor and cirrhosis associated with HCC. Acinar structures, thickened liver trabeculae, peripheral distribution of nuclei and nuclear irregularities seemed the most specific indicators of association with HCC, and cirrhotic nodules showing four or more of the assessed features were often located in the vicinity of a tumor (Ojanguren *et al.*, 1997).

Hepatocellular adenomas, most often seen in the setting of exogenous steroid hormone intake or hereditary metabolic disorders, have been shown to give rise to HCC. However, the occurrence is very infrequent.

1.10 CARCINOGENESIS

It is accepted that neoplastic development is a stepwise process which involves at least two or more genetic events cumulating in unrestrained cellular growth, tissue invasion and metastasis. These genetic changes may be inherited as germline mutations which predispose to an increased risk for the development of cancer. More often they are acquired and the result of any one or a combination of chemical, physical or biological insults to the cell (Leong *et al.*, 1995). An alternative view is that neoplastic development results from adaptive responses to environmental perturbations (Farber and Rubin, 1991).

Colonic carcinogenesis is the best characterised human cancer model. The so-called adenoma–carcinoma sequence in the colon formed the basis for studying the underlying molecular events and the responsible genes. While some animal models of hepatic carcinogenesis satisfy such a sequence of events, the situation in human HCC is not as well defined.

HCC has revealed allele losses from chromosomes 4, 5q, 11p, 13q, 16q and 17p (especially the latter). Mutations of p53 have been documented in HCC-derived cell lines and in as many as 80% of liver cancers in China and southern Africa (Bressac *et al.*, 1990, 1991; Scorsone *et al.*, 1992). These mutations have commonly consisted of a transversion of G to T to C at the third base of codon 249. While p53 mutations may have an important role in hepatocarcinogenesis, such mutations represent one of the most commonly recognized changes in human carcinomas and are generally a late event in carcinogenesis. Aflatoxin B$_1$ causes transversion of G to T almost exclusively and preferentially binds to G residues in the G-C-rich regions in codon 249 of the p53 gene, suggesting that this mycotoxin may have a carcinogenic role in a subset of patients with HCC.

Changes in DNA methylation have been proposed as an essential step in carcinogenesis as they relate to the regulation of gene expression and cellular differentiation. DNA hypomethylation has been reported in chemical hepatocarcinogenesis (Ushijima *et al.*, 1997) but increases in deoxycytosine methylation have been reported following ingestion of the hepatocarcinogen methapyriline (Hernandez *et al.*, 1989). Prolonged feeding of diets deficient in sources of transferable methyl groups such as choline and methionine induced a high incidence of HCC in rats (Locker *et al.*, 1986).

While cirrhosis is a major risk factor for liver cancer, the reason for this association is largely unknown. It has been suggested that a deficiency in the ability to repair $O(6)$-methylguanine–DNA underlies this increased risk although this may be only one of several contributory factors (Collier *et al.*, 1996).

The actions of alcohol and other chemicals in the development of HCC continue to be investigated. Alcohol cannot be considered as a *bona fide* promoting agent for HCC and appears to act through its induction of cirrhosis as well as the modulation, in an as yet ill-defined manner, of the process of carcinogenesis with other recognized carcinogenic agents such as HBV and HCV (Farber, 1996). The association of HBV and HCC is strong and in addition to the supporting arguments made earlier in this chapter, hepatoma cell lines have successfully produced HBsAg and have been demonstrated to have integrated HBV DNA. The DR1 and DR2 sequences, which form a 11-base pair nucleotide sequence at both sides of the cohesive ends of the HBV genome, are preferential sites for viral integration into the host genome. HBV DNA integration is almost invariably present in HBsAg-positive HCCs. The presence of integrated HBV DNA in the non-tumorous hepatocytes of such livers further indicates that integration precedes carcinogenesis; however, no oncogenes have yet been identified within the HBV genome. While the virus is frequently fragmented after it integrates into the hepatocyte genome, the HBx gene appears to be consistently retained in a functional form, leading to speculation of its role in carcinogenesis. In tissue cultures, the X protein acts as a transcriptional transactivator of viral genes and it is possible that this protein may alter host gene expression in a manner which leads to HCC formation. Transgenic mice harboring the HBx gene develop multifocal areas of altered hepatocytes, benign adenomas and eventually HCC (Kim *et al.*, 1991). Studies in HBx transgenic mice indicate that the HBx gene has mitogenic activity both *in vitro* and *in vivo* and suggest that the HBx gene contributes to hepatocarcinogenesis by driving cells into deregulated cell cycle control (Koike, 1995).

Finally, a causal association between HBV and HCC is supported by numerous studies of three hepadnaviruses which are phylogenetically related to the human HBV. These occur in the eastern woodchuck (*Marmota manax*), Beechey ground squirrel (*Spermophilus beecheyi*), and Peking duck (*Anas domesticus*) in which persistent antigenemia is associated with the development of HCC (Korba *et al.*, 1989).

Much important information has been accumulated on the molecular and genetic events leading up to HCC, especially in the experimental model, but the genes involved and the mutations necessary for hepatocarcinogenesis still remain largely unknown (Sherman, 1995).

REFERENCES

Anthony, P.P. (1987) Liver cell dysplasia: what is its significance? *Hepatology*, **7**, 394–6.

Austin, H., Delzell, E., Grufferman, S. *et al.* (1986) A case-control study of hepatocellular carcinoma and the hepatitis B virus, cigarette smoking and alcohol consumption. *Cancer Research*, **46**, 962–6.

Beasley, R.P. and Hwang, L.Y. (1984) Epidemiology of hepatocellular carcinoma, in *Viral Hepatitis and Liver Disease* (eds G.H. Vyas, J.L. Dienstag and J.H. Hoofnagle), Grune & Stratton, New York, pp. 209–24.

Bianchi, L. (1993) Glucogen storage disease I and hepatocellular carcinoma. *European Journal of Pediatrics*, **152(Suppl. 1)**, S63–70.

Blum, H.E., Offensperger, W.B., Walter, E. *et al.* (1987) Hepatocellular carcinoma and hepatitis B virus infection: molecular evidence for monoclonal origin and expansion of malignantly transformed hepatocytes. *Journal of Cancer Research and Clinical Oncology*, **113**, 466–72.

Bosch, X. and Munoz, N. (1989) Epidemiology of hepatocellular carcinoma, in *Liver Cell Carcinoma. Falk Symposium No. 51* (eds P. Bannasch, D. Keppler and G. Weber), Kluwer, Dordrecht, pp. 3–14.

Bressac, B., Galvin, K.M., Liang, T.J. *et al.* (1990) Abnormal structure and expression of p53 gene in human hepatocellular carcinoma. *Proceedings of the National Academy of Sciences, USA*, **87**, 1973–7.

Bressac, B., Kew, M.C., Wands, J.R. and Ozturk, M. (1991) Selective G to T mutations of p53 gene in hepatocellular carcinoma from southern Africa. *Nature*, **350**, 429–31.

Carr, B.I. and van Thiel, D.H. (1990) Hormonal manipulation of human hepatocellular carcinoma. *Journal of Hepatology*, **11**, 287–9.

Cheah, P.L., Looi, L.-M., Lim, H.P. and Yap, S.F. (1990) Childhood primary hepatocellular carcinoma and hepatitis B virus infection. *Cancer*, **65**, 174–6.

Chu, N.S. and Hung, T.P. (1993) Geographic variations in Wilson's disease. *Journal of Neurological Science*, **117**, 1–7.

Collier, J.D., Bassendine, M.F. and Burt, A.D. (1996) Characterization of the DNA repair enzyme for *O*(6)-methylguanine in cirrhosis. *Journal of Hepatology*, **25**, 158–65.

Colombo, M. (1996) The natural history of hepatitis C. *Baillieres Clinical Gastroenterology*, **10**, 275–88.

Cortes-Espinosa, T., Mondragon-Sanchez, R., Hurtado-Andrade, H. and Sanchez-Cisneros, R. (1997) Hepatocellular carcinoma and hepatitis in Mexico: a 25 year necropsy review. *Hepatogastroenterology*, **44**, 1401–3.

Craig, J.R., Peters, R. and Edmonson, H. (1989) *Tumors of the Liver and Intrahepatic Bile Ducts. Fascicle 26*, Armed Forces Institute of Pathology, Washington, DC.

Crystal, R.G. (1990) Alpha-1-antitrypsin deficiency, emphysema and liver disease. *Journal of Clinical Investigation*, **85**, 1343–52.

D'Arville, C.N. and Johnson, P.J. (1990) Growth factors, endocrine aspects and hormonal treatment in hepatocellular carcinoma – an overview. *Journal of Steroid Biochemistry and Molecular Biology*, **37**, 1007–12.

Dehner, L.P., Snover, D.C., Sharp, H.L. *et al.* (1989) Hereditary tyrosinaemia type I (chronic form). *Human Pathology*, **20**, 149–58.

Director of Hospital Services Hong Kong (1992) *Annual Departmental Report, Hong Kong.*

Eagon, P.K., Francavilla, A., Di Leo, A. *et al.* (1991) Quantitation of estrogen and androgen receptors in hepatocellular carcinoma and adjacent normal human liver. *Digestive Disease and Sciences*, **36**, 1303–8.

Eriksson, S., Carlson, J. and Velez, R. (1986) Risk of cirrhosis and primary liver cancer in alpha-1-antitrypsin deficiency. *New England Journal of Medicine*, **314**, 736–9.

Esumi, M., Aritaka, T., Arii, M. *et al.* (1986) Clonal origin of human hepatoma determined by integration of hepatitis B virus DNA. *Cancer Research*, **46**, 5767–71.

Fan, S.T. and Wong, J. (1996) Hepatocellular carcinoma in the East, in *Hepatobiliary Malignancy* (ed. J. Terblanche), Churchill Livingstone, London, pp. 169–83.

Farber, E. (1996) Alcohol and other chemicals in the development of hepatocellular carcinoma. *Clinical and Laboratory Medicine*, **16**, 377–94.

Farber, E. and Rubin, H. (1991) Cellular adaptation in the origin and development of cancer. *Cancer Research*, **51**, 2751–61.

Forman, D. (1991) Editorial. Ames, the Ames test and the causes of cancer. *British Medical Journal*, **303**, 428–9.

Gangaidzo, I.T. and Gordeuk, V.R. (1995) Hepatocellular carcinoma and African iron overload. *Gut*, **37**, 727–30.

Gerber, M.A. (1986) Recent studies on the developing human hepatocellular carcinoma. *Cancer Surveys*, **5**, 741–63.

Govindarajan, S., Craig, J.R. and Valinluck, B. (1988) Clonal origin of hepatitis B virus-associated hepatocellular carcinoma. *Human Pathology*, **19**, 403–5.

Grasso, P. (1987) Experimental liver tumours in animals, in *Liver Tumors: Bailliere's Clinical Gastroenterology* (eds R. Williams and P.J. Johnson), Bailliere, London, pp. 183–305.

Henmi, A., Uchida, T. and Shikata, T. (1985) Karyometric analysis of liver cell dysplasia and hepatocellular carcinoma. *Cancer*, **55**, 2594–9.

Hernandez, L., Allen, P.T., Poirier, L.A. and Lijinski, W. (1989) S-adenosylmethionine, S-adenosylhomocysteine and DNA methylation levels in rats fed methapyriline and analogs. *Carcinogenesis*, **10**, 557–62.

Ishii, A., Matsuoka, H., Aji, T. *et al.* (1994) Parasite infection and cancer: with special emphasis on *Schistosoma japonicum* infections (Trematoda). A review. *Mutation Research*, **305**, 273–81.

Jakobovits, A.W. (1981) Primary liver cell carcinoma complicating autoimmune chronic active hepatitis. *Digestive Disease Sciences*, **26**, 694–9.

Kauppinen, R. and Mustajoki, P. (1988) Acute hepatic porphyria and hepatocellular carcinoma. *British Journal of Cancer*, **57**, 117–20.

Kim, C.M., Koike, K., Saito, I. *et al.* (1991) HBx gene of hepatitis B virus induces liver cancer in transgenic mice. *Nature*, **351**, 317–20.

Koike, K. (1995) Hepatitis B virus HBx gene and hepatocarcinogenesis. *Intervirology*, **38**, 134–42.

Kondo, F., Hiroka, N., Wada, K. and Kondo, Y. (1987) Morphological clues for the diagnosis of small hepatocellular carcinomas. *Virchows Archives (A)*, **411**, 15–21.

Kondo, F., Wada, K., Nagato, Y. *et al.* (1989) Biopsy diagnosis of well differentiated hepatocellular carcinoma based on new morphologic criteria. *Hepatology*, **9**, 751–5.

Korba, B.E., Wells, F.V., Baldwin, B. *et al.* (1989) Hepatocellular carcinoma in woodchuck hepatitis virus-infected woodchucks: presence of viral DNA in tumor tissue from chronic carriers and animals serologically recovered from acute infections. *Hepatology*, **9**, 461–70.

Kosaka, A., Takashi, H., Yajima, Y. *et al.* (1996) Hepatocellular carcinoma associated with anabolic steroid therapy: report of a case and review of the Japanese literature. *Journal of Gastroenterology*, **31**, 450–4.

Laferia, G., Kaye, S.B. and Crean, G.P. (1988) Hepatocellular and gastric carcinoma associated with familial polyposis coli. *Journal of Surgical Oncology*, **38**, 19–21.

Lau, J.Y.-N. and Lai, C.-L. (1990) Hepatocarcinogenesis. *Tropical Gastroenterology*, **11**, 9–24.

Lefkowitch, J.H. (1981) The epidemiology and morphology of primary malignant liver tumors. *Surgical Clinics of North America*, **61**, 169–81.

Leong, A.S.-Y., Robbins, P. and Spagnolo, D.V. (1995) Tumor genes and their proteins in cytologic and surgical specimens. Relevance and detection systems. *Diagnostic Cytopathology*, **13**, 411–22.

Leuschner, I., Harms, D. and Schmidt, D. (1988) The association of hepatocellular carcinoma in childhood with hepatitis B virus infection. *Cancer*, **62**, 2363–9.

Locker, J., Reddy, T.V. and Lombardi, B. (1986) DNA methylation and hepatocarcinogenesis in rats fed a choline-devoid diet. *Carcinogenesis*, **7**, 1309–12.

Matsui, T., Takano, M., Miyamoto, K. *et al.* (1986) Nude mice bearing human primary hepatocellular carcinoma that produces hepatitis B surface, core and e antigen, as well as deoxyribonucleic acid polymerase. *Gastroenterology*, **90**, 135–42.

McGoldrick, J.P., Boston, V.E. and Glasgow, J.K.T. (1986) Hepatocellular carcinoma associated with congenital macronodular cirrhosis in a neonate. *Journal of Pediatric Surgery*, **21**, 177–9.

Melia, W.M. (1985) Hepatocellular carcinoma in primary biliary cirrhosis: detection by α-fetoprotein estimation. *Gastroenterology*, **87**, 660–5.

Melnick, J.L. (1983) Hepatitis B virus and liver cancer, in *Viruses Associated with Human Cancer* (ed. L.A. Phillips), Marcel Dekker, New York, pp. 337–67.

Moore, S.W., Hesseling, P.B., Wessels, G. and Schneider, J.W. (1997) Hepatocellular carcinoma in children. *Pediatric Surgery International*, **12**, 266–70.

Munoz, N. and Bosch, X. (1988) Epidemiology of hepatocellular carcinoma, in *Neoplasms of the Liver* (eds K. Okuda and K.G. Ishak), Springer, Berlin, pp. 3–19.

Munoz, N. and Linsell, A. (1982) Epidemiology of primary liver cancer, in *Epidemiology of Cancer in the Digestive Tract* (eds P. Correa and W. Haenzel). Nijhoff, The Hague, pp. 161–95.

Naccarato, R. and Farinati, F. (1991) Hepatocellular carcinoma, alcohol and cirrhosis: facts and hypothesis. *Digestive Disease Sciences*, **36**, 1137–42.

Nagasue, N., Kohno, H., Chang, Y. *et al.* (1990) Specificity of androgen receptors of hepatocellular carcinoma and liver in humans. *Hepatogastroenterology*, **37**, 474–9.

Nagasue, N., Ito, A., Yukaya, H. and Ogawa, Y. (1985) Androgen receptors in hepatocellular carcinoma and surrounding parenchyma. *Gastroenterology*, **89**, 643–7.

Nalpas, B., Pol, S., Thepot, V. *et al.* (1995) Hepatocellular carcinoma in alcoholics. *Alcohol*, **12**, 117–20.

National Institutes of Health (1977) National Institutes of Health Consensus Development Conference Panel Statement: Management of hepatitis C. *Hepatology*, **26 (3 Suppl. 1)**, 2S–10S.

Newberne, P.M. and Butler, W.D. (1978) *Rat Hepatic Neoplasia*. MIT Press, Cambridge, MA.

Niederau, C., Fischer, R., Sonnenberg, A. *et al.* (1985) Survival and causes of death in cirrhotic and in non-cirrhotic patients with primary hematochromatosis. *New England Journal of Medicine*, **313**, 1256–62.

Ohno, Y., Shiga, J. and Machinami, R. (1990) A histopathological analysis of five cases of adenomatous hyperplasia containing minute hepatocellular carcinoma. *Acta Pathologica Japonica*, **40**, 267–78.

Ojanguren, I., Castella, E., Ariza, A. *et al.* (1997) Liver cell atypias: a comparative study in cirrhosis with and without hepatocellular carcinoma. *Histopathology*, **30**, 106–12.

Okada, S. (1996) Iron-induced tissue damage and cancer: the role of reactive oxygen species-free radicals. *Pathology International*, **46**, 311–32.

Okuda, K., Kojiro, M. and Okuda, H. (1993) Neoplasms of the liver, in *Diseases of the Liver*, 7th edn (eds L. Schiff and E.R. Schiff), J.B. Lippincott Co., Philadelphia, pp. 1236–96.

Omata, M. (1987) Current perspectives on hepatocellular carcinoma in Oriental and African countries compared to developed Western countries. *Digestive Diseases*, **5**, 97–115.

Oon, C.J., Rauff, A. and Tan, L.K.A. (1989) Treatment of primary liver cancer in Singapore. A review of 3200 cases seen between January 1, 1977 and July 31, 1987. *Cancer Chemotherapy and Pharmacology*, **23 (Suppl.)**, S13–16.

Patterson, K., Kapur, S.P. and Chandra, R.S. (1985) Hepatocellular carcinoma in a non-cirrhotic infant after prolonged parenteral nutrition. *Journal of Pediatrics*, **27**, 734–45.

Purtilo, D.T. and Gottlieb, L.S. (1973) Cirrhosis and hepatoma occurring at Boston City Hospital (1917–1968). *Cancer*, **32**, 458–62.

Roncalli, M., Borzio, M., Brando, B. *et al.* (1989) Abnormal DNA content in liver cell dysplasia: a flow cytometric study. *International Journal of Cancer*, **44**, 204–7.

Rustgi, V.K. (1987) Epidemiology of hepatocellular carcinoma. *Gastroenterological Clinics of North America*, **16**, 545–51.

Saracci, R. and Repetto, F. (1980) Time trends of primary liver cancer: indication of increased incidence in selected cancer registry populations. *Journal of National Cancer Institutes*, **65**, 241–6.

Saunders, J.B. and Latt, N. (1993) Epidemiology of alcoholic liver disease. *Baillieres Clinical Gastroenterology*, 7, 555–79.

Schiff, E.R. (1997) Hepatitis C and alcohol. *Hepatology*, **26 (3 Suppl. 1)**, 39S–42S.

Scorsone, K.A., Zhou, Y.Z., Butel, J.S. and Slagle, B.L. (1992) P53 mutations cluster at codon 249 in hepatitis B virus-positive hepatocellular carcinomas from China. *Cancer Research*, **52**, 1635–8.

See, K.L., See, M. and Glund, C. (1992) Liver pathology associated with the use of anabolic-androgenic steroids. *Liver*, **12**, 73–9.

Sharara, A.I., Hunt, C.M. and Hamilton, J.D. (1996) Hepatitis C. *Annals of Internal Medicine*, **125**, 658–68.

Sherman, M. (1995) Hepatocellular carcinoma. *Gastroenterologist*, **3**, 55–6.

Shikata, T. (1976) Primary liver carcinoma and liver cirrhosis, in *Hepatocellular Carcinoma* (eds K. Okuda and R.L. Peters), John Wiley, New York, pp. 53–68.

Simonetti, R.G. (1989) Prevalence of antibodies to hepatitis C virus in hepatocellular carcinoma. *Lancet*, **ii**, 1338–40.

Simonetti, R.G., Camma, C., Fiorello, F. *et al.* (1991) Hepatocellular carcinoma. A worldwide problem and the major risk factors. *Digestive Disease Sciences*, **36**, 962–72.

Simpson, I.W. (1982) Membraneous obstruction of the inferior vena cava and hepatocellular carcinoma in South Africa. *Gastroenterology*, **82**, 171–8.

Sogaard, P.E. (1981) Nodular transformation of the liver, alpha fetoprotein and hepatocellular carcinoma. *Human Pathology*, **12**, 1052–4.

Stromeyer, F.W. and Ishak, K.G. (1981) Nodular transformation (nodular 'regenerative' hyperplasia) of the liver. *Human Pathology*, **12**, 60–70.

Su, D.L. (1979) Drinking water and liver cancer: an epidemiological approach to the etiology of this disease in China. *Chinese Medical Journal* (English), **92**, 748–52.

Takayama, T., Makuuchi, M., Hirohashi, S. *et al.* (1990) Malignant transformation of adenomatous hyperplasia to hepatocellular carcinoma. *Lancet*, **336**, 1150–3.

Tarao, K., Ohkawa, S., Shinmizu, A. *et al.* (1993) The male preponderance in incidence of hepatocellular carcinoma in cirrhotic patients may depend on the higher DNA synthetic activity of cirrhotic tissue in men. *Cancer*, **72**, 369–74.

Thiese, N.D. (1995) Macroregenerative (dysplastic) nodules and hepatocarcinogenesis: theoretical and clinical considerations. *Seminars in Liver Diseases*, **15**, 360–71.

Thiese, N.D. (1997) Precursor lesions of hepatocellular carcinoma, in *Pathology of liver transplantation, viral hepatitis and tumors* (eds W.M.S. Tsui, A.S.-Y. Leong, C.T. Liew and W.F. Ng), International Academy of Pathology, Hong Kong Division, Hong Kong pp. 87-92.

Thomas, R.M., Bermann, J.J., Yetter, R.A. *et al.* (1992) Liver cell dysplasia: a DNA aneuploid lesion with distinct morphologic features. *Human Pathology*, **23**, 496–503.

Tibbs, C.J. (1997) Tropical aspects of viral hepatitis. Hepatitis C. *Transactions of the Royal Society of Medicine and Hygiene*, **91**, 121–4.

Toms, J.R. (1982) *Trends in Cancer Survival in Great Britain*, Cancer Research Campaign, London.

Tong, M.J. and Hwang, S.J. (1994) Hepatitis B virus infection in Asian countries. *Gastroenterology Clinics of North America*, **23**, 523–36.

Trichopoulos, D., Day, N.E., Kaklamani, E. *et al.* (1987) Hepatitis B virus, tobacco smoking and ethanol consumption in the etiology of hepatocellular carcinoma. *International Journal of Cancer*, **39**, 45–9.

Ushijima, T., Morimura, K., Hosoya, Y. *et al.* (1997) Establishment of methylkation- sensitive-representational difference analysis and isolation of hypo- and hypermethylated genomic fragments in mouse liver tumors. *Journal of National Academy of Sciences, USA*, **94**, 2103–5.

Watanabe, S., Okita, K., Harada, T. *et al.* (1983) Morphologic studies of liver cell dysplasia. *Cancer*, **72**, 1551–6.

Waterhouse, J.A.H. (1974) *Cancer Handbook of Epidemiology and Prognosis*, Churchill Livingstone, Edinburgh.

Weinberg, A.G. and Finegold, M.J. (1983) Primary hepatic tumors in childhood. *Human Pathology*, **14**, 512–37.

Weinberg, A.G., Mize, C.E. and Worthan, H.G. (1976) The occurrence of hepatoma in the chronic form of hereditary tyrosinaemia. *Journal of Pediatrics*, **88**, 434–8.

Weinstein, S., Scottalini, A.G., Loo, S.T. *et al.* (1985) Ataxia telengiactasia with hepatocellular carcinoma in a 15 year old girl and studies of her kindred. *Archives of Pathology and Laboratory Medicine*, **109**, 1000–4.

Wild, C.P., Jensen, L.A., Cova, L. and Montesano, R. (1993) Molecular dosimetry of alfatoxin exposure: contribution to understanding the multifactorial etiopathogenesis of primary hepatocellular carcinoma with particular reference to hepatitis B virus. *Environmental Health Perspectives*, **99**, 115–22.

Willett, W.C. and MacMahon, B. (1984) Diet and cancer – an overview. *New England Journal of Medicine*, **310**, 633–8, 697–703.

Wu, P.C. (1983) Hepatocellular carcinoma: epidemiology and pathology. *Hong Kong Practitioner*, **5**, 790–5.

Yu, M.W. and Chen, C.J. (1994) Hepatitis B and C viruses in the development of hepatocellular carcinoma. *Critical Reviews in Oncology and Hematology*, **17**, 71–91.

Yu, S.Z. (1985) Epidemiology of primary liver cancer, in *Subclinical Hepatocellular Carcinoma* (ed. Z.Y. Tang), China Academic, Beijing, 189–95.

Yu, S.Z. (1995) Primary prevention of hepatocellular carcinoma. *Journal of Gastroenterology and Hepatology*, **10**, 674–82.

PRESENTATION AND APPROACH TO DIAGNOSIS

2

P.J. Johnson

2.1 INTRODUCTION

Hepatocellular carcinoma (HCC) presents at a very late stage in its natural history. If we assume that from its onset a tumor doubles in size about 30 times before it is clinically detectable, then in most cases the clinical course of HCC involves only the last one or two doubling times. This can be attributed to the large size of the liver that precludes the tumor from being readily palpated while small. The large functional reserve of the liver also delays presentation with functional disturbances due to HCC such as jaundice or ascites. This chapter concentrates on those symptoms that lead to diagnosis but mentions, in passing, other symptoms that may develop during the course of the disease. The overall approach to establishing the diagnosis is also discussed, although each of the modalities involved is described in more detail in subsequent chapters.

A high index of suspicion must be exercised in patients at increased risk of HCC. Such subjects include those who are known to be chronic carriers of the hepatitis B virus (HBV), hepatitis C virus (HCV), or those who have cirrhosis of any other cause (Johnson and Williams, 1987; Beasley, 1988; Columbo *et al.*, 1991). In these groups, the annual incidence rate for HCC is in the order of 1–5% per annum. Males are particularly at risk (the male-to-female ratio is between 4:1 and 10:1), particularly as their age increases. This having been said, it must be emphasized that in more than half the cases, HCC development is the first indication of cirrhosis or chronic viral carriage. Such patients are not known, either by themselves or their physician, to be at risk before the tumor develops (Zaman *et al.*, 1990). A high index of suspicion should also be exercised in all patients presenting with certain symptoms (outlined below) in high-incidence areas. On the other hand, delay in diagnosis can be expected in patients in low-incidence areas where experience with HCC is limited as the tumor is rare. Besides more specific complaints, most patients will, at the time of presentation, have a variable constellation of symptoms that include anorexia, nausea and lethargy.

2.2 THE COMMON MODES OF PRESENTATION

The most common mode of presentation is with the triad of abdominal pain in the right upper quadrant, weight loss and the presence of an hepatic mass (Ihde *et al.*, 1974; Lai *et al.*, 1981). The pain is usually in the form of a dull ache in the right upper quadrant, sometimes referred to as the shoulder. Sudden attacks of

Hepatocellular Carcinoma: Diagnosis, investigation and management. Edited by Anthony S.-Y. Leong, Choong-Tsek Liew, Joseph W.Y. Lau and Philip J. Johnson. Published in 1999 by Arnold, London. ISBN 0 340 74096 5.

more severe pain may be caused by spontaneous bleeding into the tumor. Hepatomegaly, often massive, is an invariable feature of symptomatic malignant liver tumors. The liver feels firm or stony hard. The combination of a vascular bruit, which can be heard in about 25% of cases, and a rub is said to be diagnostic of HCC (Sherman and Hardison, 1979). Usually the symptoms will only have been present for a few weeks in high-incidence areas or for a few months in lower-incidence areas. In any event, it is apparent that delay in seeking medical advice is seldom a reason for the late diagnosis or a factor that can be held responsible for delayed intervention. Patients who present in this manner usually have a tumor >6 cm in diameter.

2.2.1 HEPATIC DECOMPENSATION

The second most common mode of presentation is decompensation of cirrhosis. The classical picture is that of a male with previously well-controlled cirrhosis who develops ascites, recurrent variceal hemorrhage or encephalopathy. Typically the ascites becomes difficult to control with diuretic therapy and may be blood-stained. Jaundice of the hepatocellular type may also be part of this presentation and it is usually steadily progressive. Obviously, there are several other causes of this picture of hepatic decompensation, but HCC development must always enter into the differential diagnosis.

2.2.2 GASTROINTESTINAL HEMORRHAGE

About 10% of cases will present with gastrointestinal (GI) bleeding. In half of the cases the bleed will have been from esophageal varices; this is much more frequent if the patient has portal vein invasion which presumably increases the portal pressure. Nonetheless, bleeding from benign causes is also common. A rare event is direct invasion of the GI tract, stomach or duodenum, by tumor (Plate 1) (Yeo *et al.*, 1995).

In both the above-mentioned common modes of presentation, the patient may have cutaneous stigmata of chronic liver disease but this is by no means always the case. It is well documented that the majority of patients who present with HCC, as well as having no history of chronic liver disease, have no clinical signs thereof. It is also important to note that the failure to detect clinical signs of chronic liver disease does not imply its absence. In one study, only 11 of 211 HCC patients were considered as having chronic liver disease on the basis of clinical examination, but at autopsy the figure was 90% (Lai *et al.*, 1981).

2.2.3 TUMOR RUPTURE – 'HEMOPERITONEUM'

A particularly dramatic presentation is spontaneous rupture of the tumor in which there is a sudden onset of abdominal pain and swelling. Although hemoperitoneum is a frequent event late in the course of the disease, it is a presenting feature in <5% of cases. The patient presents with shock and a rigid, silent abdomen. The diagnosis is established by paracentesis which reveals blood-stained fluid (Ong and Taw, 1972; Lai *et al.*, 1981; Miyamoto *et al.*, 1991).

2.2.4 ASYMPTOMATIC PRESENTATION

Increasingly, because of screening programs, tumors are being detected before any symptoms develop (Heyward *et al.*, 1985; Lok and Lai, 1989). With current imaging procedures, tumors as small as 0.5 cm can be detected. It is even being suggested that, using tumor marker screening, tumors may be detected before they can be seen on ultrasound imaging, i.e. during a preclinical phase of the disease (Johnson *et al.*, 1997). The frequency of asymptomatic diagnosis is entirely dependent on the intensity of the screening program. In most countries those cases detected at this stage remain a small 'lucky' minority (see below). Not surprisingly, the natural history of these very early lesions is different from symptomatic tumors and apparent survival is much better (Ebara *et al.*, 1986). Surgical resection or liver transplantation is often curative in this group.

2.3   RARER MODES OF PRESENTATION

Spread to involve the hepatic vein and inferior vena cava (Fig. 2.1) is a cause of the Budd–Chiari syndrome which presents with massive tense ascites. Obstructive jaundice may be due to compression of the bile ducts by the tumor rather than by hepatocellular failure. In approximately half the cases the site of obstruction is intrahepatic and in the others extrahepatic (Lau *et al.*, 1995). Other rare causes of jaundice include direct growth of the tumor into the bile duct or bleeding from the tumor into the biliary system (hematobilia). HCC has occasionally been reported as a cause of 'pyrexia of unknown origin' (PUO). Frequently, the PUO occurs late in the disease and leads to diagnostic difficulties during management. For example, it is often difficult to know after starting chemotherapy whether a fever is due to neutropenic sepsis or the 'fever of malignant disease'. Rare metastatic presentations include spinal cord compression and mucosal deposits (Fig. 2.2).

2.3.1   ENDOCRINE AND PARANEOPLASTIC SYNDROMES

HCC has gained a reputation for unusual paraneoplastic presentations (Kew and Dusheiko, 1981) but this is largely due to highly selective reporting. In the author's experience, <1% of all cases will present with any of these syndromes, although asymptomatic cases will be detected more frequently if sought assiduously. Among the paraneoplastic syndromes, a high red cell count (erythrocytosis) is well recognized and is presumed to be related to ectopic production of erythropoietin or an erythropoietin-like substance (Kew and Fisher, 1986). Depending on diagnostic criteria, figures of up to 10 % have been given but the erythrocytosis is very seldom of any clinical significance. The diagnosis is complicated by the fact that in patients with cirrhosis the plasma volume is expanded so that the red cell mass may be increased even in the presence of a normal hematocrit.

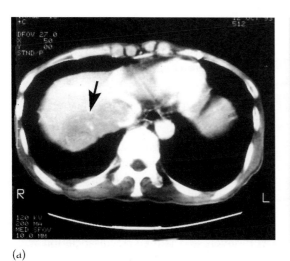

(a)

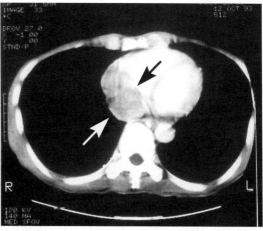

(b)

Fig. 2.1 (a) and (b)   CT scans showing tumor invasion in the inferior vena cava extending to the right atrium.

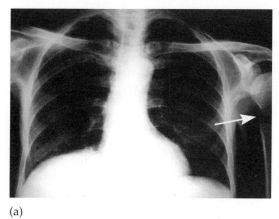

(a)

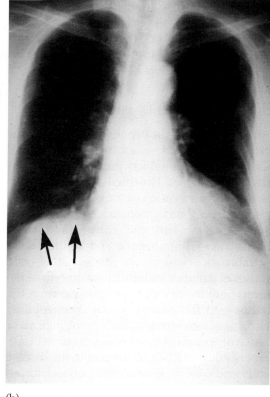

(b)

Fig. 2.2   Plain chest radiograph in HCC. (a) Humeral metastasis leading to fracture (arrow). There may also be a lytic area in the left anterior fourth rib; (b) double density over the right hemidiaphragm – the 'hump' sign is strongly suggestive of HCC (double arrows).

By contrast, hypoglycemia, although rare, is a cause of serious symptoms (Shapiro *et al.*, 1990). Two types are recognized. The first, or type A, occurs during the terminal stage of a rapidly growing tumor. This type is seldom symptomatic and is only detected if diligently searched for. A much greater clinical problem is type B disease in which severe symptomatic hypoglycemia occurs relatively early in the disease course (McFadzean and Yeung, 1969). This poses a particularly difficult management problem as the hypoglycemia does not respond consistently to any therapeutic approach and the physician usually resorts to long-term enteral glucose administration. Other even rarer presentations include gyne-

comastia, hypercalcemia and hyperthyroidism (Helzeberg *et al.*, 1985).

2.4   CLINICAL FEATURES OF SPECIFIC SUBTYPES

Three rare, histologically defined primary liver cancers deserve special consideration since they have specific clinical correlates. The fibrolamellar variant of HCC has several distinctive clinical features including a young age of presentation, normal α-fetoprotein (AFP) levels and lack of any association with cirrhosis. Patients are invariably HBV-negative. The histological picture is one of central dense fibrotic bands and eosinophilic tumor cells. The tumor is very rare in the Far East and in high-incidence areas in general (Craig *et al.*, 1980; Cooke *et al.*, 1986). Another histological variant with which fibrolamellar carcinoma may be confused has very marked sclerosis but does not carry a better prognosis. It is often associated with hypercalcemia and is easily mistakenly classified as a cholangiocarcinoma (Peters, 1976). The unusual vascular tumor, now termed 'epithelioid haemangioendothelioma' may occasionally occur in the liver. Its distinction from HCC is important as the prognosis is distinctly better. Originally described in the lung as 'intravascular bronchioloalveolar tumor', similar lesions arising in the liver were first described by Ishak *et al.* (1984) who used 'epithelioid haemangioendothelioma'. This terminology recognizes that although the lesion may, by conventional histology, appear epithelioid in origin, immunohistochemical study shows that the cells express factor VIII-associated antigen but no reactivity for epithelial markers, thereby confirming their endothelial origin (Scoazec *et al.*, 1989).

2.5   HCC IN THE NON-CIRRHOTIC LIVER

In all areas of the world 10–20% of HCC cases arise within a histologically normal liver. This group appears a distinct biological entity with distinctive clinical features. Compared with 'cirrhotic' HCC, the incidence in females is higher, the typical age of presentation is lower, the tumor is less often AFP-positive, and survival, although still poor, is relatively better (Melia *et al.*, 1984). The characteristic clinical features are detailed in Table 2.1 where they are compared with cirrhotic HCC. The distinction is important since, as the regenerative capacity of the normal liver is much greater than that of the cirrhotic liver, the surgeon can be much more aggressive in his management. However, it also follows that the normal non-tumorous liver can 'hide' a developing tumor for

Table 2.1   Clinical and laboratory features of a group of 50 patients with non-cirrhotic HCC compared with 100 patients with cirrhotic HCC. All figures are percentages except where stated otherwise.

	No cirrhosis	Cirrhosis
Demographics		
Age (years)	36 ± 14	56 ± 13*
Male	56	98*
Female	44	2*
Presentation		
Abdominal pain	50	44
Awareness of a mass	36	7*
Weight loss	32	36
Hemoperitoneum	2	2
Hepatic decompensation		
Jaundice	10	24*
Fluid retention	8	28*
Upper GI hemorrhage	0	11*
Encephaolpathy	0	3*
Laboratory features		
Elevated SAP	90	96
Elevated AST	58	93*
Elevated bilirubin	34	65*
Low serum albumin	40	73*
Prolonged PT	30	50*
AFP positive	87	46*
Median log AFP (ng/ml)	7000	7000

SAP, serum alkaline phosphatase activity. AST, aspartate aminotransferase activity. PT, prothrombin time.
The series was predominantly based on a series from a low-incidence Western area.
*Difference is statistically significant at $p < 0.05$ level.
Adapted from Melia *et al.* (1984).

longer than the cirrhotic liver and therefore non-cirrhotic HCCs tend to present later and at a larger size.

2.6   SHOULD WE BE SCREENING FOR HCC?

The answer to this difficult question depends largely on who is asking the question and what resources are available. Whole-population screening is almost certainly not an option, but HCC has the advantage over many other tumors, in that there are well-defined high-risk groups – patients with chronic liver disease and those who carry the hepatitis B or C viruses. The lifetime risk of HCC development for a male in any of these groups is in the range of 10–40%. In such an individual, who has access to the necessary resources, it seems likely that 3-monthly AFP estimation and ultrasound examinations will detect tumor development before it becomes clinically apparent. Some of these patients will go on to have a successful tumor detection and resection, and the physician will congratulate himself on a successful screening application. Disappointingly, however, such successes involve only a 'lucky minority' of those screened. The reasons why screening does not lead to a successful outcome more often are listed in Table 2.2(A).

The points listed in Table 2.2(A) also weigh heavily on those who have to give consideration to the introduction of HCC screening programs as part of a public health initiative. Each point in Table 2.2(A) will decrease the percentage of those at risk who are successfully detected and treated. When applied to a population rather than the individual additional factors need to be taken into consideration (Table 2.2(B)). On the basis of the numerous obstacles to a successful screening program listed in Table 2.2, there seems little doubt that only a small percentage of the total cases will be successfully detected and treated. Ultimately, however, each country would have to undertake a detailed cost utility\effectiveness program or model the factors in Table 2.2 as they relate to that particular country or health care system.

In addition to these depressing observations, there are other subtle 'knock on effects' for a program aimed at screening hepatitis carriers and these might make even the most beneficent of healthcare providers pause for thought. As noted in Table 2.2, it would be essential first to screen the 'normal' population to detect the high-risk subjects, usually chronic carriers of hepatitis B or C. This would

Table 2.2 Reasons for failure of a screening program for patients at high risk of HCC development

A. *The individual patient undergoing screening*
- When the tumor is detected, the liver function may be too poor for him to withstand a resection
- The tumor may already be multifocal or metastatic and is therefore unresectable
- The tumor may yet recur after apparently successful resection
- The patient may die as a complication of the operation

B. *A population*
All points listed above, plus:
- Some of those at high risk of HCC will decline to enter the program; others will default on follow-up
- Others will decline operation even if a tumor is detected that is potentially operable.

C. *Sources of additional costs (over and above the infrastructure needed for the screening program)*
- All those undergoing resection, or being considered for resection, will need further investigations; many ultimately will prove inoperable
- There is a risk of false-negative and positive results for AFP. False-positive results will necessitate further investigations
- Many of those at risk will not be aware of their risk factors. To cover the whole population there will need to be a preliminary screen, for example, to detect all HBsAg or anti-HCV-positive subjects

be relatively easy to organize, and inexpensive, but it would probably double the number of known carriers of viral hepatitis. All of these newly found carriers would then look for further (often very expensive) medical care including antiviral treatment. It should be further emphasized that in assessing the cost utility benefit of a screening program, the number of years of life saved even among those successfully screened and operated upon will be limited because these patients will still have a prognosis much poorer than that of the general population, because of their underlying chronic viral hepatitis. When we consider that there are many high HCC incidence areas in the world where universal vaccination against HBV is still not practised, it remains unlikely that a screening program for high-risk groups will be economically justified.

2.7 APPROACH TO DIAGNOSIS

Suspicion of HCC will usually arise on the basis of the symptom complexes as described above, or by the detection of a raised serum AFP level in a patient known to have cirrhosis or to be a HBV carrier.

2.7.1 INITIAL INVESTIGATIONS

This entails four parts: imaging procedures (including plain chest radiograph), serum AFP estimation, routine liver function tests and serology for chronic viral hepatitis.

The first aim is to document the presence of a space-occupying lesion within the liver. The precise techniques used will depend on regional or local availability and expertise. In most clinical units the first line investigation test will be an ultrasound examination, or less frequently a computed tomographic (CT) scan. These approaches are described in detail in Chapter 4. An ultrasound scan (USS) shows the tumor as hypoechoic while small, becoming progressively hyperechoic with ill-defined margins as it enlarges. USS can also assess the patency of the portal and hepatic veins particularly when Doppler flow studies are undertaken (Tanaka *et al.*, 1993). It permits differentiation between solid and cystic space-occupying lesions, and can allow accurate measurement of the main tumor size and daughter nodules if present. USS is particularly appropriate for regular screening of cirrhotic patients for the development of HCC, since lesions as small as 0.5 cm can be detected. Tumor and cirrhotic nodules can

often be differentiated but the entire examination is very operator-dependent. Computed tomographic (CT) scanning is equally sensitive but, in addition, a detailed search for primary or secondary lesions outside the abdomen is possible, although examination time and expense may limit applicability. HCC is seen as a hypodense lesion which does not enhance with contrast (Takayasu *et al.*, 1995).

2.7.2 DIAGNOSTIC CONFUSION CAUSED BY HEMANGIOMAS

Hemangoimas are the most common of the hepatic tumors, arising in around 5% of normal individuals. They are a frequent source of confusion in assessing patients with suspected HCC. Although hemangiomas do not cause symptoms unless very large, they are frequently encountered when screening high-risk patients by ultrasound, a technique which cannot confidently distinguish them from HCC. Hemangiomas may be solitary or multiple and to rule out the development of an HCC among them, or to determine which of several lesions is the primary tumor, which are daughter nodules and which are hemangiomas, can be extremely difficult.

There is no perfect test but if the distinction is clinically important then dynamic CT scanning is the most widely available technique and criteria for recognition of hemangiomas have been published (Ashida *et al.*, 1987). An alternative approach is to use scanning with ^{99m}Tc-labeled red blood cells, but it is likely that in the future magnetic resonance imaging (MRI) will become the definitive investigation. Although percutaneous biopsy is not advised when hemangiomas are suspected, it is the experience of those in the field that when they are biopsied by mistake, there is very seldom any more bleeding than with other liver tumors. Even at laparotomy the problem may not be solved since there may be multiple hemangiomas, not all can be inspected. In these circumstances the only option is to follow the patient over 1 month or so. HCC will continue to increase in size whereas hemangiomas will not.

The lowly plain chest radiograph should not be forgotten. Occasionally lung, or even bony, metastases will be seen at presentation and this clearly has implications for further investigation (Fig. 2.2a). Also it may be possible to see a bulge on the left diaphragm, a finding very characteristic of HCC (Fig. 2.2b).

2.7.2.1 α-Fetoprotein

Serum AFP levels are elevated above the reference range of 0–10 ng/ml in 50–80% of patients with HCC at the time of presentation (Tekata, 1990). The median value is in the order of 3000 ng/ml in low-incidence areas and 10 000–100 000 ng/ml in high-incidence areas, where levels may reach 10 000 000 ng/ ml (10 g/l) (Sawabu and Hattori, 1987). The test is primarily of value in the diagnosis of HCC developing in patients with cirrhosis where a level >500 ng/ml is, *in the presence of a liver mass*, virtually diagnostic. Levels between 10 and 500 ng/ml may occur in other non-malignant liver diseases, particularly severe untreated chronic hepatitis and fulminant liver failure (Alpert and Fuller, 1978). However, a steadily rising value, over 1–2-months, is very strongly suggestive of HCC. New approaches may help distinguish AFP derived from HCC, from that derived from benign liver disease (Sato *et al.*, 1993; Burditt *et al.*, 1994). The test is less useful in distinguishing between primary and secondary tumors in the non-cirrhotic liver. Only 50% of such cases of HCC have elevated levels, and up to 10% of patients with hepatic metastases will have elevated levels. Other tumor markers are of value in the diagnosis of the fibrolamellar variant of HCC and these include the vitamin B_{12} binding protein (Paradinas *et al.*, 1982), and neurotensin (Collier *et al.*, 1984).

2.7.2.2 The routine 'liver function tests' and viral serology

The standard liver function tests are not of diagnostic significance but form part of the initial assessment because, if grossly deranged, they may influence the degree to which the physician goes to establish the diagnosis (see below). The significance of the viral serology depends on local conditions. Thus, in low-incidence areas, its detection would be counted in favor of the diagnosis, whereas in high-incidence areas, such as Sub Saharan Africa and the Far East, where the great majority of patients are carriers, its absence would indicate that biopsy for histological confirmation would be important.

2.8 INITIAL ASSESSMENT

Following careful physical examination and with the above investigations to hand, the physician is in a position to make an initial assessment. In many instances a confident diagnosis can be established at this stage, particularly in high-incidence areas. If the following are present:

- an hepatic mass which is, in the opinion of the radiologist, consistent with HCC;
- a known history of chronic liver disease or a positive test for hepatitis B or C; and
- an AFP level >500 ng/ml,

then the diagnosis of HCC is almost certain.

2.9 FURTHER INVESTIGATIONS

If any of the preceding conditions are not fulfilled and the index of suspicion remains high, then further investigations are indicated. If doubt about the presence of a space-occupying lesion remains, CT with lipiodol or hepatic angiography may be required. If the AFP is within the reference range or <500 ng/ ml, histological proof of the tumor is usually obtained before proceeding further. However, the natural desire to confirm the diagnosis histologically, particularly in view of the gravity of the prognosis, needs to be tempered with a consideration of the benefit-to-risk ratio for the patient. For example, in a patient with severely decompensated cirrhosis, and in whom liver transplantation is not an option, it is unlikely that establishing the diagnosis will have any impact on further management and will certainly risk hemorrhage which may lead to further decompensation.

2.9.1   AT WHAT STAGE AND BY WHAT APPROACH SHOULD HISTOLOGY BE OBTAINED?

It should be remembered that there are two distinct reasons for undertaking tumor biopsy. The first is to determine whether the lesion is malignant, and the second is to determine the nature of the tumor, or at least to distinguish between a primary and a secondary tumor. The first aim is usually successful although the differentiation between a very well-differentiated HCC and a benign adenoma may, on occasion, prove difficult. However, the pathologist will often have difficulty in confidently diagnosing or excluding HCC on histological grounds when the tumor is poorly differentiated. This distinction may be important in clinical management when, for example, deciding whether to proceed to further investigation with a view to resection. Under these circumstance the serum AFP level may be of help. Another strategy is to biopsy the non-tumorous part of the liver. If this is cirrhotic, then a primary lesion becomes much the most likely diagnosis.

If it is decided that histological confirmation of the diagnosis is necessary, the stage of the investigation at which biopsy should be undertaken still requires careful consideration because of the small risk of tumor dissemination along the needle track. Provided that the prothrombin time is not more than 3 s prolonged, and the patient is not deeply jaundiced, the conventional percutaneous approaches using Menghini, Trucut or fine-needle (the latter depending on the availability of expert cytological opinion) are usually safe. The frequency with which tumor tissue can be obtained can be increased by using ultrasound to guide the operator or by combining biopsy with laparoscopy. The former approach is now routine practice in most institutions. When there is reason to believe that the lesion may be resectable, many surgeons prefer to avoid preoperative biopsy, and the possible risks of tumor dissemination, and await frozen section confirmation at the time of operation.

2.10   APPROACH TO THE DIAGNOSIS OF RECURRENT DISEASE AFTER SURGICAL RESECTION OR TRANSPLANTATION

A small percentage of so-called 'recurrences' after resection will, in fact, be 'new tumors' (the distinction between 'new' and 'recurrent' tumor can only be made confidently if, for example, it can be shown that the insertion site of HBV sequences is the same in the original and the subsequent tumor) but in most cases they will represent true recurrences of the original tumor. Ninety per cent of recurrences will be clinically apparent within 2 years of the operation. The approach to diagnosis of recurrence is broadly similar to that of the *de novo* tumor. Certain characteristics of the original tumor predict an increased likelihood of recurrence and these include, tumor size >5 cm in diameter, histological evidence of vascular invasion and lack of encapsulation. The AFP status of the original tumor and the recurrence do not change so that if the original tumor secreted AFP then the recurrence will, and vice versa. It should be noted *that normalization of AFP does not necessarily imply complete tumor removal*, and should not decrease the physician's index of suspicion for recurrence. It may simply mean the volume of tumor remaining is too small to synthesize sufficient AFP to raise the serum levels above the upper limit of reference range; recurrence may still occur.

The site of relapse is invariably intrahepatic after conventional surgical resection and will be readily screened for, and detected by, ultrasound examination. After transplantation the sites of recurrence may be more widespread and unusual. CT scanning of areas suggested on the basis of clinical examination and symptoms will need to be undertaken. In those who had raised AFP levels preoperatively, a rising AFP in the postoperative period invariably means impending clinical recurrence which it may precede by several months.

2.11   CONCLUSIONS

It is not so long ago that diagnostic options were so limited that HCC was considered a diagnosis that could only be established at a post-mortem examination. While it is true that progress in finding effective treatment has been slow, there is no doubt that major strides have been made in diagnosis. A confident diagnosis can now be established in the great majority of patients presenting with compatible symptoms. With the era of presymptomatic or even preclinical diagnosis, small, surgically resectable tumors are becoming increasingly diagnosed. It is not beyond the bounds of possibility that these small tumors may be significantly more amenable to medical therapy than their massive symptomatic counterparts.

REFERENCES

Alpert, E. and Fuller, E.R. (1978) Alpha-fetoprotein (AFP) in benign liver disease: evidence that normal liver regeneration does not induce AFP synthesis. *Gastroenterology*, **74**, 856–8.

Ashida, C., Fishman, E.F., Zerhouni, E.A. *et al.* (1987) Computed tomography of hepatic cavernous haemangioma. *Journal of Computer Assisted Tomography*, **11**, 455.

Beasley, R.P. (1988) Hepatitis B virus the major etiology of hepatocellular carcinoma, *Cancer*, **61**, 944–56.

Burditt, L., Johnson, M., Johnson, P.J. *et al.* (1994) Detection of hepatocellular carcinoma-specific alpha fetoprotein by isoelectric focusing. *Cancer*, **74**, 25–9.

Collier, N.A., Weinbren, K., Bloom, S.R. *et al.* (1984) Neurotensin secretion by fibrolamellar carcinoma of the liver. *Lancet*, **i**, 538–40.

Columbo, M., de Franchis, R., Del Ninno, E. *et al.* (1991) Hepatocellular carcinoma in Italian patients with cirrhosis. *New England Journal of Medicine*, **325**, 675–80.

Cooke, C., Mooy, N. and Matz, L.R. (1986) Fibrolamellar carcinoma of the liver. *Pathology*, **8**, 281–9.

Craig, J.R., Peters, R.L. and Omata, M. (1980) Fibrolamellar carcinoma of the liver: a tumor of adolescents and young adults with distinctive clinicopathologic features. *Cancer*; **46**, 372–9.

Ebara, M., Ohto, M., Shinagawa, T. *et al.* (1986) Natural history of minute hepatocellular carcinoma smaller than three centimeters complicating cirrhosis. A study of 22 patients. *Gastroenterology*, **90**, 289–98.

Helzeberg, J.H., McPhee, M.S., Zarling, E.J. *et al.* (1985) Hepatocellular carcinoma: an unusual course with hyperthyroidism and inappropriate thyroid-stimulating hormone production. *Gastroenterology*, **88**, 181–4.

Heyward, W., Lanier, A., McMahon, B. *et al.* (1985) Early detection of primary hepatocellular carcinoma. *Journal of the American Medical Association*, **254**, 191–4.

Ihde, D.C., Sherlock, P., Winawer, S.J. *et al.* (1974) Clinical manifestations of hepatoma. A review of 6 years experience at a cancer hospital. *American Journal of Medicine*, **56**, 83–91.

Ishak, K., Sesterhenn, I.A., Goodman, M.Z.D. *et al.* (1984) Epithelioid haemangioendothelioma of the liver: a clinical pathologic and follow-up study of 32 cases. *Human Pathology*, **15**, 839–52.

Johnson, P.J., Leung, N., Cheng, P. *et al.* (1997) 'Hepatoma-specific' alphafetoprotein may permit preclinical diagnosis of malignant change in patients with chronic liver disease. *British Journal of Cancer*, **75**, 236–40.

Johnson, P.J. and Williams, R. (1987) Cirrhosis and the aetiology of hepatocellular carcinoma. *Journal of Hepatology*, **4**, 140–7.

Kew, M.C. and Dusheiko, G.M. (1981) Paraneoplastic manifestations of hepatocellular carcinoma, in *Frontiers in Liver Disease* (eds P.D. Berk and T.C. Chalmers), Thieme-Stratton, New York, pp. 305–19.

Kew, M.C. and Fisher, J.W. (1986) Serum erythropoietin concentrations in patients with hepatocellular carcinoma. *Cancer*, **58**, 2485–8.

Lai, C.L., Lam, K.C., Wong, K.P. *et al.* (1981) Clinical features of hepatocellular carcinoma: review of 211 patients in Hong Kong. *Cancer*, **47**, 2746–55.

Lai, E.C.S., Wu, K., Choi, T.K. *et al.* (1989) Spontaneous ruptured hepatocellular carcinoma. An appraisal of surgical treatment. *Annals of Surgery*, **210**, 24–5.

Lau, W.Y., Leung, W.Y., Ho, S. *et al.* (1995) Obstructive jaundice secondary to hepatocellular carcinoma. *Surgical Oncology*, **4**, 303–8.

Lok, A.S.F. and Lai, C.L. (1989) Alpha-fetoprotein monitoring in Chinese patients with chronic hepatitis B virus infection: role in the early detection of hepatocellular carcinoma. *Hepatology*, **9**, 110–15.

McFadzean, A.J.S. and Yeung, R.T.T. (1969) Further observations on hypoglycaemia in hepatocellular carcinoma. *American Journal of Medicine*, **47**, 220–35.

Melia, W.M., Wilkinson, M.L., Portmann B.C. *et al.* (1984) Hepatocellular carcinoma in the non-cirrhotic liver: a comparison with that complicating cirrhosis. *Quarterly Journal of Medicine*, new series LIII, **211**, 391–400.

Miyamoto, M., Sudo, T. and Kuyama T. (1991) Spontaneous rupture of hepatocellular carcinoma: a review of 172 Japanese cases. *American Journal of Gastroenterology*, **86**, 68–71.

Ong, B.G. and Taw, J.L. (1972) Spontaneous rupture of hepatocellular carcinoma. *British Medical Journal*, **4**, 146–9.

Paradinas, F.J., Melia, W.M., Wilkinson, M.L. *et al.* (1982) High serum levels of vitamin B12 binding capacity as a marker of the fibrolamellar variant of hepatocellular carcinoma. *British Medical Journal*, **285**, 840–2

Peters, R.L. (1976) Pathology of hepatocellular carcinoma, in *Hepatocellular Carcinoma* (eds K. Okuda and R. L. Peters), John Wiley, New York.

Sato, Y., Nakata, K., Kao, Y. *et al.* (1993) Early recognition of hepatocellular carcinoma based on altered profiles of alpha-fetoprotein. *New England Journal of Medicine*, **25**, 1802–6.

Sawabu, N. and Hattori, N. (1987) Serological tumor markers in hepatocellular carcinoma, in *Neoplasms of the Liver* (eds K. Okuda and K.G. Ishak), Springer, Tokyo, pp. 227–38.

Scoazec, J.Y., Degott, C., Reynes, M. *et al.* (1989) Epithelioid hemangioendothelioma of the liver: an ultrastructural study. *American Journal of Pathology*, **131**, 38–47.

Shapiro, E.T., Bell, G.I., Polonsky, K.S. *et al.* (1990) Tumor hypoglycemia: relationship to high molecular weight insulin-like growth factor II. *Journal of Clinical Investigation*, **85**, 1672–9.

Sherman, H.I. and Hardison, J.F. (1979) The importance of a coexistent hepatic rub and bruit. *Journal of the American Medical Association*, **241**, 1495.

Takayasu, K., Furukawa, H., Wakao, F. *et al.* (1995) CT diagnosis of early hepatocellular carcinoma: sensitivity, findings, and CT-pathologic correlation. *American Journal of Roentgenology*, **164**, 885–90.

Tanaka, S., Kitamura, T., Fujita, M. *et al.* (1993) Color Doppler flow imaging of liver tumors. *American Journal of Roentgenology*, **160**, 515–21.

Tekata, K. (1990) Alpha-fetoprotein: re-evaluation in hepatology. *Hepatology*, **12**, 1420–32.

Yeo, W., Sung, J.Y., Ward, S.C. *et al.* (1995) A prospective study of upper gastrointestinal haemorrhage in patients with hepatocellular carcinoma. *Digestive Diseases and Sciences*, **40**, 2516–20.

Zaman, S.N., Johnson, P.J. and Williams, R. (1990) Silent cirrhosis in patients with hepatocellular carcinoma: implications for screening in high- and low-incidence areas. *Cancer*, **65**, 1607–11.

TUMOR MARKERS

3

S.K.W. Ho and P.J. Johnson

3.1 INTRODUCTION

Tumor markers are substances that can be measured quantitatively by biochemical or immunochemical methods, in tissue or body fluids such as plasma and have some degree of specificity for cancer in general or specific tumors. Tumor markers are useful in (1) identifying the presence of a cancer, possibly the tissue of origin, (2) establishing the extent of the tumor burden before treatment and (3) monitoring the response to therapy.

An ideal tumor marker should be specific for a particular type of cancer. It should be produced only by that type of tumor and not by any non-neoplastic condition. It should be absent or only present in quantitatively indistinct amounts in the normal population. The marker should also be highly sensitive so that the amount produced by a very small tumor is measurable by available laboratory methods. The quantity of the marker should correlate with the tumor load so that it may be used in staging the disease and monitoring response to therapy. The biological half-life of the marker must be short enough so that when the production drops/or ceases, the level falls off rapidly. It should also have prognostic relevance and predict the outcome of symptomatic patients. If an ideal tumor marker fulfilling all these requirements exists then invasive procedures for histological diagnosis and other invasive diagnostic manipulations can be avoided.

The tumor markers that have been used in patients with hepatocellular carcinoma (HCC) will be reviewed to examine their clinical relevance and usefulness.

3.2 α-FETOPROTEIN (AFP)

α-fetoprotein (AFP) was first identified by electrophoresis of fetal serum in 1956 (Bergstrand and Czar, 1956). Its association with liver cancer was discovered when AFP was detected by immunodiffusion in serum from mice, and later from patients, with HCCs (Abelev *et al.*, 1963; Tatarinov, 1964). Based on the study of AFP levels in a small number of patients, it was suggested that AFP was a diagnostic marker for HCC (Tatarinov, 1964). However, the subsequent detection of AFP in patients with various types of hepatitis and cirrhosis made the picture more complicated (O'Conor *et al.*, 1970). At that time the method for detection was insensitive and suitable only at concentrations $>2.5 \,\mu g/ml$. Radioimmunoassay for AFP with a sensitivity to $0.25 \,ng/ml$ was developed in the early 1970s (Rouslahti and Seppala, 1971) and allowed the demonstration and quantitative estimation of AFP levels in normal human serum. The increase

Hepatocellular Carcinoma: Diagnosis, investigation and management. Edited by Anthony S.-Y. Leong, Choong-Tsek Liew, Joseph W.Y. Lau and Philip J. Johnson. Published in 1999 by Arnold, London. ISBN 0 340 74096 5.

in sensitivity resulted in a reduction in the specificity of AFP as a diagnostic marker for HCC since modestly raised serum levels of AFP were frequently demonstrated in patients with hepatitis and liver cirrhosis, the latter a predisposing factor of HCC. Other pathological conditions in which raised AFP levels are detected include yolk sac tumors and gastrointestinal tumors (up to 9%).

3.2.1   DIAGNOSTIC SIGNIFICANCE

The reference range of serum AFP in normal adults depends on the assay used. A range between 0.1 and 5.8 ng/ml (mean 2.6 ± 1.6 ng/ml) has been determined by radioimmunoassay (Masseyeff *et al.*, 1974). Cut-offs of 5 or 10 ng/ml are commonly adopted.

3.2.1.1   Clinico-pathological features and AFP levels

It has been reported that 34.0–45.5% of patients with HCC have AFP levels >1000 ng/ml (The Liver Study Group of Japan, 1987). In small HCCs (<3 cm), serum AFP levels <20 ng/ml have been found in 25–46% of patients (Okuda, 1986). Well-differentiated small HCCs (<2 cm) mostly do not show detectable serum AFP (Kondo *et al.*, 1989) and the tumor cells do not show AFP by immunostaining (Brumm *et al.*, 1989). Thus, small tumors tend to have lower levels of AFP although there is no clear relation between AFP levels and tumor size (Sawabu and Hattori, 1987). Male patients with HCCs have been found to have slightly higher serum AFP concentrations than females (Mawas *et al.*, 1970; O'Conor *et al.*, 1970). It has also been observed that there is a general increase of mean serum AFP levels with younger patients (Mawas *et al.*, 1970; Namieno *et al.*, 1995).

Hepatitis B surface antigen (HBsAg) seropositive patients with HCC have a greater frequency of high AFP levels, but they also overlap to a greater extent with the AFP levels in HBsAg-positive patients with cirrhosis and/or chronic active hepatitis. The specificity of AFP for the detection of HCC in this serologically defined subgroup is thus decreased (Lee *et al.*, 1991). Several studies have found a significantly higher percentage of patients with high AFP levels among HCC patients with underlying cirrhosis when compared with those without (Johnson *et al.*, 1981; Trevisani *et al.*, 1995).

The percentage of patients in Japan with HCC who showed serum AFP levels <20 ng/ml at presentation increased from 3.6 to 29% during the 9 years from 1978 to 1986. On the other hand, HCC patients with serum AFP >10 000 ng/ml decreased from 53.5 to 6.4% during the same period (Nomura *et al.*, 1989). It was suggested that a larger number of HCCs with low AFP levels, presumably small tumors, were detected by more sensitive imaging techniques such as ultrasound and computed tomography. A similar observation from 1975 to 1984 was reported in another study (Sawabu and Hattori, 1987).

3.2.1.2   Diagnosis of HCC from benign liver disease

Significant but small AFP rises between 10 and 1000 ng/ml are frequently seen in adult patients with hepatitis and liver cirrhosis. The frequency of elevation (>10 ng/ml) in chronic hepatitis and cirrhosis has been reported to 22 and 40% respectively, although these figures depend on the stage and the serological activity of the disease (Sawabu and Hattori, 1987). AFP elevations may be associated with the seroconversion from HBe antigenemia to HBe antibody positivity accompanied by bridging necrosis in the liver (Liaw *et al.*, 1986). Thus, AFP concentrations between 10 and 1000 ng/ml represent a 'grey area' since both benign conditions such as chronic hepatitis and cirrhosis and small HCCs may show values within this range.

The sensitivity and specificity of AFP as a diagnostic marker for HCC depend on the cut-off levels chosen. An evaluation on 239 cases of chronic hepatitis, 277 cases of cirrhosis and 95 cases of HCC at varying clinical stages demonstrated a sensitivity of 78.9% and a specificity of 78.1% when adopting >20 ng/ml as the cut-off level for diagnosis of HCC (Taketa, 1989). On increasing the cut-off level for HCC to >200 ng/ml, the specificity of the test rose to 99.6% at the expense of the sensitivity which dropped to 52.6%.

The poor specificity of serum AFP at low levels for HCC severely limits its practical application in the detection of small HCCs when curative resection is a feasible option. Several approaches have been used to improve the specificity of AFP as a diagnostic test for HCC.

3.2.1.3   Monitoring time trends of AFP levels

In a patient with cirrhosis, a steadily rising AFP level is considered good evidence for HCC development. However, by the time a confident diagnosis can be made after a serial determination of AFP levels, the tumor may be too large for resection. Conversely, if levels fall or fluctuate, then HCC is less likely (Sawabu and Hattori, 1987) but an unexplained decline in serum AFP level has been seen in a patient with untreated HCC (Chen et al., 1984) and drops in AFP levels have also been observed in the preterminal stage of HCC patients.

In another study, six patients had persistent or progressive increase in AFP levels and were confirmed to have HCC, whereas HCC was not identified in patients with elevations >200 ng/ml, persisting >6 months (Lok and Lai, 1989). This led to the conclusion that monitoring time-trends of AFP levels alone is not a satisfactory method for early diagnosis of HCC.

However, steadily increasing levels of serum AFP >1000 ng/ml are generally accepted as an indication of AFP-producing tumors (Sell, 1990).

3.2.1.4   Lectin-binding affinities of AFP variants

The second approach is based on the variable affinity of different AFP variants for lectins. Human AFP is a glycoprotein with a molecular mass of 72 000 containing 4% of carbohydrate by weight. It has one asparagine-linked biantennary complex-type oligosaccharide per molecule as a fundamental structure, with additional major and minor sugar chain heterogeneities, depending on its origin (Yoshima et al., 1980). AFP purified from ascitic fluid from HCC patients has a sugar structure which readily binds to concanavalin A (Con A) while that produced by yolk sac tumors is characterized by a glycolinkage with N-acetyl-glucosamine in the mannose part which inhibits binding of the molecules to Con A. The Con A-bound fraction accounts for the larger proportion of AFP in liver cirrhosis and HCC, while the Con A-unbound fraction occurs with yolk sac tumors and metastatic liver cancers of gastrointestinal origin. Thus, HCC can be distinguished from AFP-producing metastatic liver cancer by the binding to Con A.

The presence or absence of fucose attached to N-acetyl-glucosamine, adjacent to asparagine, is thought to account for the difference in binding to another type of lectin, lentil lectin (Du et al., 1991). The unbound fraction eluted from the lentil lectin column contains the majority of AFP molecules found in benign liver disease, whereas AFP from HCC has a lower unbound fraction and the bound fraction is variably increased. These differing affinities for the lentil lectin allow differentiation of HCC from benign liver diseases. However, these tests are tedious and the results are sometimes not reproducible.

3.2.1.5   Detection of HCC-specific isoforms of AFP by isoelectric focusing

Isoelectric focusing (IEF) as a technique for separating and identifying the HCC-specific AFP isoforms based on charge heterogeneities has been developed as an alternative to testing lectin affinities. Up to five isoforms of AFP with different isoelectric points are visible through chemiluminescence (Burditt *et al.,* 1994). Two of these isoforms have been shown to be HCC-specific and may be detected up to 19 months before radiological evidence of the tumor.

The technique has been simplified by using anti-AFP conjugated with horse-radish peroxidase and up to nine different isoforms of AFP have been resolved by using a much higher voltage of 2000 V (Ho *et al.,* 1996). Eight different banding patterns of AFP have been identified in serum samples from 110 HCC patients with modestly raised AFP levels of 50–500 ng/ml. Either one or both of two characteristic bands (+II and +III) (Fig. 3.1) were found in 96% of the HCC patients. These bands were not observed in 10 patients with uncomplicated cirrhosis and were therefore considered as HCC-specific.

The specificity of these AFP isoforms was assessed by studying 53 patients attending an out-patient clinic for chronic liver diseases (Johnson *et al.,* 1997). All 53 patients had AFP levels >50 ng/ml at entry into the study. The HCC-specific AFP isoform (+II) was detected in the sera from 26 of these patients taken at the time of enrolment. During an 18-month follow-up (median 12 months) a diagnosis of HCC was established in 19 of the 26 patients (Fig. 3.2). Ultrasound evidence of tumor development was found in only two cases at the time AFP was found to be elevated. In the remaining 17 patients, the diagnosis was established at a median of 3.6 months (range 1–18 months) after the HCC-specific isoform of AFP was first detected. On the other hand, among those 27 patients without the HCC-specific isoform, only three developed tumors within the follow-up period (Fig. 3.2). Thus the HCC-specific AFP may permit the malignant change in patients with chronic liver disease to be inferred before it becomes detectable by routine ultrasound examination. Detection of HCC-specific isoforms in patients with chronic liver disease necessitates more careful and focused screening by imaging investigations such as computed tomography or hepatic

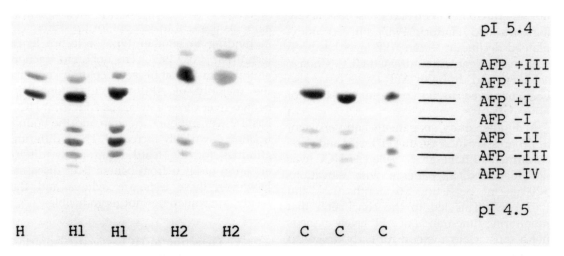

Fig. 3.1 Isoforms of AFP. Each lane represents the banding pattern obtained from serum samples from different patients. The presence of isoform +II constitutes a positive 'hepatoma-specific' AFP test. H and H1 are the commonest patterns in cases of established HCC. Examples H2 are the less common 'HCC-specific' patterns. Examples C are the patterns seen in patients with cirrhosis who did not develop HCC. (Reproduced from Johnson *et al.,* 1997.)

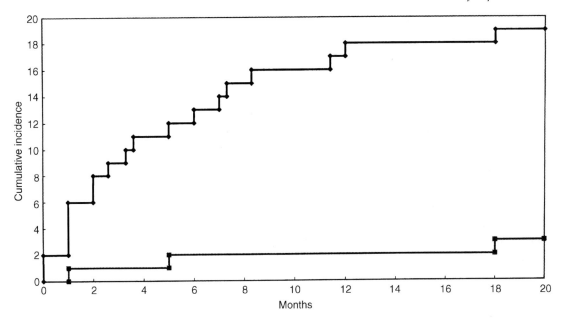

Fig. 3.2 Cumulative incidence of HCC with time in two groups of patients with chronic liver disease and raised AFP levels. The first group (26 patients) showed the 'hepatoma-specific' isoform of AFP, and the second group (27 patients) did not. The difference between the two curves is statistically highly significant (p <0.0001, log-rank test). With 'hepatoma-specific band (◆); without 'hepatoma-specific band (■). (Reproduced from Johnson *et al.*, 1997.)

angiography, in addition to ultrasound scan. By doing so, more early cases of HCC may be identified for treatment by curative resection.

3.2.2   PROGNOSTIC SIGNIFICANCE

Patients with raised serum AFP levels at the time of diagnosis have been reported to have a poorer prognosis compared with AFP-negative cases with matched tumor sizes (Nomura *et al.*, 1989).

3.2.2.1   Monitoring response to surgical treatment

It has been shown that complete excision of tumors produces an immediate fall in serum levels of AFP which parallels its catabolic decay rate at a half-life of 3.5–4 days (Sell, 1981). Poor survival rates were observed in patients showing longer half-lives of AFP.

However, the achievement of a normal level does not necessarily imply complete clearance of the disease as demonstrated in two patients with recurrence of tumor after transplantation who initially returned to normal levels of AFP (Urabe *et al.*, 1990).

Re-elevation of AFP level is a strong indication of recurrence although there are always exceptions. A gradual rise in serum AFP levels was observed in seven patients without any evidence of postoperative recurrence (Ezaki *et al.*, 1988) and patients having residual disease may not reveal a rise (Curtin *et al.*, 1989). The changes of serum AFP levels after liver transplantation for HCC follow a similar pattern (Andorno *et al.*, 1989). Such rises are attributed either to recurrence of tumor or to damage of liver cells from replication of HBV in the transplanted liver. During the phase of graft rejection, AFP levels have not been observed to increase.

3.2.2.2   Monitoring response to chemotherapy

The various forms of chemotherapy available in the 1970s were considered ineffective for HCC and they caused only minor and transient decreases in serum AFP levels (McIntire *et al.*, 1976). However, the serum AFP in nine of 26 patients was found to decrease by >50% after chemotherapy in one study (Matsumoto *et al.*, 1974). The decrease continued for >3 months and patients had either a good or a fair clinical response. Nine other patients showed a transient decrease of <50% and gradually returned to the pretreatment level or slightly above, until death. Among these cases, eight had fair clinical response and one showed a progressive increase in tumor size. The last subgroup of patients had continuous increase in AFP and did not respond to chemotherapy at all.

It was found that patients who failed to respond to chemotherapy or had recurrence after initially successful chemotherapy and surgery showed AFP levels rising exponentially, with a doubling time of 6.5–112 days (mean 41 days). The doubling times correlated positively with patient survival (Johnson and Williams, 1980).

3.2.2.3   Monitoring response to radiotherapy

Response rates to radiotherapy, as measured by the decrease in tumor markers, were much higher than those based on changes in tumor size/volumes from CT images (Barone *et al.*, 1982; Nauta *et al.*, 1987; Lau *et al.*, 1997). Also, the reduction in tumor volumes appeared much later than the fall in tumor marker levels. In a number of patients with hepatic metastases, no change in size of the liver defects on CT scanning was noted, yet at the time of exploration no viable tumor cells were found in the liver (Barone *et al.*, 1982). We have had a similar experience with a patient treated by selective internal radiation (SIR) therapy using yttrium-90 microspheres (Lau *et al.*, 1998). The patient presented with an inoperable HCC of 12 cm and an AFP level of 2972 ng/ml. After two SIR treatments the AFP level was normalized (<10 ng/ml) but a tumor nodule of 5 cm was still apparent on the CT images. The 'tumor' was resected and was found to contain no viable HCC cells. Thus, the normalization of the AFP level seems to be a more sensitive indicator of tumor response than CT images.

The discrepancy between the tumor marker levels and CT images has been attributed to fibrosis produced by the radiotherapy (Barone *et al.*, 1982). It has also been suggested that the size of tumor nodules on CT scans after treatment depends on a number of other factors including the rate of the tumor cell death and reparative process, and the extent to which the repair and re-organization of cells is visible on CT images (Nauta *et al.*, 1987). It is therefore not surprising that tumor marker production ceases completely following the killing or damage of the tumor cells, while abnormalities persist on the CT images.

The possibility that radiation might have eradicated the clone of tumor cells producing the tumor marker, with the residual tumor shown on the CT representing marker-negative clones cannot be ruled out. Thus, it will be ideal to compare serum tumor markers such as AFP with an imaging modality such as position emission tomography, which is capable of differentiating viable tumor from necrotic tissue by measuring metabolic utilization of radiolabeled glucose.

3.3   SERUM FERRITIN

Serum ferritin was found to have no role in the differential diagnosis of HCC (Melia *et al.*, 1983) because raised levels were found in 34 of 35 (97%) patients with HCC and in 20 of 23 (87%) with uncomplicated cirrhosis. However, both its sensitivity (88 versus 59%) and specificity (85 versus 68%) were found to be superior to AFP as a diagnostic marker for HCC in another study (Giannoulis *et al.*, 1984).

Values of serum ferritin obtained in patients with HCC were significantly higher than those with cirrhosis. Furthermore, high ferritin levels were found to occur more frequently in low AFP-producing HCC. Thus, the simultaneous determination of both markers in serial samples has been recommended to increase the diagnostic sensitivity (Nakano *et al.*, 1984). This is supported by the results of another study (Tatsta *et al.*, 1986) which showed that the diagnostic rate for lesions <3 cm in diameter was raised from 75% by measuring AFP alone to 100% when both serum ferritin and AFP were measured.

Although serum ferritin has been found to be of no diagnostic value by Melia *et al.* (1983) because of the poor specificity, it has been suggested to be a useful marker for monitoring response to treatment, particularly in the AFP-negative patients (Nakano *et al.*, 1984). Unlike AFP, there is always an initial transient rise following treatment before the level falls with tumor regression, but ferritin continues to rise if disease progresses.

3.4 γ-GLUTAMYLTRANSPEPTIDASE (γ-GTP) ISOENZYME

γ-glutamyltranspeptidase (γ-GTP) isoenzyme is a fetal isoenzyme. Similar to AFP, its activity is quite low in the adult liver but is extremely high in the fetal liver and HCC (Fiala *et al.*, 1972). Three types of serum γ-GTP isoenzymes appear to be specific for HCC. They stand out as distinctive bands among a total of 13, which appear during electrophoresis on polyacrylamide gradient gel (Sawabu *et al.*, 1983). At least one or more of the three specific bands were detected in 109 of 200 patients with HCC. They were detected in only one of 57 patients with liver cirrhosis and one of 43 patients with chronic hepatitis.

Although the HCC-specific γ-GTP occurred more frequently in patients with higher AFP levels, it was also found in 29 of 76 (38%) patients with AFP <400 ng/ml and in 11 of 41 (27%) patients with AFP <100 ng/ml. These

HCC-specific isoenzymes may thus serve as a diagnostic marker to complement AFP. The presence of HCC-specific γ-GTP was found to be independent of the stage of the disease. They have been identified in 53% of stage I disease which was below the detection limit of liver scanning. Thus, these isoenzymes appear to be useful for the detection of relatively early HCC. Attempts to characterize these HCC-specific isoenzymes suggested, as with AFP, that their specificity is largely due to structural differences in the carbohydrate moieties resulting from altered post-ribosomal processing of the glycoproteins in the tumor cells. These structural differences give rise to distinct molecular weights, electrophoretic mobility and lectin affinity.

3.5 ALKALINE PHOSPHATASE (ALP)

Among the various organ-specific isoforms of alkaline phosphatase (ALP) discovered, one named variant ALP (VAALP) was found to be highly specific for HCC (Szuki *et al.*, 1975). It was present in 31% of 51 patients. It is less sensitive than AFP and γ-GTP but it has a much higher specificity as it is negative in patients with other types of cancer and in patients with benign hepatobiliary diseases. Furthermore, since its prevalence is independent of the AFP level and the presence of γ-GTP, it may serve as a marker complementary to AFP or γ-GTP.

3.6 DES-γ-CARBOXY PROTHROMBIN (DCP)

Des-γ-carboxy prothrombin (DCP) is an abnormal prothrombin released into the blood when vitamin K-dependent carboxylase activity of the liver is inhibited, due to either the absence of vitamin K or the presence of a vitamin K antagonist. It is hardly detectable in normal subjects. Moderately raised levels were found in some patients with acute hepatitis, liver cirrhosis and metastatic liver cancer (Blanchard *et al.*, 1981). Sixty-nine of 76 patients (91%) with HCC showed high levels. At a cut-off value of 300 ng/ml, the test was positive in 67% of 76 patients with HCC and in one of 17 patients with metastatic liver cancer, but it was negative in all 28 patients with chronic active hepatitis. Again, there was no correlation between levels of AFP and DCP. Raised DCP levels were detected in 16 of 28 patients (57%) with HCC whose AFP levels were <400 ng/ml (Liebmen *et al.*, 1984). Furthermore, DCP is useful for monitoring the response to treatment by surgery or chemotherapy. A recent study of 147 patients who underwent curative resection for HCC concluded that positivity of both DCP (>0.1 AU/ml) and AFP (>50 ng/ml) is one of the independent factors of poor prognosis for both overall survival and disease free interval (Shimada *et al.*, 1996).

3.7   α-1-ANTITRYPSIN (AAT)

α-1-antitrypsin (AAT) is a glycoprotein, of molecular mass of 54 000, synthesized by the liver. It consists of a single polypeptide chain with four oligosaccharide side chains of two different types. The activity of AAT was found to be significantly higher in HCC than in benign liver diseases (Chio and Don, 1979). There was no correlation between levels of AAT and AFP, suggesting that AAT may be a useful maker to aid the diagnosis of AFP-negative HCC.

Serum AAT levels in stage I HCC were significantly lower than those in stage II or III (Tu and Wu, 1989). Patients with proven underlying cirrhosis had slightly higher levels than non-cirrhotic patients. Among cases of AFP-negative HCC, AAT levels in HBsAg-positive patients were slightly higher than in HBsAg-negative patients. AAT levels increased with tumor size. HCC patients with well-encapsulated tumors and without tumor thrombus were found to have lower AAT levels than those with unencapsulated tumors or with capsular penetration, and also in those with vascular thrombi. Furthermore, tumor resectability was higher in patients with lower preoperative AAT levels.

3.8   ALDOLASE A

High activity of aldolase, one of the key enzymes in the glycolytic pathway responsible for catalysing the cleavage of fructose 1,6-diphosphate and frutose 1-phosphate, has been found in patients with HCC (Asaka *et al.*, 1983). Its serum level in benign liver disease such as cirrhosis and hepatitis was lower than in HCC. A positive aldolase A level was found in 11 of 17 patients (64.71%) with tumors ≤5 cm and in 23 of 29 patients (79.31%) with stage I tumors (Zong and Wu, 1989) suggesting that the marker may be useful in early diagnosis. No parallel relationship between levels of aldolase A and AFP was found and the two markers appeared complementary. Aldolase A level returned to normal after complete resection of HCC and increased when there was recurrence.

3.9   5′-NUCLEOTIDE PHOSPHODIESTERASE V (5′-NPD)

5′-nucleotide phosphodiesterase V (5′-NPD) is an enzyme that hydrolyzes a nucleotide to form a nucleoside and phosphoric acid. It was positive in 83.2% of 95 patients with HCC (Lu *et al.*, 1980) and was detected in 8.3% of cases of cirrhosis and 13.3% of hepatitis (Lu and Chen, 1989). The positivity rate was 85.7% among AFP-positive HCC patients and 76.0% in AFP-negative cases. In a Japanese study, the diagnostic value of this enzyme for HCC was found to be relatively high, especially in patients with low or negative AFP levels (Fujiyama *et al.*, 1990). It was noted that jaundice gave a non-specific false-positive reaction in the assay for this enzyme so that it should not be used in patients with jaundice.

3.10   TISSUE POLYPEPTIDE ANTIGEN (TPA)

Tissue polypeptide antigen (TPA) has been investigated for detection of HCC in cirrhotic patients (Leandro *et al.*, 1990). The study involved two groups of cirrhotic patients, 35 with and 90 without HCC. There was a significant difference between the mean TPA levels in the two groups and the best diagnostic accuracy for HCC with 48.6% sensitivity and 85.6% specificity was found at a cut-off value of 240 U/L. However, there is a significant correlation between TPA levels and liver enzymes so that great caution must be exercised when using TPA as a diagnostic aid as liver dysfunction may cause its elevation.

3.11 α-L-FUCOSIDASE

The serum α-L-fucosidase activity level in patients with HCC (575.76 ± 272.86 nmol/ml/h) was significantly higher than that in patients with cirrhosis (274.55 ± 138.97 nmol/ml/h; $p<0.001$) or other neoplasms (257.91 ± 128.12 nmol/ml/h; $p<0.001$) (Giardina *et al.*, 1992). With a sensitivity of 76% and a specificity of 90.9% at a cut-off of 443 nmol/ml/h, α-L-fucosidase is considered a useful marker for detecting HCC when used in conjunction with AFP and ultrasound scan of the liver. We have found that the levels of the enzyme in Chinese patients with chronic liver diseases overlapped to a much greater extent with the levels in HCC. Thus, its usefulness for the diagnosis of HCC requires further evaluation.

3.12 CONCLUSIONS

In conclusion, although AFP can only fulfil part of the requirements of an ideal tumor marker, it is superior to all the other nine markers presently available and still remains the most commonly used test to aid the diagnosis and monitoring of HCC. A serum level >500 ng/ml is considered almost diagnostic of HCC in high-incidence areas. Detection of HCC-specific isoforms by isoelectric focusing techniques is recommended for levels between 50 and 500 ng/ml. The absence of such bands suggests that the patient is unlikely to have HCC whereas the presence of the HCC-specific isoforms should prompt more frequent and focused radiological screening with the intent of early detection of the cancer.

REFERENCES

Abelev, G.I., Perova, S.D., Khramkova, N.I. *et al.* (1963) Production of embryonal α-globulin by transplantable mouse hepatomas. *Transplant Bulletin*, **1**, 174–80.

Andorno, E., Salizzoni, M., Schieroni, R. *et al.* (1989) Role of serum alpha-fetoprotein in pre- and post-orthotopic liver transplantation (OLT) for malignant disease. *Journal of Nuclear Medicine and Allied Science*, **33** (Suppl. to no. 3), 132–4.

Asaka, M., Nagasue, K., Miyazaki. *et al.* (1983) Aldolase A isoenzyme levels in serum and tissue of patients with liver diseases. *Gastroenterology*, **84**, 155–60.

Barone, R.M., Byfield, J.E., Goldfarb, P.B. *et al.* (1982) Intra-arterial chemotherapy using an implantable infusion pump and liver irradiation for treatment of hepatic metastases. *Cancer*, **50**, 850–62.

Bergstrand, C.G. and Czar, B. (1956) Demonstration of new protein fraction in serum from the human fetus. *Scandinavian Journal of Clinical Laboratory Investigation*, **8**, 174–6.

Blanchard, R.A., Furie, B.C., Jorgensen, M. *et al.* (1981) Acquired vitamin K-dependent carboxylation deficiency in liver disease. *New England Journal of Medicine*, **305**, 242–5.

Brumm, C., Schulze, C., Charels, K. *et al.* (1989) The significance of alpha-fetoprotein and other tumour markers in differential immunocytochemistry of primary liver tumours. *Histopathology*, **14**, 503–13.

Burditt, I.J., Johnson, M.M., Johnson, P.J. *et al.* (1994) Detection of hepatocellular carcinoma-specific alphafetoprotein by isoelectric focussing. *Cancer*, **74**, 25–9.

Chio, L.F. and Don, C.J. (1979) Changes in serum alpha-antitrypsin, alpha acid glycoprotein and beta glycoprotein I in patients with malignant hepatocellular carcinoma. *Cancer*, **43**, 596–604.

Curtin, J.P., Rubin, S.C., Hoskins, W.J. *et al.* (1989) Second-look laparotomy in endodermal sinus tumour : a report of two patients with normal levels of alpha-fetoprotein and residual tumour at re-exploration. *Obstetrics and Gynecology*, **73**, 893–5.

Du, M.-Q., Hutchinson, W., Johnson, P.J. *et al.* (1991) Differential alpha fetoprotein lectin binding in hepatocellular carcinoma. *Cancer*, **67**, 476–80.

Ezaki, T., Hirofumi, Y., Ogawa, Y. *et al.* (1988) Elevation of alphafetoprotein level without evidence of recurrence after hepatectomy for hepatocellular carcinoma. *Cancer*, **61**, 1880–3.

Fiala, S., Fiala, A.E. and Dixon, B. (1972) γ-Gluta-myl transpeptidase in transplantable chemically induced rat hepatomas and 'spontaneous' mouse hepatomas. *Journal of the National Cancer Institutes*, **48**, 1393–401.

Fujiyama, S., Tsude, K., Sakai, M. *et al.* (1990) 5'-Nucleotide phosphodiesterase isozyme-V in hepatocellular carcinoma and other liver diseases. *Hepatogastroenterology*, **37**, 469–73.

Giannoulis, E., Arvanitakis, C., Nikopoulous, A. *et al.* (1984) Diagnostic value of serum ferritin in primary hepatocellular carcinoma. *Digestion*, **30**, 236–41.

Giardina, M.G., Matarazzo, M., Varriale, A. *et al.* (1992) Serum alpha-1-fucosidase. A useful marker for the diagnosis of hepatocellular carcinoma. *Cancer*, **70**, 1044–8.

Ho, S., Cheng, P., Yuen, J. *et al.* (1996) Isoelectric focusing of alphafetoprotein in patients with hepatocellular carcinoma-frequency of specific banding patterns at non-diagnostic serum levels. *British Journal of Cancer*, **73**, 985–8.

Johnson, P.J., Leung, N., Cheng, P. *et al.* (1997) 'Hepatoma-specific' alphafetoprotein may permit preclinical diagnosis of malignant change in patients with chronic liver disease. *British Journal of Cancer*, **75**, 236–40.

Johnson, P.J., Melia, W.M., Palmer, M.K. *et al.* (1981) Relationship between serum alpha-fetoprotein, cirrhosis and survival in hepatocellular carcinoma. *British Journal of Cancer*, **44**, 502–5.

Johnson, P.J. and Williams, R. (1980) Serum alphafetoprotein estimation and doubling time in hepatocellular carcinoma: influence of therapy and possible value in early detection. *Journal of the National Cancer Institutes*, **64**, 1329–32.

Kondo, F., Wada, K., Nagato, Y. *et al.* (1989) Biopsy diagnosis of well-differentiated hepatocellular carcinoma based on new morphologic criteria. *Hepatology*, **9**, 751–5.

Lau, W.Y., Ho, S., Leung, T.W.T. *et al.* (1998) Selective internal radiation therapy for non-resectable hepatocellular carcinoma with intra-arterial infusion of yttrium-90 microspheres. *International Journal of Radiation Oncology, Biology and Physics*, **40**, 583–92.

Leandro, G., Zizzari, S., Piccoli, A. *et al.* (1990) The serum tissue polypeptide antigen in the detection of hepatocellular carcinoma in cirrhotic patients. *Hepatogastroenterology*, **37**, 449–51.

Liaw, Y.-F., Tai, D.-I., Chen, T.-J. *et al.* (1986) Alpha-fetoprotein changes in the course of chronic hepatitis: relation to bridging hepatic necrosis and hepatocellular carcinoma. *Liver*, **6**, 133–7.

Liebmen, H.A., Furie, B.C., Tong, M.J. *et al.* (1984) Des-γ-carboxy (abnormal) prothrombin as a serum marker for primary hepatocellular carcinoma. *New England Journal of Medicine*, **310**, 1427–31.

Lok, A.S.F. and Lai, C.L. (1989) α-Fetoprotein monitoring in Chinese patients with chronic hepatitis B virus infection: role in early detection of hepatocellular carcinoma. *Hepatology*, **9**, 110–15.

Lu, H.M. and Chen, Q. (1989) 5'-Nucleotide phosphodiesterase V and hepatocellular carcinoma, in *Primary Liver Cancer* (eds Z.-Y. Tang, M.-C. Wu and S.-S. Xia), China Academic, Beijing, pp. 269–76.

Lu, H.M., Chen, Q., Sze, P.C. *et al.* (1980) The significance of 5'-nucleotide phosphodiesterase isoenzymes in the diagnosis of liver carcinoma. *International Journal of Cancer*, **26**, 21–35.

Masseyeff, R., Bonet, C., Drouet, J. *et al.* (1974) Radioimmunoassay of α-fetoprotein: I. Technique and serum level in normal adult. *Digestion*, **10**, 17–28.

Matsumoto, Y., Suzuki, T., Ono, H. *et al.* (1974) Response of alpha-fetoprotein to chemotherapy in patients with hepatoma. *Cancer*, **34**, 1602–6.

Mawas, C., Buffe, D. and Burtin, P. (1970) Influence of age on alphafetoprotein incidence. *Lancet*, **i**, 1292.

McIntire, K.R., Vogel, C.L., Primack, A. *et al.* (1976) Effect of surgical and chemotherapeutic treatment on alpha-fetoprotein levels in patients with hepatocellular carcinoma. *Cancer*, **37**, 677–83.

Melia, W.M., Bullock, S., Johnson, P.J. *et al.* (1983) Serum ferritin in hepatocellular carcinoma, comparison with alphafetoprotein. *Cancer*, **51**, 2112–15.

Nakano, S., Kumada, T., Sugiyama, K. *et al.* (1984) Clinical significance of serum ferritin determination for hepatocellular carcinoma. *American Journal of Gastroenterology*, **79**, 623–7.

Namieno, T., Kawata, A., Sato, N. *et al.* (1995) Age-related, different clinicopathologic features of hepatocellular carcinoma patients. *Annals of Surgery*, **221**, 308–14.

Nauta, R.J., Heres, E.K., Thomas, D.S. *et al.* (1987) Intraoperative single-dose radiotherapy. Observations on staging and interstitial treatment of unresectable liver metastases. *Archives of Surgery*, **122**, 1392–5.

Nomura, F., Ohnishi, K. and Tanabe, Y. (1989) Clinical features and prognosis of hepatocellular carcinoma with reference to serum alpha-feto-protein levels. *Cancer*, **64**, 1700–7.

O'Conor, G., Tatarinov, Y.S., Abelev, G.I. *et al.* (1970) A collaborative study for the evaluation of a serological test for primary cancer. *Cancer*, **25**, 1091–8.

Okuda, K. (1986) Early recognition of hepatocellular carcinoma. *Hepatology*, **6**, 729–38.

Rouslahti, E. and Seppala, M. (1971) Studies of carcino-fetal protein III. Development of a radio-immunoassay of alpha-fetoprotein. Demonstration of alpha-fetoprotein in serum of healthy human adults. *International Journal of Cancer*, **8**, 374–83.

Sawabu, N. and Hattori, N. (1987) Serological tumour markers in hepatocellular carcinoma, in *Neoplasms of the Liver* (eds K. Okuda and K.G. Ishak), Springer, Tokyo, pp. 227–38.

Sawabu, N., Nakagen, M., Ozaki, K. *et al.* (1983) Clinical evaluation of specific γ-GTP isoenzyme in patients with hepatocellular carcinoma. *Cancer*, **51**, 327–31.

Sell, S. (1981) Diagnostic applications of alpha-fetoprotein, government regulations prevent full application of a clinically useful test. *Human Pathology*, **12**, 959–63.

Sell, S. (1990) Cancer markers of the 1990's. *Clinical Laboratory Medicine*, **10**, 1–37.

Shimada, M., Takenaka, K., Fujiwara, Y. *et al.* (1996) Des-γ-carboxy prothrombin and α-fetoprotein status as a new prognostic indicator after hepatic resection for hepatocellular carcinoma. *Cancer*, **78**, 2094–100.

Szuki, H., Iino, S., Endo, Y. *et al.* (1975) Tumor-specific alkaline phosphatase in hepatoma. *Annals of the New York Academy of Science*, **259**, 307–16.

Taketa, K. (1989) AFP. *Journal of Medical Technology* **33**, 1380–4.

Tatarinov, Y.S. (1964) Presence of embryospecific α-globulin in the serum of patients with primary hepatocellular carcinoma. *Vopi Medica Khimia*, **10**, 90–1.

Tatsta, M., Yamamura, H., Iishi, H. *et al.* (1986) Value of serum alpha-fetoprotein and ferritin in the diagnosis of hepatocellular carcinoma. *Oncology*, **43**, 306–10.

The Liver Study Group of Japan (1987) Primary liver cancer in Japan. Sixth Report. *Cancer*, **60**, 1400–11.

Trevisani, F., D'Intino, P.E., Caraceni, P. *et al.* (1995) Etiologic factors and clinical presentation of hepatocellular carcinoma. Differences between cirrhotic and noncirrhotic Italian patients. *Cancer*, **75**, 2220–32.

Tu, Z.-X. and Wu, M.-C. (1989) Clinical significance of serum alpha-1-antitrypsin determination in AFP-negative primary liver cancer. In *Primary Liver Cancer* (eds Z.-Y. Tang, M.-C. Wu and S.-S. Xia), China Academic, Beijing, pp. 262–8.

Urabe, T.S., Hayashi, S., Terasaki, M. *et al.* (1990) An assessment of therapeutic effect of hepatocellular carcinoma by the serial change of serum AFP value. *Japanese Journal of Gastroenterology*, **87**, 100–8.

Yoshima, H., Mizuochi, T., Ishii, M. *et al.* (1980) Structure of the asparagine-linked sugar chains of α-fetoprotein purified from human ascites fluid. *Cancer Research*, **40**, 4276–81.

Zong, M. and Wu, M.-C. (1989) Clinical study of aldolase A in primary liver cancer, in *Primary Liver Cancer*, (eds Z.-Y. Tang, M.-C. Wu and S.-S. Xia), China Academic, Beijing, pp. 269–76.

S.C.-H. Yu, M.S.Y. Chan and J.W.Y. Lau

4.1 OVERVIEW

4.1.1 GROSS PATHOMORPHOLOGICAL CHARACTERISTICS OF HEPATOCELLULAR CARCINOMA

The gross morphology of hepatocellular carcinoma (HCC) can be classified into three categories: (1) solitary massive expansive tumor with or without daughter nodules, (2) multifocal or nodular tumor and (3) diffuse or multiple small tumors. External fibrous capsule (pseudocapsule) and internal septae are present in 50% of HCC of 1.5–2 cm diameter (Kanai *et al.*, 1987), they are more common in larger size tumors, and the overall occurrence is 80% for all sizes of HCC (Liver Cancer Study Group of Japan, 1990). Tumor capsular invasion occurs in up to 38% of HCC (Liver Cancer Study Group of Japan, 1990). When the tumor is not encapsulated, usually in the non-cirrhotic liver, the tumor boundary is poorly demarcated and is irregular. The typical mosaic pattern, which represents the nodule in nodule phenomenon, occurs in 63% of massive expansive and nodular tumors (Honda *et al.*, 1992a). The tumor may exhibit intratumoral necrosis, hemorrhage and fatty change, which progress as the tumor grows in size. Calcification occurs in 2–12% of tumors. The massive expansive and nodular type of HCC is typically hypervascular, with the blood supply being predominantly derived from the hepatic artery. Arterioportal shunting occurs within the tumor. The massive expansive tumor may proliferate in an extrahepatic direction to produce a pedunculated mass. Spontaneous rupture of the tumor through the liver capsule with intraperitoneal hemorrhage occurs in 2.9–14.5% of cases.

Cirrhosis is a common accompanying condition, especially in Asia where it is present in 67–96% of patients with HCC. In the West, the proportion is 38–50% (Okuda, 1992).

There is a great tendency for HCC to invade the portal vein, occurring in up to 62% of autopsy cases (Liver Cancer Study Group of Japan, 1990), so providing a channel for spread to the rest of the liver and rarely in a retrograde fashion into the superior mesenteric vein (Plate 3). The presence of a portal vein tumor is an important clue to the diagnosis of HCC as <8% of portal vein tumors are due to other malignancies. Tumor invasion of the hepatic vein is also frequent, occurring in up to 26% of autopsy cases, and it opens a pathway for systemic spread. Extension into the right atrium via the hepatic vein and inferior vena cava may be complicated by pulmonary embolism (Fig. 4.1). Bile duct obstruction may occur as a

Hepatocellular Carcinoma: Diagnosis, investigation and management. Edited by Anthony S.-Y. Leong, Choong-Tsek Liew, Joseph W.Y. Lau and Philip J. Johnson. Published in 1999 by Arnold, London. ISBN 0 340 74096 5.

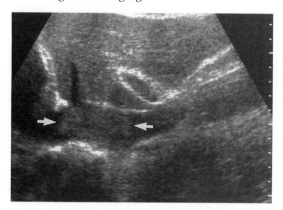

Fig. 4.1 HCC extension into the inferior vena cava near the right atrium on ultrasonography.

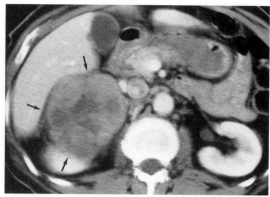

Fig. 4.2 Retroperitoneal extension of a pedunculated HCC mimicking an adrenal tumor on computed tomography.

result of compression by massive intrahepatic tumors or enlarged nodes at the porta hepatis. It may also be due to direct tumor invasion with or without complicating hemobilia. Intrabiliary tumor fragmentation may also obstruct the common bile duct with tumor emboli, sometimes in the absence of an obvious intrahepatic tumor.

Direct invasion of the diaphragm, abdominal wall, pancreas, peritoneum, mesentery and omentum may occur. Retroperitoneal extension through the bare area of liver into the superior aspect of perirenal spaces in the form of a pedunculated mass may mimic an adrenal tumor (Fig. 4.2). The lung is the commonest site of distant metastasis. Lymph node metastasis is the second commonest, usually occurring at the porta hepatis, celiac axis and around the pancreatic head. Other sites of metastasis include the spleen and other intraperitoneal organs, peritoneum, adrenal gland, bone, skin, breast and rarely brain (Fig. 4.3). Peritoneal spread of HCC is quite different from the usual carcinomatosis peritonei. They occur as single or multiple discrete hypervascular masses in the omentum or peritoneum (Fig. 4.4). Intracranial metastasis may be due to brain metastasis or skull metastasis without brain involvement.

The majority of cases of brain metastasis have simultaneous lung metastasis but without skull or other bone metastasis. Brain deposits are hypervascular. They may very rarely present as intracranial hemorrhage, the likelihood increasing with the size of the tumor. Skull metastasis is rare, and it may be multiple and quite large with brain invasion or extradural extension causing compression of the brain (Fig. 4.5). Skull metastasis is often associated with extracranial bone metastasis without lung metastasis.

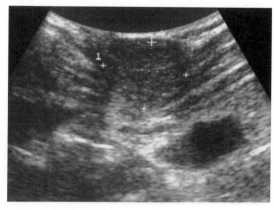

Fig. 4.3 Subcutaneous metastasis of HCC on ultrasonography (crosses).

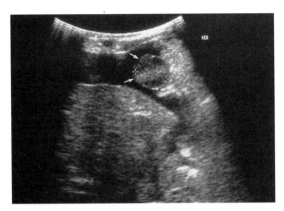

Fig. 4.4 A discrete omental mass of HCC on ultrasonography.

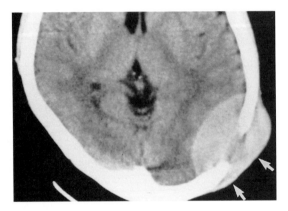

Fig. 4.5 Skull metastasis of HCC with extradural and extracranial extension on computed tomography.

4.1.2 ROLE OF DIAGNOSTIC IMAGING

Diagnostic imaging is mandatory in the clinical management of HCC. First, it is necessary for detection of the primary or recurrent tumor. Second, it enables a specific radiological diagnosis to be made in some instances. Third, it allows for staging with respect to the operability and the postresection prognosis in terms of recurrence and survival rate. This forms the basis for selection of treatment options. Fourth, it provides guidance for percutaneous biopsy and local therapy such

as ethanol injection, laser therapy or microwave coagulation. Fifth, it allows the determination of tumor vascularity and the degree of lung shunting as a pre-procedure work up for transcatheter intra-arterial treatment. Sixth, it offers an avenue for transcatheter intra-arterial treatment with various radioactive, chemotherapeutic or embolizing agents through the technique of angiographic catheterization. Finally, it allows post-treatment assessment of tumor changes and the evaluation of the effectiveness of treatment.

Determining the size, location and number of tumors, and also identifying whether there is encapsulation, vascular invasion, lymph node or distant metastases, involvement of adjacent organs or structures, and coexistence of cirrhosis, accomplish the staging of HCC. Tumors are best localized to specific subsegments according to Bismuth's nomenclature which is a slightly modified Couinaud's system, to offer a level of anatomical detail sufficient for hepatic surgery and radiology. In Bismuth's nomenclature, all hepatic segments except for the caudate lobe are defined vertically by the three hepatic veins and transversely by the right and left portal branches (Fig. 4.6). Segment I corresponds to the caudate lobe, II and III correspond to the left lateral superior and inferior subsegment, IVa and IVb to the left medial superior and inferior subsegment, and V, VIII, VI, VII to the right anterior inferior, anterior superior, posterior inferior and posterior superior subsegments (Soyer, 1993).

The role of the individual imaging modalities will be discussed in the respective sections of this chapter.

4.2 RADIOGRAPHY

Plain radiography can reveal hepatomegaly in the presence of a huge tumor, and, rarely, tumor calcification. However, these findings are non-specific and of limited clinical value. More importantly, metastatic disease to the

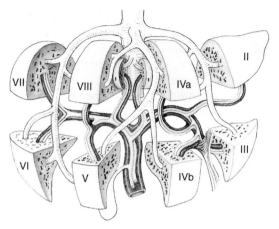

Fig. 4.6 A diagrammatic representation of sub-segmental hepatic anatomy according to Bismuth's nomenclature. (Reproduced with permission from Nelson, R.C., Chezmar, J.L., Sugarbaker, P.H. *et al.* [1990] Preoperative localization of focal liver lesions to specific liver segments: utility of CT during arterial portography. *Radiology* **176**, 89–94.)

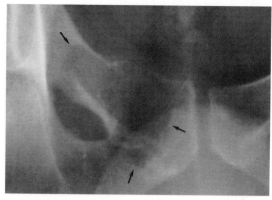

Fig. 4.8 An expansile osteolytic metastasis of HCC in right pubic bone on plain radiography.

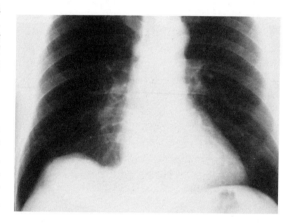

Fig. 4.9 A diaphragmatic hump due to HCC on chest radiography.

lung and bone may be detected (Figs 4.7 and 4.8). The presence of a diaphragmatic hump on chest radiography is a specific sign which is more sensitive than ultrasonography, computed tomography and hepatic angiography for diagnosing tumor invasion of the diaphragm (Lau *et al.*, 1995) (Fig. 4.9).

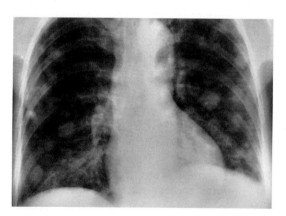

Fig. 4.7 Bilateral multiple lung metastases of HCC on chest radiography.

4.3   ULTRASONOGRAPHY

4.3.1   ADVANTAGES, APPLICATIONS AND LIMITATIONS

Ultrasonography (US) offers a non-invasive, convenient and radiation-free means of obtaining an immediate three-dimensional perception of HCC and related anatomical structures, with a reasonable sensitivity for detecting small tumors. It is widely used for mass screening in the high-risk population. It is effective in identifying blood vessels and bile ducts, differentiating solid and cystic lesions, and in elucidating cirrhosis and evidence of portal hypertension. It is also a very useful tool to guide percutaneous needle biopsy or local therapy. Color and duplex US may allow characterization of liver masses as well as identification of hemodynamic disturbances and venous invasion.

Adequate ultrasonographic examination of the liver may sometimes be impossible due to intervening bone, lung or bowel gas, especially in the presence of dense fatty tissue in the body wall or when the liver is small and cirrhotic. Potential blind spots may occur in segments II, IV, VII and VIII of a shrunken liver. The tumor size may be underestimated. In cirrhotic livers, the sensitivity of tumor detection is compromised due to the diminished liver size and inhomogeneous echogenic echotexture, it also does not provide good distinction between regeneration nodules and small HCC.

The detection sensitivity of US for small (< 3 cm) HCC is 63–84% (Sheu, 1984; Matsui *et al.*, 1985; Takayasu *et al.*, 1990; Santis *et al.*, 1992). It decreases to 38% for tumors < 1 cm (Takayasu, 1990). The overall detection sensitivity for all sizes is 58.9–81% (Tanaka *et al.*, 1986; Miller *et al.*, 1991; Santis *et al.*, 1992). In end-stage cirrhotic livers, the overall sensitivity decreases to 42% (Dodd *et al.*, 1992). US is less accurate than computed tomography (CT) and magnetic resonance imaging (MRI) for detecting the fibrous capsule and fibrous septae of HCC, but it is more accurate in detecting the mosaic appearance (Honda *et al.*, 1992b) (Fig. 4.10). Owing to its high specificity, a US-diagnosed HCC should be considered as such until proven otherwise (Tanaka, 1986). When compared with CT, US is less accurate in assessing resectability as it tends to underestimate the extent of parenchymal involvement: but it is more sensitive in detecting vascular invasion. US may identify small hypovascular, well-differentiated HCC not detectable with angiography and lipiodol CT.

Contrast-enhanced US with intra-arterial carbon dioxide microbubbles allows the sonographic detection of small hypervascular lesions. Intravenous Levovist-enhanced color Doppler US may be useful in diagnosing hypervascular HCC and distinguishing it from other benign liver lesions. Intraoperative ultrasound of the liver can identify tumors not detected preoperatively, allowing the surgeon to determine intraoperatively the feasibility and extent of liver resection. Demonstration of the topography of tumors and the relationship to adjacent hepatic vascular structures can be invaluable in planning the plane of resection and the safety margin. Laparoscopic US also shows promising early results.

4.3.2   TRANSABDOMINAL ULTRASONOGRAPHY

Transabdominal ultrasonographic examination of the liver and its adjacent organs is usually performed with an electronic curvilinear 3.5 MHz real-time transducer, scanning subcostally and intercostally with the patient lying in a supine, and then a left decubitus, position. Cooperation from the patient with breath-holding at deep inspiration or expiration helps to avoid image obscuration by the lung, gut or ribs. Scanning with the patient in a standing posture may enable a more thorough examination of segments VII and VIII.

The solitary or multifocal nodular HCC is usually round or oval, with a well-defined regular boundary and a thin hypoechoic peripheral zone which represents the tumor capsule (Figs 4.10 and 4.11). Posterior echo-enhancement is uncommon and may also occur in hemangioma and metastases. Bilateral acoustic shadows occur only occasionally but they are quite specific to HCC. The majority of small HCC ≤ 1 cm in diameter are of homogeneous and hypoechoic echotexture, which is non-specific and may not be distinguishable from the echo pattern of regeneration nodules in cirrhosis. Histologic examination at this stage reveals a solid cell

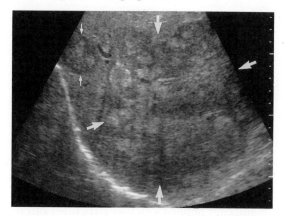

Fig. 4.10 A massive expansive HCC (big arrows) and a daughter nodule (small arrows) on ultrasonography. Note the hypoechoic external pseudocapsule and hyperechoic internal nodules separated by hypoechoic fibrous septae.

mass without necrosis. The tumor becomes non-homogeneous and more hyperechoic or isoechoic when it grows in size, due to fatty degeneration, clear cell change, sclerotic change or coagulation necrosis. The characteristic mosaic pattern and fibrous septae of HCC are well demonstrated with US, so is the star-shaped central hypoechoic area (Fig.

4.10). The less common type of nodular HCC that appears ultrasonographically to be homogeneous and diffusely hyperechoic is probably due to fatty change or dilated sinusoids. It is usually surrounded by a thin peripheral hypoechoic halo and does not change in appearance when the tumor grows (Fig. 4.11).

In the absence of a definite ultrasonographic finding of a liver mass, indirect evidence such as compression, interruption or irregularity of the wall of a blood vessel, localized bulging of the hepatic surface, or a dilated intrahepatic bile duct due to extrinsic compression by a tumor mass or intraductal tumor infiltration, should raise the suspicion of a liver tumor (Figs 4.12 and 4.13). In the diffuse type of HCC, US may show diffuse distortion of the normal internal architecture of liver parenchyma in which multiple areas of increased echogenicity may be recognized (Figs 4.12 and 4.13). However, as no definite tumor mass can be identified, an isoechoic diffuse HCC may be completely missed. In a background of cirrhosis with regeneration nodules, the detection of small HCC by US is much more difficult than the detection of metastases in a normal liver.

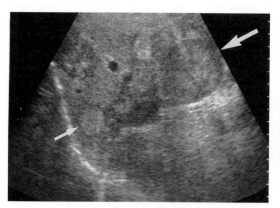

Fig. 4.11 Multifocal nodular HCCs with hypoechoic external pseudocapsules on ultrasonography. Some nodules show the mosaic pattern (big arrow) and some are diffusely hyperechoic (small arrow).

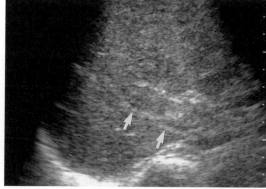

Fig. 4.12 An isoechoic diffuse HCC without a tumor margin on ultrasonography. Note the distortion of liver parenchymal architecture and portal vein invasion.

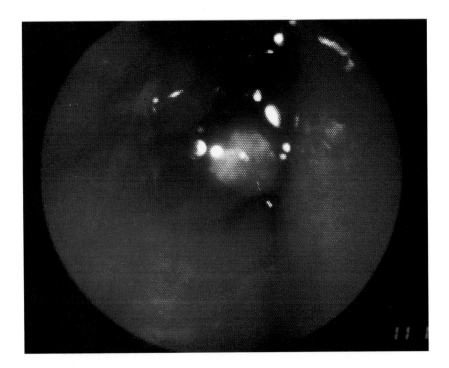

Plate 1 Endoscopic view of direct duodenal invasion by HCC causing gastrointestinal hemorrhage.

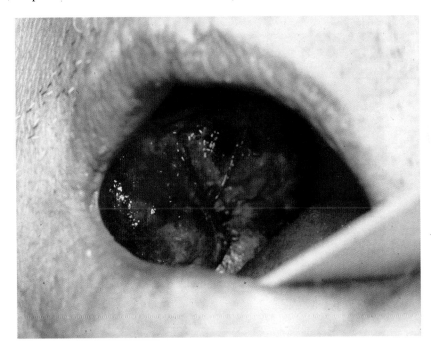

Plate 2 HCC metastatic to the oral mucosa.

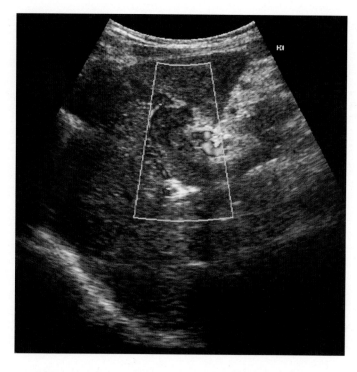

Plate 3 HCC invasion of the portal vein on power Doppler ultrasonography.

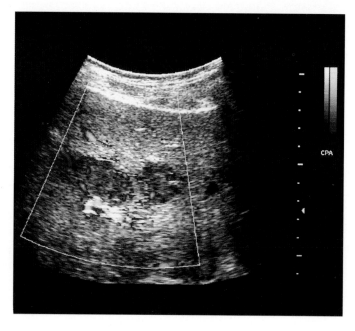

Plate 4 Two nodular HCC on power Doppler ultrasonography.

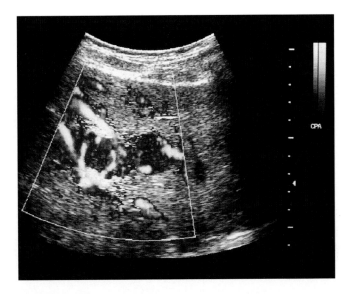

Plate 5 Note the enhancement of power Doppler signals and better depiction of vascularization pattern after Levovist administration.

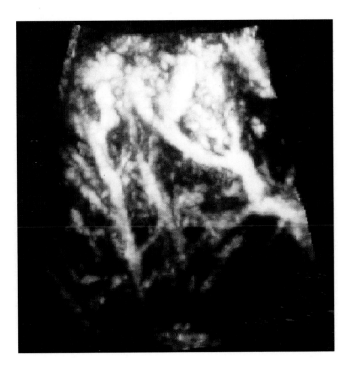

Plate 6 The same lesions on three-dimensional Levovist enhanced power Doppler ultrasonography.

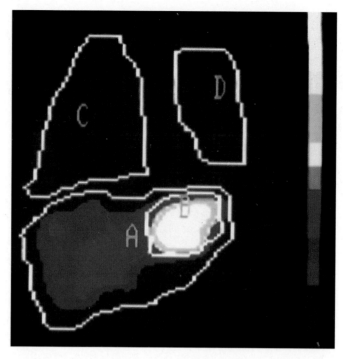

Plate 7 Hepatic arterial perfusion scintigraphy with technetium-99m macroaggregated albumin showing preferential activity over the HCC due to tumor vascularity.

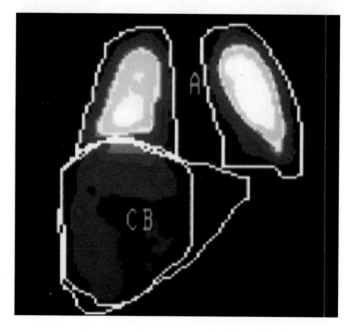

Plate 8 Activity over the lungs due to tumor-to-lung vascular shunting.

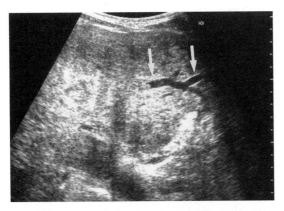

Fig. 4.13 An ill-defined diffuse HCC with hyperechoic texture on ultrasonography. Note the distorted liver architecture and also obstruction of the intrahepatic bile duct due to tumor invasion.

4.3.3 DOPPLER ULTRASONOGRAPHY

Duplex Doppler US can aid in the characterization of focal liver lesions, with a high degree of specificity but low sensitivity. A Doppler shift ≥ 4.5 KHz gives a 70% sensitivity, 95% specificity and 89% positive predictive value in distinguishing hepatoma from metastases. A Doppler shift ≥ 1.75 KHz gives a 68% sensitivity, 94% specificity and 96% positive predictive value in distinguishing malignant tumors from hemangiomas. The detection of pulsatile flow in portal vein thrombi with Doppler US in patients with cirrhosis is a moderately sensitive (62%) but highly specific (95%) sign for the diagnosis of malignant portal vein thrombus. However, continuous flow can be detected in benign and malignant portal vein thrombus and is thus not useful in differentiating between the two (Dodd *et al.*, 1995).

Color Doppler US is a useful means of evaluating the hemodynamics of hepatic tumors. The peak systolic flow velocity seen in HCC and other malignant hepatic tumors significantly exceeds that seen in hemangiomas. Peak systolic flow velocities ≥ 0.4 and ≥ 0.8 m/s suggest a malignant hepatic tumor rather than a hemangioma, with specificities

of 91 and 100%, and accuracy of 71 and 92% respectively (Numata *et al.*, 1993). Demonstration of internal vascularity with color Doppler US may differentiate HCC and metastatic tumors from hemangiomas, but it does not help in distinguishing HCC from metastatic tumors (Nino-Murcia *et al.*, 1992). Qualification of the intratumoral color signals with a three-step grading system may be valuable in diagnosing HCC which shows a higher grade of signals than do metastases and hemangiomas (Lee *et al.*, 1996). The depiction of an arterial pulsating afferent tumor vessel or a constant flow efferent tumor vessel continuing to a portal branch with color Doppler US is useful in distinguishing HCC from adenomatous hyperplastic nodules (Tanaka *et al.*, 1992).

Power Doppler US is a new technology that displays the total, integrated Doppler power in color. It is superior to conventional color Doppler US in demonstrating tumor vascularity in HCC, with an increased dynamic range and sensitivity. The detection rate is unaffected by the small size and deep location of the lesion.

4.3.4 CONTRAST-ENHANCED ULTRASONOGRAPHY WITH INTRAARTERIAL CARBON DIOXIDE MICROBUBBLES

Carbon dioxide- (CO_2) enhanced US can be performed with transcatheter injection of CO_2 microbubbles in the hepatic artery. The solution of CO_2 microbubbles can be prepared by mixing gaseous CO_2 with either heparinized saline and patient's blood, or with 20% glucose solution and 25% albumin. Contrast-enhanced US is more sensitive (86%) than conventional angiography (63%), digital subtraction angiography (70%) and lipiodol CT (82%) in detecting small hypervascular HCC (≤ 3 cm), especially those <1 cm in diameter. It allows classification of the tumor vascularity into hypervascular, isovascular and hypovascular, which may help in guiding the subsequent treatment strategy (Masatoshi *et al.*,

1992). Contrast-enhanced US may be a useful tool for detecting minute HCC nodules developing within an adenomatous hyperplastic nodule, which can be depicted as hyperechoic foci in an area of hypoechoic change (Nomura *et al.*, 1993). As small additional nodules and characteristic vascularization patterns of HCC, hemangioma, metastases, focal nodular hyperplasia and regeneration nodules can be shown, it may help to improve the staging and characterization of hepatic tumors (Veltri *et al.*, 1994).

4.3.5 INTRAVENOUS LEVOVIST-ENHANCED COLOR DOPPLER ULTRASONOGRAPHY

The ultrasound contrast agent Levovist (Schering AG, Germany) is a suspension of micrometer-sized particles of galactose and gaseous bubbles which can pass through the lungs without any noteworthy side effects (Dodd *et al.*, 1995). Intravenous administration of Levovist enhances the color Doppler signals and allows for an easier and better depiction of vascularization patterns of liver lesions than with conventional color Doppler US (Plates 4–6). Levovist-enhanced color Doppler US has proved to be effective in the evaluation of HCC vascularity and it correlates well with angiographic findings. Thus it may be useful in diagnosing hypervascular HCC (Fujimoto *et al.*, 1994), especially the deeply located lesions that cannot be assessed by color Doppler US alone. HCC shows intratumoral color signals and tumor-margin enhancement related to cardiac contractions, whereas hemangioma may show tumor margin enhancement with or without intratumoral signals which are unrelated to cardiac contractions. Focal fatty change in contrast, does not give intratumoral nor tumor margin enhancement. Levovist-enhanced color Doppler US may thus help to differentiate hyperechoic HCC from other hyperechoic lesions including hemangiomas and focal fatty change (Tano *et al.*, 1997).

4.3.6 INTRAOPERATIVE ULTRASONOGRAPHY

Intraoperative US (IUS) is usually performed with a low profile 5 or 7.5 MHz linear array transducer applied onto the moist liver surface. Direct examination of the liver allows the use of high-frequency transducers that produces US images of high resolution. In the absence of interposing organs or structures, image degradation and artifacts are minimized. As a result, it is more sensitive than any other modality for detecting primary or secondary liver cancers (96–100%), including computerized tomographic arterial portography (65–89%) (Parker *et al.*, 1989; Soyer *et al.*, 1993; Fortunato *et al.*, 1995). IUS is more accurate than computerized tomography for assessing portal vein or hepatic vein invasion and determining the feasibility and extent of liver resection (Parker *et al.*, 1989). IUS adds new information in 23–29% of cases (Fortunato *et al.*, 1995; Kokudo *et al.*, 1996). The surgical plan is modified by the intraoperative findings in 41–51% of cases (Parker *et al.*, 1989; Kane *et al.*, 1994; Haider *et al.*, 1995). Additional uses include the provision of guidance for cryoablation, ethanol injection and biopsy. Without intraoperative ultrasonography modern liver surgery cannot be performed.

4.3.7 LAPAROSCOPIC ULTRASONOGRAPHY

Laparoscopic US performed with a 5–7.5 MHz transducer is a safe and expeditious technique that permits examination of all liver segments through a single cannula site (Marchesa *et al.*, 1996). It can identify liver tumors not visible during laparoscopy, provides additional staging information and optimizes patient selection for liver resection with a curative intent (John *et al.*, 1994). Staging of liver tumors with laparoscopy and laparoscopic ultrasound to assess resectability prior to a major laparotomy is useful to avoid unnecessary surgery (Barbot *et al.*, 1997).

4.4 COMPUTED TOMOGRAPHY

4.4.1 ADVANTAGES, APPLICATIONS AND LIMITATIONS

Compared with US, computed tomography (CT) is much less limited by operator performance and the body build of patients. It allows objective display of the cross-sectional anatomy of the liver and its adjacent organs with virtually no blind spots and a remarkable spatial resolution. With the administration of intravenous contrast material, CT enables accurate evaluation of the location and extent of disease and it may help in differentiating HCC from the other liver tumors. The topographic relationship between the tumor and the adjacent vascular and biliary structures can be demonstrated, as well as the evidence of extrahepatic extension and metastatic spread. CT can identify biliary dilatation, portal and hepatic venous invasion, tumor extension into inferior vena cava and right atrium, and also lymph node and adrenal metastasis (Figs 4.14 and 4.15).

The drawback of CT compared with US is that it is more expensive and not mobile. Contrast-enhanced CT is inferior to US for detection of small HCC (< 3 cm) (Matsui *et al.*, 1985; Santis *et al.*, 1992). A difference of 10 Hounsfield units is required for recognizing an intraparenchymal lesion. Small lesions may not be depicted or only partially demonstrated due to the partial volume effect, especially in segments II, III, VII and VIII. CT is not sensitive for the detection of diffuse-type HCC and intrabiliary HCC, as well as lymphadenopathy at the porta hepatis. Artifacts due to ribs and contrast media in the stomach may arise.

Spiral CT, also known as helical or volume-acquisition CT, involves continuous patient translation during X-ray source rotation and data acquisition. A continuous spiral volumetric data set can be acquired within 20–30 s, allowing the whole liver to be scanned within a single breath hold to coincide with the

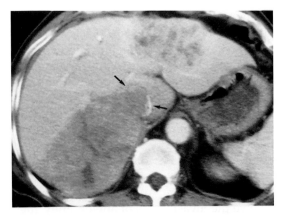

Fig. 4.14 Tumor invasion of a right hepatic vein with extension into the inferior vena cava (arrows) on contrast-enhanced computed tomography.

arterial and portal venous phase of hepatic enhancement. The volumetric data set enables retrospective image reconstruction at selected locations along the z-axis with reduced inter-scan interspace or overlapping slices to minimize partial volume averaging without additional radiation doses or scanning time. These factors, in conjunction with the ability to eliminate respiratory section misregistration and motion artifacts, result in improved lesion conspicuity. Multiplanar and three-dimensional reconstruction of the volumetric data are useful in localizing and defining the extent

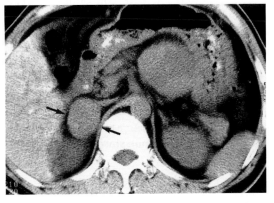

Fig. 4.15 An adrenal metastasis from HCC on computed tomography.

of the liver tumor in and demonstrating optimally the porta hepatis which is a difficult area to examine with standard CT due to its complicated anatomy and oblique orientation. The limitations of spiral CT include increased image noise, decreased longitudinal resolution, increased time for image processing and increased requirements for data storage.

CT arteriography (CTA), CT arterial portography (CTAP) and lipiodol CT are sensitive in depicting focal liver lesions, including those < 2 cm in diameter. As these investigations involve the invasiveness of angiography, they should be reserved as a preoperative staging and planning procedure for candidates with a known liver tumor that is potentially resectable. CTAP provides excellent delineation of the hepatic vasculature and allows for accurate segmental localization of liver tumors. Lipiodol CT is valuable for preoperative staging of HCC and detecting small HCC in patients with elevated α-fetoprotein. A major limitation on the use of CTA is the requirement of suitable vascular anatomy, with the proper hepatic artery supplying all parts of the liver, a finding which occurs only in approximately 50% of patients. A significant limitation of CTAP is the frequent occurrence of non-tumorous perfusion defects. The accuracy of CTAP in detecting HCC is further diminished in patients with cirrhosis, as the reduced or reversed portal blood flow in portal hypertension with concomitant porto-systemic collaterals will result in decreased and inhomogeneous portal perfusion of the liver. However, a combined study of CTAP and CTA may be valuable to improve tumor detection and may allow differentiation of malignant from benign nodules in cirrhotic liver. CTAP and CTA have been utilized much less frequently for HCC assessment than for the investigation of metastases.

4.4.2   CONTRAST-ENHANCED CT

HCC may appear as hypodense or isodense lesions on precontrast CT. With the admin-istration of intravenous contrast material, contrast-enhanced CT (CECT) improves the detection and characterization of liver lesions. The use of CECT alone for liver examination with the omission of precontrast CT has been advocated for the sake of cost effectiveness; however, with this approach those HCCs that become isodense with the liver following contrast administration may be missed. Dynamic incremental scanning is the preferred CECT technique for routine liver scanning with conventional CT. A bolus of 150 ml 30% contrast material is usually administered intravenously as either a uniphasic (2–3 ml/s) or biphasic (50 ml at 3–5 ml/s, followed by 100 ml at 1 ml/s) injection. Using a fast scanner with scanning time of 2–3 s and repetition rates of 7–10 scans per min, contiguous axial scanning of the whole liver with 10 mm collimation can be completed in 2 min. With an aim to optimize lesion conspicuousness by rapid incremented scanning when the liver–lesion contrast difference is maximal, scanning usually commences at about 45 s after the start of contrast administration so that liver scanning is initiated and completed within the bolus and non-equilibrium phases of the time–density curve of hepatic enhancement (Foley, 1989; Walkey, 1991).

The enhancement pattern depicted with dynamic incremental CECT scanning at early (45–110 s) and late (6–7 min) phase is useful in characterizing HCC. HCC constitutes 86% of the tumors that appear totally hyperdense in the early phase, 92% of tumors that appear totally hyperdense in the early phase and totally hypodense in the delayed phase, 82% of tumors that appear totally isodense in the early phase, 100% of tumors that appear totally isodense in the early phase and totally hypodense in the delayed phase (Honda *et al.*, 1992a). Hyperattenuation of the large HCCs (≥ 5 cm) at CECT appears a function of dilated sinusoids within the tumor (peliotic changes) as well as vascularity. In patients with advanced cirrhosis, hypovascular HCCs can be hyperattenuating at CT. With dynamic incremental CECT, the mosaic pattern is demonstrated in 46% of HCC, venous invasion in 33% and tumor encapsulation in 31%. These characteristic CT features of HCC occur with similar frequencies in Asian and non-Asian populations. The previously reported CT morphologic differences of HCC between Asian and non-Asian patients may be due to differences in underlying liver disease, tumor size and histologic grade (Stevens *et al.*, 1994). CECT is more accurate than US in evaluating the fibrous capsule and septae of HCC, but it is less accurate than MRI in demonstrating the capsule, septae and mosaic pattern (Honda *et al.*, 1992b) (Figs 4.16 and 4.17). The CT appearance of the characteristic mosaic pattern of HCC comprises enhancing nodules, low attenuation areas and internal septa. Histologic correlation of the enhancing tissue corresponds to viable tumor, and the low attenuation areas correspond to areas of necrosis, fibrosis and hemorrhage (Stevens *et al.*, 1996). On CECT large portal venous thrombus of HCC may be enhanced, whereas HCC thrombus in the peripheral portal branches of the third and more distal orders may appear as punctate or linear low density structures.

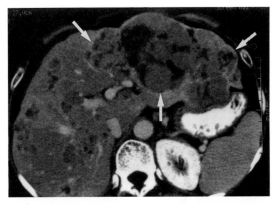

Fig. 4.17 Internal structures of a massive expansive HCC on contrast-enhanced computed tomography. Note the nodules, septae and hypoattenuating areas.

Triphasic spiral CT performed at 25–30 s (arterial phase), 60–70 s (portal venous phase) and 300–360 s (delayed phase) after the commencement of a uniphasic bolus injection of 120 ml 30% contrast material at 3 ml/s with data acquisition time within 20 s at each phase, 10 mm collimation and 10 mm/s table incrementation detected 86% of nodular HCC at the arterial phase, 67% at the portal venous phase and 72% at the delayed phase. Spiral CT at the arterial phase is significantly superior to the other two phases for HCC detection. The addition of portal venous phase is superior to the arterial phase alone. The best result is achieved by the combination of all three phases (Cho *et al.*, 1996; Choi *et al.*, 1997). Arterial phase spiral CT in addition to delayed phase CT also significantly improves detection of small HCC (≤ 3 cm) for which portal venous phase CT is of limited value (Mitsuzaki *et al.*, 1996). Reconstruction of 8 mm thick spiral CT images with interscan spacing reduced from 8 to 4 mm is shown to increase the confidence in detection and the detection rate of liver lesions, especially those with size < 1 cm (Urban *et al.*, 1993).

In one study, 87% of HCC showed moderate to marked hyperattenuation in the arterial

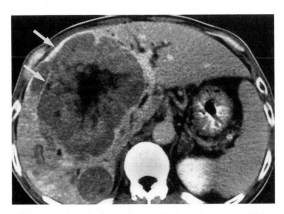

Fig. 4.16 A massive expansive HCC with a daughter nodule on contrast-enhanced computed tomography. Note the enhancing pseudocapsule and fibrous septae.

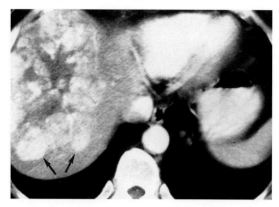

Fig. 4.18 Arterial-phase spiral computed tomography of a massive expansive HCC. Note the marked hyperattenuation of internal nodules.

phase (Fig. 4.18). In the portal venous phase 54% of HCC were isoattenuated and 39% were hypoattenuated. In the delayed phase 80% of HCC showed hypoattenuation (Cho *et al.*, 1996). Evaluation of the contrast enhancement pattern of spiral CT at arterial and delayed phases is useful in the differential diagnosis of liver tumors. Total or peripheral nodular high attenuation in the late phase is the most useful pattern in distinguishing hemangiomas from malignant tumors (96 versus 0%). A combination of totally high attenuation in the arterial phase and low attenuation in the late phase is useful in the differentiation of HCC from metastases (42 versus 0%) (Choi *et al.*, 1995).

4.4.3   CT ARTERIOGRAPHY

CTA consists of axial hepatic CT scanning with 10–15 s delay after the start of intra-arterial injection of contrast material at the proper hepatic artery. Artifacts may arise from the angiographic catheter and over-concentrated contrast material. The use of contrast material with reduced concentration at 15% and increased injection rate at 3–5 ml/s improves the quality of CTA scans without layering of contrast material along the artery

and avoids differential enhancement of the right and left hepatic lobes.

Non-pathological focal enhancements of various shapes is a common finding in CTA and may cause interpretation difficulties. They are especially frequent in segment III, V and VI with a tendency to locate at the edge of liver (Kanematsu *et al.*, 1997) (Fig. 4.19). As HCC nodules are typically hyperattenuating in CTA whereas regeneration nodules are not, CTA is therefore helpful in distinguishing between the nodules in cirrhotic liver in conjunction with CTAP in which HCC nodules are typically hypoattenuating and regeneration nodules are typically isoattenuating (Fig. 4.19). Tumor conspicuousness and recognition of tumors sites are significantly better on three-dimensional CTA images reconstructed from spiral CT data than on conventional angiography, as well as depiction of tumour-feeding arteries (Fig. 4.20). Maximum-intensity projection is the preferred technique for three-dimensional CTA reconstruction (Kanematsu *et al.*, 1996).

4.4.4   CT ARTERIAL PORTOGRAPHY

CTAP is performed by intra-arterial injection of 100–150 ml 60% contrast material into the superior mesenteric (SMA) or splenic artery at 3–5 ml/s and obtaining axial hepatic CT scans during portal vein and the subsequent hepatic parenchymal enhancement. Spiral CT is preferable for scanning the liver within the narrow time window, when the liver–lesion contrast difference is optimal, with a scanning delay of 20–40 s after the commencement of contrast injection. Injection at the splenic artery has been preferred for CTAP because of greater parenchymal enhancement and fewer non-tumoral perfusion defects, unlike SMA injections which more commonly also produce greater enhancement in the dependent portions of the liver (Little *et al.*, 1994). The overall sensitivity of CTAP in detecting HCC ranges from 68–95% (Matsui *et al.*, 1985; Marine *et al.*, 1990; Takayasu *et al.*, 1990). For

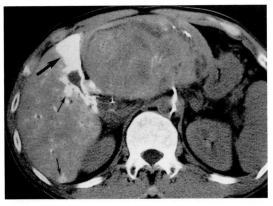

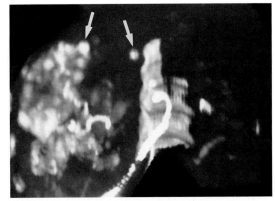

Fig. 4.19   **Fig. 4.20**

Figs 4.19 and **4.20** CT arteriographgy. The focal enhancement of liver parenchyma to the right (patient's left) of the gallbladder is non-pathological (big arrow). The small HCCs in the right lobe are well depicted as discrete hyperattenuating nodules (small arrows) (Fig. 19). Three-dimensional CT arteriography. The right lobe nodules are well demonstrated (Fig. 20).

small lesions ≤ 2 cm, the sensitivity varies from 29 to 54% (Marine *et al.*, 1990). A double-phase spiral CTAP with the two phases separated by 10–18 s may improve the detection rate for HCC (Ichikawa *et al.*, 1996).

As the tumors are predominantly supplied by the hepatic artery, 95% of HCC are hypoattenuated on spiral CTAP, the rest being isoattenuated. Vascular invasion and encapsulation are depicted in 50% of patients. The detection of a homogeneously hypoattenuating liver mass with associated vascular invasion on spiral CTAP should raise the possibility of HCC (Soyer *et al.*, 1995). There is a high false-positive rate of up to 42% per lesion basis (Peterson *et al.*, 1992) due to non-tumorous perfusion defects which may result from systemic vascular communication or aberrant venous drainage. They may also represent focal fibrosis, focal fatty change, cirrhotic nodule, regeneration nodule, cyst or benign tumors. Wedge-shaped or flat perfusion defects located peripherally, and defects characteristically located anterior to the porta hepatis or adjacent to the intersegmental fissure in left lobe are nearly always benign (Peterson *et al.*, 1992). It has been advocated that delayed CT and CTA following CTAP should be utilized to evaluate further the CTAP findings to reduce the false-positive rates.

4.4.5 DELAYED CT

High-dose delayed CT is usually performed as an adjunctive examination 4–6 h after CTAP with contiguous CT scanning through the entire liver at 7–10 mm collimation. By this time about 1–2% of the iodinated contrast material administered for the CTAP is normally excreted by the functioning hepatocytes into the biliary tract, providing sufficient hepatic parenchymal enhancement for lesion detection without additional contrast material. As it relies on the normal excretory function of hepatocytes, this technique is often suboptimal in patients with cirrhosis or hepatocellular damage secondary to chronic biliary obstruction. Delayed CT does not improve tumor detection but it may be useful in differentiating tumors from non-tumorous perfusion defects on CTAP. It is most useful for larger (>1 cm) wedge-shaped perfusion defects and least useful for smaller (< 1 cm) round defects (Nazarian *et al.*, 1994).

4.4.6 LIPIODOL CT

Lipiodol CT is usually performed with contiguous CT scanning of the whole liver at 10 mm collimation 10–14 days after intra-arterial administration of 5–10 ml lipiodol into the entire hepatic arterial circulation.

Lipiodol CT is the most sensitive preoperative imaging technique for detecting HCC (Takayasu *et al.*, 1990; Santis *et al.*, 1992; Choi *et al.*, 1997) with a sensitivity of 93% for small HCC ≤ 3 cm and 83–100% for HCC ≤1 cm (Takayasu *et al.*, 1990; Santis *et al.*, 1992). It is therefore highly valuable in the detection of small lesions undetectable by other imaging techniques and is used for HCC screening in patients with elevated α-fetoprotein, as well as preoperative assessment of tumor resectability.

HCC typically takes up intra-arterially administered lipoidol for various postulated reasons with variable retention patterns such as solid, patchy, mixed, thin rim and thick irregular rim (Fig. 4.21). Hypovascular HCC or small HCC of a few millimeters in size may produce false-negative results. Daughter nodules adjacent to large (> 5 cm) hypervascular HCC may also be missed due to a 'steal' phenomenon. As lipiodol may be washed out from HCC within 23 days, a CT

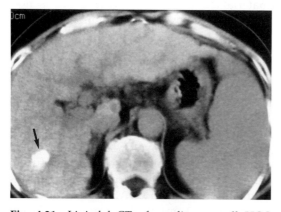

Fig. 4.21 Lipiodol CT of a solitary small HCC among the nodularity of a cirrhotic liver. Note the solid pattern of lipiodol retention.

scan performed after this time may contribute to the false-negative rate. Lipiodol accumulation is not a specific finding for HCC, it may also occur in hemangioma, focal nodular hyperplasia, regeneration nodules and biopsy sites. Lipiodol retention in hemangioma is slowly washed out but it persists for at least 3 months and up to 38 months, with a spotty, nodular or mixed retention pattern (Moon *et al.*, 1996).

4.5 MAGNETIC RESONANCE IMAGING

4.5.1 ADVANTAGES, APPLICATIONS AND LIMITATIONS

Magnetic resonance imaging (MRI) provides multiplanar images with excellent contrast resolution without the need for radiation exposure or iodinated contrast material injection. As the intensities of individual elements in a MR image is determined by their proton density, longitudinal relaxation time (T_1), transverse relaxation time (T_2), flow or motion, chemical shift, and magnetic susceptibility, instead of the tissue densities, MRI provides alternative information to CT in tumor imaging. MR images of the liver are not affected by bone or bowel gas, and allow distinctive demonstration of intrahepatic vascular structures.

MRI is a non-invasive means useful for detecting HCC and superior in demonstrating the characteristic internal details of HCC. It is valuable in screening for tumor recurrence after liver resection, and evaluation of response after percutaneous ethanol injection or transcatheter arterial embolization. MRI is slightly superior to conventional CT for detection of small HCC (< 3 cm), with a detection rate of 63%; however, it is significantly inferior to lipiodol CT (93%) (Santis *et al.*, 1992).

The expensive instrumentation and running cost of MRI may limit its extensive use. A major source of image degradation in the liver is motion artifacts which may arise from respiratory or gross patient movement, cardiac or vascular pulsation and bowel peristalsis, especially in sequences requiring long acquisition time. Patients with ferromagnetic implants and claustrophobia are not suitable for MRI examination.

4.5.2 CONVENTIONAL SPIN-ECHO PULSE SEQUENCE

MRI of the liver is usually performed with a superconducting system operating at 1.5 Tesla to obtain 5–10 mm-thick sections with 0–5 mm intersection gaps with or without respiratory and cardiovascular motion compensation. T_1-weighted (T_{1W}) conventional spin-echo (CSE) pulse sequence with short repetition time and echo time (T_R/T_E) and multiple signal acquisitions produces images with excellent spatial resolution, good information density and high signal- to-noise ratio, offering fine morphological detail of the liver optimal for the study of HCC, although the contrast resolution between normal and pathological tissue is poor (Fig. 4.22). The T_2-weighted (T_{2W}) CSE sequence with long T_R/T_E and multiple acquisitions is much more sensitive to pathological tissue with good contrast resolution. However, it provides much less informa-

tion density and requires longer acquisition time.

On T_{1W} images about one-half of HCCs are hypointense, one-third hyperintense and one-sixth isointense. HCC is almost always hyperintense and never hypointense on T_{2W} images, although it can be isointense (Itoh *et al.*, 1987). The majority of small HCCs (< 3 cm) are hyperintense on T_{1W} and T_{2W} images (Santis *et al.*, 1992). In one study, all the HCCs with the histologic differentiation classified as grade 1 according to the Edmondson and Steiner classification were hyperintense on T_{1W} images (Kadoya *et al.*, 1992), regardless of whether intracellular fat deposits were present. However, signal intensity alone may not be a reliable sign of low-grade HCC because the paramagnetic ions copper and iron in HCC contribute to the signal intensity patterns (Honda *et al.*, 1997).

Although regeneration nodules in cirrhotic liver are commonly hypointense on T_{1W}, and isointense or hypointense on T_{2W} images, benign liver lesions are usually identified on a morphological basis due to the variability and non-specificity of their MR signal intensity. The demonstration of characteristic pathomorphological internal features of HCC on MR images

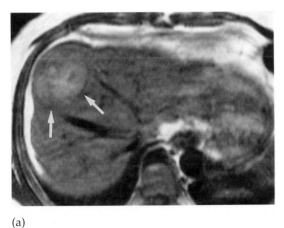

(a)

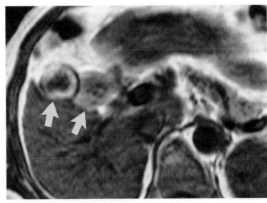

(b)

Fig. 4.22 (a) and (b) T_1-weighted spin-echo pulse sequence with respiratory compensation showing the hypointense pseudocapsule and mosaic pattern of HCC.

is of great help in distinguishing HCC from the other liver masses, including metastatic tumors, as the MR signal intensities of HCC and the other masses closely resemble each other and it may not be possible to differentiate HCC from the other lesions on the basis of signal intensities. MRI is excellent for depicting the structural details of HCC, especially the pseudocapsule, which is the commonest characteristic of HCC (Itoh *et al.*, 1987; Honda *et al.*, 1992b). The pseudocapsule appears as a distinctive hypointense peripheral rim better seen on T_{1W} images (Fig. 4.22). Occasionally it may be surrounded by a hyperintense external ring. Fibrous septae are also hypointense. The mosaic pattern is visualized as a collection of multiple nodular compartments of various signal intensities separated by fibrous septae. Venous tumor thrombi may be well demonstrated in major portal branches and hepatic veins as hyperintense lesions causing local abnormal dilatation of the venous structure.

After percutaneous ethanol injection or transcatheter arterial embolization, residual viable tumor tissue can be identified by their hyperintense appearance on T_{2W} images, whereas necrotic tissue appears as hypointense areas on T_{2W} images (Bartolozzi *et al.*, 1994).

4.5.3   OTHER MAGNETIC RESONANCE IMAGING TECHNIQUES

While the conventional SE pulse sequence has been a standard technique, new, fast acquisition sequences and techniques have been developed that aim towards an improvement in lesion detection, lesion conspicuousness, signal-to-noise ratio (S/N), lesion-to-liver contrast-to-noise ratio (C/N), spatial resolution, phase artifacts and overall image quality as well as great reduction in acquisition time, enabling ultrafast, motion-free scanning within a single breath-hold and application of dynamic contrast studies. When compared with T_{2W}-CSE sequence, fat-suppressed T_{2W} SE sequence is shown to improve the S/N and C/N ratios, and depicts better hepatic lesions. It is therefore recommended for routine use in T_{2W} SE imaging of the liver (Lu *et al.*, 1994). Fast spin-echo (FSE) sequence, also known as turbo spin-echo (TSE), derived from rapid acquisition with relaxation enhancement produces T_{2W} images with better subjective image quality and reduced artifacts, superior for the characterization of focal liver masses (Reimer *et al.*, 1996) (Fig. 4.23). It may also improve lesion detection if combined with T_{1W} gradient-echo sequence with the breath-hold

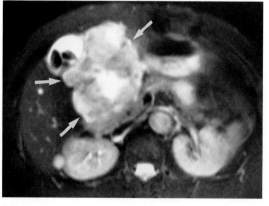

(a)

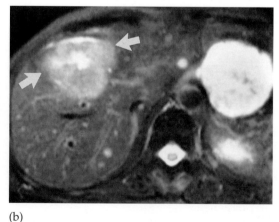

(b)

Figs 4.23 (a) and (b) T_2-weighted respiratory triggered turbo spin-echo pulse sequence with spectral presaturation inversion recovery showing the hyperintense massive HCC.

technique. T_{2W} breath-hold sequences are more sensitive for liver masses than CSE sequence, especially inversion recovery (IR)-FSE sequence which is the most sensitive with highest C/N ratio for solid masses, significantly better than IR-SE-echo-planar sequence. Fat-suppressed-half-Fourier-single-shot-T_{2W}-FSE imaging is also highly sensitive and is particularly useful in patients who are unable to hold their breath (Gaa *et al.*, 1996). Respiratory triggered FSE sequence (RT-FSE) designed with data acquisition at end expiration is superior to CSE and significantly better than inversion recovery (STIR) in lesion detection. It is also more favorable than STIR in terms of conspicuity of lesion structure, image sharpness and reduction of artifact (Keogan *et al.*, 1996) (Fig. 4.23). It is also better than non-triggered FSE for evaluation of liver masses with sharper anatomic detail and improved C/N ratio (Low *et al.*, 1997).

4.5.4 CONTRAST-ENHANCED MAGNETIC RESONANCE IMAGING

Gadolinium DTPA (Gadopentate), gadodiamide and gadoteridol are paramagnetic chelates of gadolinium (Gd) that distribute to the extracellular fluid space after intravenous administration. As a MR contrast agent, Gd predominantly shortens T_1, thus enhancing signal intensity on T_{1W} images, with a behavior analogous to that of iodinated contrast material in CT images. Gd-DTPA offers no advantage in the detection or characterization of liver lesions compared with CSE imaging due to the long acquisition time. Multi-slice dynamic MRI of the liver with single breath-hold and Gd-enhancement is more sensitive than CSE (91 versus 73%) in detecting untreated HCC that demonstrates rapid enhancement at the arterial dominant phase, and isointensity or hypointensity on delayed images (Ito *et al.*, 1993). It is an accurate technique for tumor evaluation after transcatheter arterial embolization, and can identify the false-positive findings of T_{2W} SE images. Dynamic Gd-enhanced MRI with a fast spoiled gradient-echo sequence and multiple acquisition at arterial and portal venous phases enabled increased HCC detection by 21% over CSE images (Peterson *et al.*, 1996). Multi-slice Gd-DTPA-enhanced dynamic MRI (67%) has been shown to be comparable with arterial phase spiral CT (50%) and significantly superior to SE MRI (26%) for detection of HCC (< 1 cm) (Kim *et al.*, 1995); it may be the most sensitive non-invasive means of detecting small HCC. Early enhancement of HCC and no enhancement of adenomatous hyperplasia (AH) on dynamic Gd-enhanced MRI with breath-hold T_{1W} FSE sequence allows a reliable distinction between small HCC and AH (Lencioni *et al.*, 1996). Differentiation between HCC and hemangioma is also facilitated with dynamic Gd-enhanced MR using the inversion recovery snapshot fast low angle shot (FLASH) technique, as 90% of HCC and 82% of hemangiomas show their characteristic enhancement patterns in the early and delayed phases (Murakami *et al.*, 1992).

Apart from the development of ultrafast, motion-free imaging sequences and techniques, the introduction of liver-specific contrast agents is the other trend for technical progress in MR liver imaging. Superparamagnetic iron oxide (SPIO) is a potent class of MR contrast agent selectively taken up by reticuloendothelial cells (Kupffer cell-targeted agent) after intravenous administration. SPIO has a T_2-shortening MR effect manifested as a marked reduction in signal intensity of the normal liver on proton density and T_{2W} images, resulting in elevation of lesion-to-liver contrast. SPIO produces excellent hepatic enhancement on T_{2W}-CSE image and high lesion-to-liver C/N ratio on STIR images, with an increase in lesion conspicuousness and a reduction in detectability threshold of liver tumours (Halavaara *et al.*, 1994). Although SPIO offers no benefits in T_{1W}-GE and SE sequences in terms of detectability of malignant liver lesions, it is helpful in characterizing hemangiomas and their differentiation from malignant tumors. Side effects such as hypotension are not common and are usually mild.

Gd-EOB-DTPA and Gd-BOPTA/Dimeg are newer chelates of gadolinium that are selectively taken up by hepatocytes (hepatocyte-targeted agent), producing selective enhancement of the liver parenchyma on T_{1W} images, with a marked increase of liver S/N ratio and lesion-to-liver C/N ratio. Both agents have demonstrated a safe pharmacologic and toxicologic profile with an advantage of the availability of a wide imaging time window provided by the sustained enhancement achieved after injection, allowing flexibility in selecting imaging sequences. Gd-EOB-DTPA-enhanced T_{2W} and T_{1W} MR images obtained with CSE and FLASH sequences during the hepatobiliary phase 1.5 min to 4 h after Gd-EOB-DTPA administration yields a dose-independent, statistically significant improvement in the detection of liver tumors, while providing comparable differential diagnostic information, when compared with unenhanced and Gd-DTPA-enhanced images (Vogl *et al.*, 1996). It has been shown recently that hepatic enhancement with Gd-EOB-DTPA is reduced in fatty livers and is unchanged in cirrhotic livers, whereas enhancement with SPIO (ferumoxides) is excellent in fatty livers but impaired in cirrhotic livers (Kuwatsuru *et al.*, 1997). Therefore, the knowledge of the type of diffuse liver disease is necessary prior to the choice of contrast agent for tumor detection.

Manganese (Mn) DPDP is a paramagnetic chelate that is actively extracted from blood by hepatocytes and partly excreted into the biliary tree (hepatobiliary-targeted agents). Its MR effect manifests as increased signal intensity on T_{1W} images in hepatocyte-containing areas and is maximal at about 30 min after administration and persists for 2–4 h, providing an extended time window for imaging. Focal lesions that contain hepatocytes such as HCC, focal nodular hyperplasia and regenerative nodules have been shown to take up Mn-DPDP. An improved capability for HCC

detection has been demonstrated with Mn-DPDP-enhanced MRI. The degree of HCC enhancement has been shown to correlate well with histologic differentiation, significantly greater enhancement seen in better differentiated HCC. Compared with T_{1W} gradient echo and SE, the T_{1W} fat-suppressed SE sequence provides the greatest liver enhancement and C/N ratio and is recommended for Mn-DPDP enhanced MR imaging (Slater *et al.*, 1996).

4.6   HEPATIC ANGIOGRAPHY

4.6.1   ADVANTAGES, APPLICATIONS AND LIMITATIONS

Although CT, US and MRI are widely used in the investigation of HCC, angiography still remains a very important and useful tool in the management of the disease. It provides not only additional diagnostic information that occasionally cannot be obtained from non-invasive imaging techniques, but also an avenue for transcatheter treatment. The mapping out of the hepatic arterial, portal venous and hepatic venous anatomy is often useful in the planning of the surgical operation. It is also essential for the interventional radiologist who has to navigate guidewires and catheters into the hepatic circulation. Superselective catheterization of the hepatic artery proper and its branches is necessary in any form of transcatheter treatment. Its success depends a great deal on the skill and experience of the angiographic interventional radiologist.

4.6.2   HEPATIC ARTERY ANOMALIES

Anomalies of the celiac axis and hepatic artery are very common. In a study of 200 cadavers, about 40% had some form of arterial anomalies involving the hepatic arterial circulation (Michels 1955, 1966). An anomalous artery may either be a replaced artery or an accessory. A replaced hepatic artery is a substitute for the normal hepatic artery which is absent whereas an accessory hepatic artery is a supernumerary hepatic artery in addition to the normal hepatic artery. The more common anomalies are (a) right hepatic artery arising from the superior mesenteric artery and (b) left hepatic artery arising from the left gastric artery (Figs 4.24 and 4.25). Some anomalous arteries are of surgical relevance because their abnormal courses can sometimes cause confusion during operation. Many anomalies, including some seemingly minor ones, are important to the angiographic interventional radiologists who have to deliver the treatment substance precisely to the desired sites. An example is a gastroduodenal artery arising from the right hepatic artery instead of normally from the common hepatic artery. This is a relatively minor anomaly but it causes problems in transcatheter treatment. In such a situation, any treatment substance introduced into the hepatic artery proper will perfuse not only the liver but also the areas supplied by the gastroduodenal artery, i.e. stomach, duodenum, pancreas and the greater omentum. To overcome this, the left and right hepatic arteries need to be separately catheterized for administration of treatment substances. Alternatively, the proximal portion of the gastroduodenal artery can be occluded with metallic

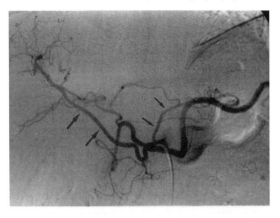

Fig. 4.25 An anomalous left hepatic artery (big arrows) arising from the left gastric artery (small arrows) on angiogram.

coils prior to injection of treatment substances into the common hepatic artery or hepatic artery proper. In the transcatheter treatment of HCC this is of vital importance to prevent complications. Many of the problems resulting from anomalous arteries can be overcome by superselective catheterization, or by embolization techniques that produce hepatic arterial flow redistribution (Chuang and Wallace, 1980).

4.6.3 ANGIOGRAPHIC APPROACHES

Access to the arterial system is usually via the femoral artery using a method based on the classical Seldinger technique (Seldinger, 1953). Very rarely when both femoral arteries are diseased, catheterization of the arterial system has to be performed through the brachial artery using a high brachial approach. This approach is similar to but safer than the axillary approach. A celiac axis arteriogram is usually performed first. A superior mesenteric arteriogram is, in most cases, also performed in view of the additional information it will provide regarding the presence or absence of anomalous hepatic arteries and the status of the portal vein. Intra-arterial administration of a vasodilator such as tolazoline or papaverine

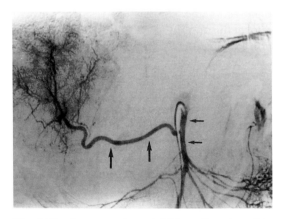

Fig. 4.24 An anomalous right hepatic artery (big arrows) arising from the superior mesenteric artery (small arrows) on angiogram.

into the superior mesenteric artery, immediately prior to contrast injection, will augment visualization of the portal vein. In some cases, when the celiac axis arteriogram can already provide all the necessary information, and one is satisfied that there is no anomalous artery arising from the superior mesenteric artery by giving test injections into the artery and viewing it under fluoroscopy, a formal superior mesenteric arteriogram can be omitted. The principle of introducing contrast medium with the catheter tip as close as possible to the organs being studied holds true in hepatic arteriography. Superselective injection into the hepatic artery proper, or the right or left hepatic artery, produces images of higher diagnostic value because it eliminates the superimposing shadows of the spleen, pancreas and stomach. Diagnostic accuracy is improved, particularly for left hepatic lobe lesions. The advantage of superselective hepatic arteriogram over coeliac axis arteriogram is also due to the hepatograms they produce. The hepatogram from a superselective hepatic arteriogram is a 'pure' arterial hepatogram, whereas that from a celiac axis arteriogram is a 'mixed' arterial and portal hepatogram. Details of the liver parenchyma in a 'pure' arterial hepatogram are far superior to those in a 'mixed' arterial and portal hepatogram. For the above reasons, tiny lesions that do not show up in coeliac axis arteriogram can often be demonstrated in superselective hepatic arteriograms. If there is doubt as to the presence or nature of a lesion, superselective intra-arterial administration of lipiodol is often helpful (Nakakuma *et al.*, 1985; Yumoto *et al.*, 1985). Lipiodol is an oily contrast medium which, in the majority of cases, will accumulate and stay in the HCC for long periods. Lipiodol that enters normal liver parenchyma will be cleared by Kupffer cells in a few days. A lipiodol CT (about 10 days after intra-arterial administration) is very useful in assessing HCC. Intra-arterial technetium-99m macroaggregated albumen (Tc-99m-MAA) can demonstrate radioactive uptake by the tumor as compared with the adjacent normal liver parenchyma (Lau *et al.*, 1994), and the percentage of radioactivity passing to the lungs via the arteriovenous shunts in the liver tumor (Leung *et al.*, 1994c). The data obtained are important in the selection of patients with inoperable disease for selective internal radiotherapy.

4.6.4   CATHETERS AND CATHETERIZATION TECHNIQUES

Catheterization of the celiac axis and superior mesenteric artery can be readily performed with a simple single-curved 5F catheter in the majority of cases. The catheter is advanced over a guidewire to just above the level of the coeliac axis (usually T12-L1) and then rotated so that its tip points anteriorly. Next, it is gradually pulled downwards. On reaching the origin of the celiac axis the catheter will simply move into it. The superior mesenteric artery can be similarly catheterized. Occasionally, when the aorta is markedly tortuous and rotated due to hypertensive diseases and arteriosclerosis, or the celiac axis or superior mesenteric artery are displaced or compressed by large tumors, a slightly more complex double-curved catheter has to be used. The double curve is reformed in the contralateral common iliac artery over the aortic bifurcation. Other methods have been described but this seems the simplest and safest way to reform the double curve. Selective catheterization of hepatic arterial branches is more demanding on the skill and experience of the angiographic radiologist. In the past, various catheters with different tip configurations have been manufactured to facilitate superselective catheterization of the hepatic circulation, and various techniques have been described (Chuang *et al.*, 1983). Some of these catheters and techniques are still occasionally useful. However, with the development in the mid-1980s of microcatheters that can be easily used coaxially within an ordinary 5F catheter, highly superselective catheterization has been made much simpler, faster and safer.

4.6.5 GENERAL ANGIOGRAPHIC APPEARANCES

Most HCCs are hypervascular (Reuter *et al.*, 1970). The hepatic arteries feeding the tumor are often dilated, tortuous, distorted and displaced. Neovasculatures show a chaotic and disorganized pattern. There is often an intense tumor stain. Vascular lakes or venous pools are common (Fig. 4.26). On the other end of the spectrum, some tumors are only mildly hypervasacular with mild tumor staining which can only be demonstrated in a good-quality superselective arteriogram. Central necrosis is not uncommon in large hypervascular tumors and it is represented angiographically by a hypovascular area. HCC can be descriptively divided into three main forms on hepatic angiogram: (1) a solitary mass, (2) a multi-nodular form with tumors of different sizes and (3) a diffuse infiltrative lesion with poorly defined margins.

4.6.6 PORTAL VEIN INVASION

Invasion of the portal trunk and its major branches is not uncommon in HCC (Fig. 4.27). The 'thread and streaks' appearance seen in hepatic arteriograms is due to tumor invasion of the vasa vasorum of the portal vein (Okuda

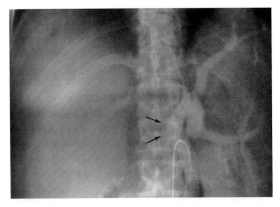

Fig. 4.27 Complete obliteration of the right branch of portal vein due to a right lobe HCC on angiogram.

et al., 1975). Arterio-portal shunting (Okuda *et al.*, 1977a) is also common with premature opacification of the portal venous system during the arterial phase. Because the normal portal vein is a low pressure system, arterioportal shunting often causes retrograde filling of the superior mesenteric vein and splenic vein. Dilated gastroesophageal varices are sometimes present. If the tumor grows into the portal vein, complete or partial obstruction of the main portal trunk or its branches can occur, and the tumor cast can be seen as a filling defect within the contrast filled portal vein during hepatic angiography (Fig. 4.28).

4.6.7 HEPATIC VEIN INVASION

The hepatic veins are usually not opacified during hepatic arteriography unless there is a change in hemodynamics. Tumor invasion of the major hepatic veins produces such a change. It has similar angiographic appearances to portal vein invasion apart from their difference in location (Okuda *et al.*, 1977b). The 'thread and streaks' sign of tumor invasion is seen in the region of the major hepatic veins (Fig. 4.29). Often tumor casts can be seen within the hepatic veins, causing complete or partial obstruction. They can even extend into the inferior vena cava or right atrium. Hepatic

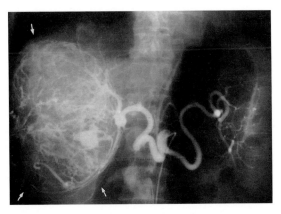

Fig. 4.26 Typical angiographic features of HCC. Note the distorted arteries, neovasculature and vascular lakes.

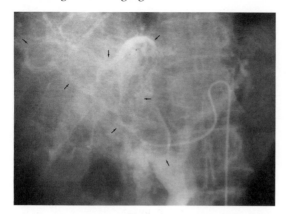

Fig. 4.28 A tumor cast of an HCC within the main trunk, and bifurcated branches of the portal vein demonstrated on the portal venous phase of hepatic angiogram.

vein invasion is an ominous sign and carries a bad prognosis. It often heralds tumor dissemination. A chest radiograph may often show the presence of pulmonary metastases.

4.6.8   SPONTANEOUS RUPTURE

If the carcinoma is situated at the surface of the liver and is hypervascular with abnormally dilated vessels, it can occasionally rupture spontaneously. It usually presents with acute abdominal pain and shock due to

hemoperitoneum. This condition can be managed either surgically or by embolization (Corr *et al.*, 1993). Angiographic demonstration of extravasation is not common (Fig. 4.30). If present, it always indicates massive bleeding and active intervention is required. In general, it is often much simpler and easier to treat spontaneous rupture through the angiographic catheter. In most cases, extravastion or the actual site of bleeding cannot be angiographically demonstrated, but an experienced angiographic interventional radiologist can almost always judge the possible bleeding site from the angiographic appearances of the tumor and selectively embolize the feeding vessel. The type of embolizing agent used and the desirable degree of embolization depend a great deal on the clinical conditions. The size and extent of the tumor, amount of normal liver tissue present, portal and hepatic vein status, and liver functions are important factors. Particulate matter such as polyvinyl alcohol foam (Chuang *et al.*, 1982) or gelfoam produce distal tumor embolization, whereas metallic coils are used for proximal occlusion. Depending on the clinical conditions, it has to be decided if distal embolization or proximal embolization alone, or a combination, is most suitable. Post-embolization syndrome (pain, nausea, vomiting, fever) can occur but it can be

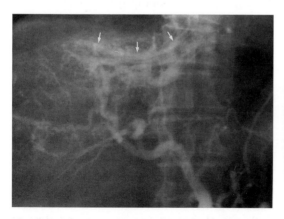

Fig. 4.29 Tumor invasion of a right hepatic vein on hepatic angiogram. Note the 'thread and streaks' sign.

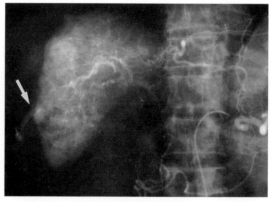

Fig. 4.30 Active contrast extravasation from a ruptured HCC on hepatic angiogram.

minimized if a limited embolization is performed with the sole aim of controlling the hemorrhage, without producing too much tissue ischemia.

4.6.9 TRANSCATHETER TREATMENT

Apart from embolization in the treatment of spontaneous rupture of HCC described above, the angiographic catheter can be used in numerous other forms of transcatheter treatment. Treatment substances such as chemotherapeutic agents (intra-arterial infusion), chemotherapeutic agents emulsified with lipiodol (chemoembolization) (Leung *et al.*, 1989), radioactive Iodine-131-lipiodol (Leung *et al.*, 1994b) and radioactive yttrium-90 microspheres (selective internal radiotherapy) (Lau *et al.*, 1994) can be readily administered via a selectively placed catheter. These will be dealt with in depth in Chapter 10.

4.7 NUCLEAR IMAGING

4.7.1 ADVANTAGES, APPLICATIONS AND LIMITATIONS

Radionuclide scintigraphy is unique in utilizing specific physiological functions of the liver and the biochemical properties of the pathological entity to offer alternative information for the characterization of liver masses and evaluation of their metabolic activities. It is therefore a valuable non-invasive and potent adjunct to the other structural imaging techniques. A major limitation of planar imaging is the poor spatial resolution.

4.7.2 PLANAR IMAGING

Technetium-99m-labeled sulfur colloid scintigraphy depicts HCC as a photopenic defect which is non-specific and may represent any solid or cystic lesion. Sulfur colloid scans may be misleading in cirrhotic livers as multiple photopenic defects may appear in up to 20% of cases (Kudo *et al.*, 1986). Focal lesions that may take up sulfur colloid include focal nodular hyperplasia (FNH), regeneration nodules and focal fatty change, due to the presence of Kupffer cells in such lesions. A sulfur colloid scan therefore is potentially useful in distinguishing FNH and HCC. However, its detection sensitivity is low for superficial lesions < 2 cm and deep lesions of size up to 4 cm, especially those located within the right lobe.

Gallium-67 scintigraphy may demonstrate neoplastic or inflammatory activity. Uptake of gallium-67 occurs in up to 88% of HCC, with activity equal to or greater than that of the adjacent liver. Other liver lesions that may show increased uptake of gallium-67 include lymphoma, metastases and abscess.

Radionuclides bound to specific molecules with a HCC-receptor targeting property, such as iodine123-Tyr-(A14)-insulin, may improve the identification of HCC and be of potential diagnostic value. It may be coupled with another liver-receptor-specific radioisotope as a double-tracer technique, such as technetium-99m-galactosyl-neoglycoalbumin for which HCCs do not express any specific receptors (Kurtaran *et al.*, 1995).

Selective increased uptake of technetium-99m (Sn)-*N*-pyridoxyl-5-methyltryptophen (99 mTc-PMT) by HCC has been demonstrated, with a specificity of 51%. A correlation has been shown between increased survival and increased 99 mTc-PMT uptake, which probably reflects a better differentiated tumor (Hasegawa *et al.*, 1991).

Iodine-123 IMP is more sensitive than gallium-67, and is more sensitive and more specific than technetium-99m-MDP for the detection of bone metastases from HCC (Suto *et al.*, 1994).

4.7.3 SINGLE PHOTON EMISSION COMPUTED TOMOGRAPHY AND POSITRON EMISSION TOMOGRAPHY

Single photon emission computed tomography (SPECT), with a three-headed high-resolution system, is a major advance in scintigraphic imaging. It provides much improved spatial resolution and therefore detection sensitivity than that offered by the planar imaging techniques. Lesions as small as 0.5–1 cm can be detected. Thallium-201 SPECT is a promising technique capable of demonstrating abnormal increased uptake in HCC with high sensitivity and specificity. It has a great potential role in the detection and characterization of HCC, particularly in patients with cirrhosis (Kampf *et al.*, 1996). Differences in liver function among different hepatic segments in cirrhosis and HCC may be quantified with technetium-99m GSA SPECT imaging.

Positron emission tomography (PET) is a non-invasive functional method useful for evaluating the perfusion and metabolism of liver tumors and for the response to different therapeutic agents. Dynamic 18F-labeled 2-fluoro-2-deoxy-D-glucose (FDG) PET enables the assessment of the activity of glucose metabolism in HCC, which correlates closely with the histologic grading. Higher degrees of activity correspond to higher-grade HCCs (Torizuka *et al.*, 1995). FDG-PET is also valuable in assessing tumor viability after transcatheter treatment of HCC (Torizuka *et al.*, 1994).

4.7.4   HEPATIC ARTERIAL PERFUSION SCINTIGRAPHY

Hepatic arterial perfusion scintigraphy with technetium-99m macroaggregated albumin (Tc-99m-MAA) is capable of providing a quantitative measurement of HCC vascularity by determining the ratio of the count rates of radioisotope activity over the tumorous and non-tumorous tissue (T/N ratio) (Plate 7). This has been shown to be more accurate in reflecting the true vascularity of HCC than selective hepatic angiography and correlates well with intraoperative beta probe dosimetry as well as liquid scintillation count of biopsy specimens (Lau *et al.*, 1994a; Leung *et al.*, 1994a). Tc-99m-MAA scintigraphy also allows

the determination of the degree of tumor-to-lung vascular shunting, which is dependent on neoplastic vascularity and not on tumor size (Leung *et al.*, 1994c) (Plate 8). The knowledge of T/N uptake ratio and degree of lung shunting is mandatory for the selection of patients with unresectable tumors for intra-arterial therapy with chemotherapeutic or radioactive agents. Hepatic arterial Tc-99m-MAA scintigraphy in combination with a high-resolution SPECT, with or without SPECT sulfhur colloid scan, may improve the sensitivity of detecting liver tumors and reduce the size of smallest detectable lesion.

4.8   IMAGE-GUIDED PERCUTANEOUS BIOPSY

4.8.1   BIOPSY OF THE LIVER TUMOR

Percutaneous needle biopsy is important as a preoperative staging procedure for excluding the malignant nature of suspicious lesions locating at critical sites in patients with otherwise resectable known or highly probable HCC. It is also useful for confirming the diagnosis of HCC and for evaluating the histologic subtype in inoperable patients, which may affect the choice of non-surgical treatment options (Yamashita *et al.*, 1995). Percutaneous biopsy should not be employed in HCC patients who are potential candidates for liver resection or transplantation (unless the diagnosis remains equivocal after extensive preoperative investigations), because needle track or intraperitoneal tumor seeding and recurrence, which are always possible following biopsy, may render the disease incurable. Biopsy can be performed under US or CT guidance with US being preferable since it provides a real-time guidance and allows much more precise sampling of small lesions ≤ 1 cm. Guidance by color Doppler US facilitates the avoidance of needle passage through hepatic or tumor vessels, which is of particular importance in patients known to be at high risk of post-biopsy bleeding.

Suspicious lipiodol-accumulating lesions demonstrated after selective hepatic arterial administration of lipiodol can be biopsied under US guidance (Lau *et al.*, 1993). Fine needles (20–22 gauge) are generally utilized for the biopsy procedure. While the larger caliber needles (18–19 gauge) may provide better preservation of tissue architecture important for histological diagnosis and subtyping of HCC, they are not preferred by most because of the possibly higher risk of serious bleeding complications compared with the finer needles, especially in patients with cirrhosis and HCC. Specimens obtained with fine-needle aspiration biopsy (FNAB) are usually submitted for cytology assessment. A combined cytological and histological approach with the FNAB specimen also prepared for histological evaluation may improve the sensitivity and specificity of HCC diagnosis (Rapaccini *et al.*, 1994). A panel of immunocytochemical stains applicable to FNAB specimens is an effective adjunct to the cytological diagnosis of HCC (Chapter 5).

Bleeding from the liver is the most frequent serious complication and is the main cause of death associated with liver biopsy. Biopsy of HCC in the cirrhotic liver is always potentially dangerous and should be performed with extra care and precautions, which include correction of bleeding tendency, patient cooperation to avoid excessive respiratory movements, and ensuring that the needle track passes through an adequate thickness of interposing liver parenchyma. Percutaneous biopsy of HCC is contraindicated if a non-tumorous intrahepatic needle track of ≥ 1 cm cannot be secured to avoid the risk of tumor laceration (Yu *et al.*, 1997). Post-biopsy embolization of the intrahepatic needle track through the outer needle of a coaxial system may offer protection to high risk patients but it also requires an adequate length of non-tumorous intrahepatic needle tract.

Recurrence of HCC at the needle track due to tumor seeding during needle biopsy is rare and may be treated by surgical excision. It usually follows FNAB and presents as a subcutaneous hard nodule in the abdominal or chest wall at the insertion site of the biopsy needle, 13–40 months after the biopsy. Elevation of α-fetoprotein level may precede the clinical presentation of needle tract tumor recurrence.

4.8.2 BIOPSY OF THE PORTAL VEIN TUMOR AND EXTRAHEPATIC METASTASES

The accurate diagnosis of tumor invasion of portal vein in the preoperative staging of HCC is important as involvement of the main branch of the portal vein is a contraindication for liver transplantation. However, portal vein thrombus detected with diagnostic imaging techniques in patients with cirrhosis can be either benign or malignant, which may not be distinguishable from one another with imaging techniques. Percutaneous biopsy of portal vein thrombus is a safe, accurate and well-tolerated procedure (Dodd and Carr, 1993) highly valuable for establishing the nature of portal vein thrombus. When utilized as the initial biopsy procedure in selected patients or when biopsy of the liver tumor fails, it can offer diagnosis and staging information simultaneously. The portal vein thrombus is usually biopsied with a FNAB technique and care should be taken not to biopsy the wall of portal vein. No procedure-related complication has been reported.

Percutaneous FNAB of HCC at the extrahepatic metastatic sites allows the diagnosis to be made even without a history of the primary liver cancer, and it also provides valuable information for staging.

4.9 DIAGNOSTIC ALGORITHM

In our institution, patients with hepatitis B viral cirrhosis and known HCC patients treated with liver resection are routinely screened at 3-month intervals for newly developed or recurrent HCC (Fig. 4.31). US is used as the first imaging technique for screening because

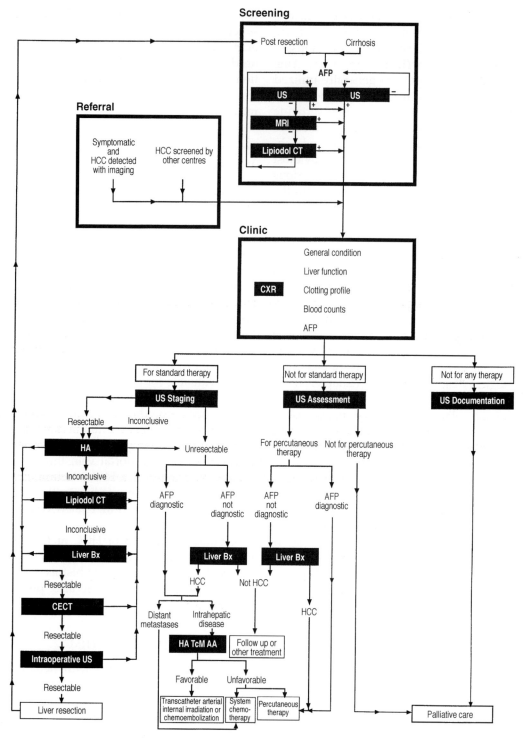

Fig. 4.31 Diagnostic algorithm.

it is radiation-free, quick and associated with a reasonable sensitivity for detecting small tumors. When US does not reveal any evidence of liver tumor and the serum α-fetoprotein level is elevated, MRI is utilized as the second line investigation since it is non-invasive and more sensitive than CECT. As lipiodol CT is superior in detection sensitivity, it is valuable as a third line of study when MRI does not provide a clue. The screening process will be repeated in 3 months if lipiodol CT is negative. All patients with imaging manifestation of liver tumor, whether screened locally or referred, are seen in a joint clinic by a multidisciplinary team of hepatologist, surgeon, clinical oncologist and radiologist. A chest radiograph (CXR) is routinely taken for every patient at the first visit to evaluate the cardiopulmonary status and to exclude metastases in the lung, which is the commonest site of distant metastasis. Based on the assessment of patient's general condition, liver function and CXR findings, an initial plan of management is determined for each patient as to whether they are suitable for undergoing standard therapy, percutaneous therapy or palliative care (Fig. 4.31).

US is performed for each patient to obtain a radiological diagnosis of the liver tumor and also for disease staging and assessment of the feasibility of percutaneous therapy. No further imaging investigations, except for image-guided liver biopsy, is performed in patients who are not suitable for standard therapy such as surgery, radiotherapy or chemotherapy. Those patients who are considered potential resection candidates after US staging are examined with hepatic angiogram (HA) for resectability. They are subsequently evaluated with CECT for anatomy and topography, prior to surgery, if the HA findings are favorable. Intraoperative US is performed at surgery for further information. If a decision cannot be reached at HA as to tumor resectability, a lipiodol CT is performed at day 10. CTAP is not routinely performed due to its limitations in liver cirrhosis. With a similar

degree of invasiveness, lipiodol CT is preferable due to its superlative sensitivity for HCC, and because of the prevalence of cirrhosis among our patients (Fig. 4.21). When it is necessary to confirm the nature of suspicious lesions depicted on lipiodol CT, an image-guided percutaneous liver biopsy is indicated. Biopsy is also performed in patients with unresectable tumors and those considered unsuitable for standard therapy, in whom the serum α-fetoprotein is below the diagnostic level of 500 ng/dl. Histologic confirmation of HCC is necessary before the contemplation of systemic chemotherapy, transcatheter arterial therapy or percutaneous therapy. Patients with unresectable HCC are assessed with Tc-99m-MAA hepatic arterial perfusion scintigraphy. Those who show favorable tumor vascularity and lung shunting ratios are treated with transcatheter arterial internal irradiation or chemoembolization. The others are treated with systemic chemotherapy or percutaneous therapy.

Those patients with unresectable HCC considered unfavorable for transcatheter therapy and those who are not fit for standard therapy are selected for percutaneous therapy such as ethanol injection. This is based on the favorable size and number of tumors.

Patients with biopsy-proven benign tumors are followed up with US. Those with other liver malignancies are managed accordingly. Palliative care is provided to those patients who are unfit for any therapy as well as those who are not suitable for standard therapy and percutaneous therapy. No further diagnostic imaging, including percutaneous biopsy, is performed after the initial US examination.

REFERENCES

Barbot, D.J., Marks, J.H., Feld, R.I. *et al.* (1997) Improved staging of liver tumors using laparoscopic intraoperative ultrasound. *Journal of Surgical Oncology*, **64**, 63–7.

Bartolozzi, C., Lencioni, R., Caramella, D. *et al.* (1994) Hepatocellular carcinoma: CT and MR features after transcatheter arterial embolization and percutaneous ethanol injection. *Radiology,* **191**, 123–8.

Cho, J.S., Kwag, J.G., Oh, Y.R. *et al.* (1996) Detection and characterization of hepatocellular carcinoma: value of dynamic CT during the arterial dominant phase with uniphasic contrast medium injection. *Journal of Computer Assisted Tomography,* **20**, 128–34.

Choi, B.I., Han., J.K., Cho, J.M. *et al.* (1995) Characterization of focal hepatic tumours. Value of two-phase scanning with spiral computed tomography. *Cancer,* **76**, 2434–42.

Choi, B.I., Lee, H.J., Han, J.K. *et al.* (1997) Detection of hypervascular nodular hepatocellular carcinomas: value of triphasic helical CT compared with iodized-oil CT. *American Journal of Roentgenology,* **168**, 219–24.

Chuang, V.P., Soo, C.S., Carrasco, C.H. *et al.* (1983) Superselective catheterisation techniques in hepatic angiography. *American Journal of Roentgenology,* **141**, 803–11.

Chuang, V.P. and Wallace, S. (1980) Hepatic arterial redistribution for intra-arterial infusion of hepatic neoplasms. *Radiology,* **135**, 295–9.

Chuang, V.P., Wallace, S., Soo, C.S. *et al.* (1982) Therapeutic Ivalon embolisation of hepatic tumors. *American Journal of Roentgenology,* **138**, 289–94.

Corr, P., Chan, M., Lau, W.Y. *et al.* (1993) The role of hepatic arterial embolisation in the management of ruptured hepatocellular carcinoma. *Clinical Radiology,* **48**, 163–5.

Dodd, G.D., Memal, D.S., Baron, R.L. *et al.* (1995) Portal vein thrombosis in patients with cirrhosis: does sonographic detection of intrathrombus flow allow differentiation of benign and malignant thrombus? *American Journal of Roentgenology,* **165**, 573–7.

Dodd, G.D. III, Miller, W.J., Baron, R.L. *et al.* (1992) Detection of malignant tumours in end-stage cirrhotic livers: efficacy of sonography as a screening technique. *American Journal of Roentgenology,* **159**, 727–33.

Foley, W.D. (1989) Dynamic hepatic CT. *Radiology,* **170**, 617–22.

Fortunato, L., Clair, M., Hoffman, J. *et al.* (1995) Is CT portography (CTAP) really useful in patients with liver tumors who undergo intraoperative ultrasography (IOUS)? *Annals of Surgery,* **61**, 560–5.

Fujimoto, M., Moriyasu F., Nishikawa, K. *et al.* (1994) Color Doppler sonography of hepatic tumors with a galactose-based contrast agent: correlation with angiographic findings. *American Journal of Roentgenology,* **163**, 1099–104.

Gaa, J., Hatabu, H., Jenkins, R.L. *et al.* (1996) Liver masses: replacement of conventional T_2-weighted spin-echo MR imaging with breath-hold MR imaging. *Radiology,* **200**, 459–64.

Haider, M.A., Leonhardt, C., Hanna, S.S. *et al.* (1995) The role of intraoperative ultrasonography in planning the resection of hepatic neoplasms. *Canadian Association of Radiologists Journal,* **46**, 98–104.

Halavaara, J.T., Lamminen, A.E., Bondestam, S. *et al.* (1994) Detection of focal liver lesions with superparamagnetic iron oxide: value of STIR and SE imaging. *Journal of Computer Assisted Tomography,* **18**, 897–904.

Hasegawa, Y., Nakano, S., Hiyama, T. *et al.* (1991) Relationship of uptake of technetium-99m-(Sn)-N-pyridoxyl-5-methyltryptophan by hepatocellular carcinoma to prognosis. *Journal of Nuclear Medicine,* **32**, 228–35.

Honda, H., Kanako. K., Kanazawa. Y. *et al.* (1997) MR imaging of hepatocellular carcinomas: effect of Cu and Fe contents on signal intensity. *Abdominal Imaging,* **22**, 60–6.

Honda, H., Matsuura, Y., Onitsuka, H. *et al.* (1992a) Differential diagnosis of hepatic tumours (hepatoma, haemangioma and metastases) with CT: value of two-phase incremental imaging. *American Journal of Roentgenology,* **159**, 735–40.

Honda, H., Onitsuka, H., Murakami, J. *et al.* (1992b) Characteristic finding of hepatocellular carcinoma: an evaluation with comparative study of US, CT and MRI. *Gastrointestinal Radiology,* **17**, 245–9.

Ichikawa, T., Ohtorno, K. and Takahashi, S. (1996) Hepatocellular carcinoma: detection with double-phase helical CT during arterial portography. *Radiology,* **198**, 284–7.

Ito, K., Choji, T., Nakada, T. *et al.* (1993) Multislice dynamic MR of hepatic tumors. *Journal of Computer Assisted Tomography,* **17**, 390–6.

Itoh, K., Nishimura, K., Togashi, K. *et al.* (1987) Hepatocellular carcinoma: MR imaging. *Radiology,* **164**, 21–5.

John, T.G., Greig, J.D., Crosbia, J.L. *et al.* (1994) Superior staging of liver tumours with laparoscopy and laparoscopic ultrasound. *Annals of Surgery,* **220**, 711–19.

Kadoya, M., Matsui, O., Takashima, T. *et al.* (1992) Hepatocellular carcinoma: correlation of MR imaging and histopathologic findings. *Radiology,* **183**, 819–25.

Kampf, J.S., Hudak, R., Abdel-Dayem, H.M. *et al.* (1996) Tl-201 chloride SPECT image of hepatocellular carcinoma. *Clinical Nuclear Medicine*, **21**, 953–7.

Kanai, T., Hirohashi, S., Upton, M.P. *et al.* (1987) Pathology of small hepatocellular carcinoma. A proposal for a new gross classification. *Cancer*, **60**, 810–9.

Kane, R.A., Hughes, L.A., Cua, E.J. *et al.* (1994) The impact of intraoperative ultrasonography on surgery for liver neoplasms. *Journal of Ultrasound in Medicine*, **13**, 1–6.

Kanematsu, M., Hoshi, H., Imaeda, T. *et al.* (1997) Non-pathological focal enhancements on spiral CT hepatic angiography. *Abdominal Imaging*, **22**, 55–9.

Kanematsu, M., Imaeda, T., Mizuno, S. *et al.* (1996) Value of three-dimensional spiral CT hepatic angiography. *American Journal of Roentgenology*, **166**, 585–91.

Keogan, M.T., Spritzer, C.E., Paulson, E.K. *et al.* (1996) Liver MR imaging: comparison of respiratory triggered fast spin-echo with T_2-weighted spin-echo and inversion recovery. *Abdominal Imaging*, **21**, 433–9.

Kim, T., Murakami, T., Oi, H. *et al.* (1995) Detection of hypervascular hepatocellular carcinoma by dynamic MRI and dynamic spiral CT. *Journal of Computer Assisted Tomography*, **19**, 948–54.

Kokudo, N., Bandai, Y., Imanishi, H. *et al.* (1996) Management of new hepatic nodules detected by intraoperative ultrasonography during hepatic resection for hepatocellular carcinoma. *Surgery*, **119**, 634–40.

Kudo, M., Hirasa, M., Takakucoa, H. *et al.* (1986) Small hepatocellular carcinoma in chronic liver disease: detection with SPECT. *Radiology*, **159**, 697–703.

Kurtaran, A., Li, S.R., Raderer, M. *et al.* (1995) Technetium-99m-galactosyl-neoglycoalbumin combined with iodine-123-Tyr-(A14)-insulin visualizes human hepatocellular carcinoma. *Journal of Nuclear Medicine*, **36**, 1875–81.

Kuwatsuru, R., Brasch, R.C., Muhler, A. *et al.* (1997) Definition of liver tumors in the presence of diffuse liver disease: comparison of findings at MR imaging with positive and negative contrast agents. *Radiology*, **202**, 131–8.

Lau, W.Y., Arnold, M., Leung, N.W. *et al.* (1993) Hepatic intra-arterial lipidol ultrasound guided biopsy in the management of hepatocellular carcinoma. *Surgical Oncology*, **2**, 119–24.

Lau, W.Y., Leung, K.L., Leung, T.W. *et al.* (1995) Resection of hepatocellular carcinoma with diaphragmatic invasion. *British Journal of Surgery*, **82**, 264–6.

Lau, W.Y., Leung, T.W., Ho, S. *et al.* (1994a) Diagnostic pharmaco-scintigraphy with hepatic intra-arterial technetium-99m macroaggregated albumin in the determination of tumour to non-tumour uptake ratio in hepatocellular carcinoma. *British Journal of Radiology*, **67**, 136–9.

Lau, W.Y., Leung, W.T., Ho, S.K. *et al.* (1994b) Treatment of inoperable hepatocellular carcinoma with intra-hepatic arterial yttrium-90 micro-spheres: a phase I and II study. *British Journal of Cancer*, **70**, 994–9.

Lee, M.G., Auh, Y.H., Cho, K.S. *et al.* (1996) Color Doppler flow imaging of hepatocellular carcinomas: comparison with metastatic tumors and haemangiomas by three-step grading for color hues. *Clinical Imaging*, **20**, 199–203.

Lencioni, R., Mascalchi, M., Caramella, D. *et al.* (1996) Small hepatocellular carcinoma: differentiation from adenomatous hyperplasia with color Doppler US and dynamic Gd-DTPA-enhanced MR imaging. *Abdominal Imaging*, **21**, 41–8.

Leung, W.T., Lau, W.Y., Ho, S.K. *et al.* (1994a) Determination of tumour vascularity using selective hepatic angiography as compared with intrahepatic-arterial technetium-99m macroaggregated albumin scan in hepatocellular carcinoma. *Cancer Chemotherapy and Pharmacology*, **335**, 33–6.

Leung, W.T., Lau, W.Y., Ho, S. *et al.* (1994b) Selective internal radiation therapy with intra-arterial iodine-131-lipiodol in inoperable hepatocellular carcinoma. *Journal of Nuclear Medicine*, **35**, 1313–8.

Leung, W.T., Lau, W.Y., Ho, S.K. *et al.* (1994c) Measuring lung shunting in hepatocellular carcinoma with intrahepatic-arterial technetium-99m macroaggregated albumin. *Journal of Nuclear Medicine*, **35**, 70–3.

Leung, W.T., Shiu, W.C.T., Chan, M. *et al.* (1989) Treatment of inoperable hepatocellular carcinoma by intra-hepatic arterial chemo-therapy with lipiodol and 4-epidoxorubicin. *Regional Cancer Treatment*, **2**, 145–8.

Little, A.F., Baron, R.L., Peterson, M.S. *et al.* (1994) Optimizing CT portography: a prospective comparison of injection into the splenic versus superior mesenteric artery. *Radiology*, **193**, 651–5.

Liver Cancer Study Group of Japan. (1990) Primary liver cancer in Japan. Clinicopathologic features and results of surgical treatment. *Annals of Surgery*, **211**, 277–87.

Low, R.N., Alzata, G.D. and Shimakawa, A. (1997) Motion suppression in MR imaging of the liver: comparison of respiratory-triggered and non-triggered fast spin-echo sequences. *American Journal of Roentgenology*, **168**, 225–31.

Lu, D.S., Saini. S., Haln. P.F. *et al.* (1994) T_2-weighted MR imaging of the upper part of the abdomen: should fat suppression be used routinely? *American Journal of Roentgenology*, **162**, 1095–100.

Marchesa, P., Milsom, J.W., Hale, J.C. *et al.* (1996) Intraoperative laparoscopic liver ultrasonography for staging of colorectal cancer, initial experience. *Diseases of the Colon and Rectum*, **39**, 73–8.

Marine, D., Takayasu, K. and Wakao, F. (1990) Detection of hepatocellular carcinoma: comparison of CT during arterial portography with CT after intraarterial injection of iodized oil. *Radiology*, **175**, 707–10.

Masatoshi, K., Shusuke, T. and Hitoshi, T. (1992) Small HCC diagnosis with US angiography with intraarterial CO_2 microbubbles. *Radiology*, **182**, 155 60.

Matsui, O., Takashima. T., Kadoya. M. *et al.* (1985) Dynamic computed tomography during arterial portography: the most sensitive examination for small hepatocellular carcinoma. *Journal of Computer Assisted Tomography*, **9**, 19–24.

Michels, N.A. (1955) *Blood Supply and Anatomy of the Upper Abdominal Organs*, J.B. Lippincott, Philadelphia.

Michels, N.A. (1966) Newer anatomy of the liver and its variant blood supply and collateral circulation. *American Journal of Surgery*, **112**, 337–47.

Miller, W.J., Federla, M.P. and Campbell, W.L. (1991) Diagnosis and staging of hepatocellular carcinoma: comparison of CT and sonography in 36 liver transplantation patients. *American Journal of Roentgenology*, **157**, 303–6.

Mitsuzaki. K., Yamashita, Y., Ogata. I. *et al.* (1996) Multiple-phase helical CT of the liver for detecting small hepatomas in patients with liver cirrhosis: contrast-injection protocol and optimal timing. *American Journal of Roentgenology*, **167**, 753–7.

Moon, W.K., Choi, B.I., Han, J.K. *et al.* (1996) Iodized-oil retention within hepatic haemangioma: characteristics on iodized-oil CT. *Abdominal Imaging*, **21**, 420–6.

Murakami, T., Baron, R.L., Peterson, M.S. *et al.* (1992) Hepatocellular carcinoma: MR imaging with mangafodipir trisodium (Mn-DPDP). *Radiology*, **200**, 69–77.

Murakami, T., Mitani, T., Nakamura, H. *et al.* (1992) Differentiation between hepatoma and hemangioma with inversion-recovery snapshot FLASH MRI and Gd-DTPA. *Journal of Computer Assisted Tomography*, **16**, 198–205.

Nakakuma, K., Tashiro, S., Hiraoka, T. *et al.* (1985) Hepatocellular carcinoma and metastatic cancer detected by iodized oil. *Radiology*, **154**, 15–7.

Nazarian, L.N., Wechsler, R.J., Grady, C.K. *et al.* (1994) CT done 4–6 hours after CT arterial portography: value in detecting hepatic tumors and differentiating from other hepatic perfusion defects. *American Journal of Roentgenology*, **163**, 851–5.

Nelson, R.C., Chezmar, J.L., Sugarbaker, P.H. *et al.* (1990) Preoperative localization of focal liver lesions to specific liver segments: utility of CT during arterial portography. *Radiology*, **176**, 89–94.

Nino-Murcia, M., Ralls, P.W., Jeffrey, R.B. *et al.* (1992) Color flow Doppler characterization of focal hepatic lesions. *American Journal of Roentgenology*, **159**, 1195–7.

Nomura, Y., Matsuda, Y., Yabuuchi, I. *et al.* (1993) Hepatocellular carcinoma in adenomatous hyperplasia: detection with contrast-enhanced US with carbon dioxide microbubbles. *Radiology*, **187**, 353–6.

Numata, K., Tanaka, K., Mitsuik *et al.* (1993) Flow characteristics of hepatic tumours at colour Doppler sonography: correlation with arteriographic findings. *American Journal of Roentgenology*, **160**, 515–21.

Okuda, K. (1992) Hepatocellular carcinoma: recent progress. *Hepatology*, **15**, 948–63.

Okuda, K., Jinnouchi, S., Nagasaki, Y. *et al.* (1977b) Angiographic demonstration of growth of hepatocellular carcinoma in the hepatic vein and inferior vena cava. *Radiology*, **124**, 33–6.

Okuda, K., Musha, H., Yamasaki, T. *et al.* (1977a) Angiographic demonstration of intrahepatic arterio-portal anastomoses in hepatocellular carcinoma. *Radiology*, **122**, 53–8.

Okuda, K., Musha, H., Yoshida, T. *et al.* (1975) Demonstration of growing casts of hepatocellular carcinoma in the portal vein by coeliac angiography: the thread and streaks sign. *Radiology*, **117**, 303–9.

Parker, G.A., Lawrence, W., Horsley, J.S. III *et al.* (1989) Intraoperative ultrasound of the liver affects operative decision making. *Annals of Surgery,* **209**, 569–77.

Pattern, R.M., Byun, J.Y. and Freeny, P.C. (1993) CT of hypervascular hepatic tumors: are unenhanced scans necessary for diagnosis? *American Journal of Roentgenology,* **161**, 979–84.

Peterson, M.S., Baron, R.L., Dodd, G.D. *et al.* (1992) Hepatic parenchymal perfusion defects detected with CTAP: imaging-pathologic correlation. *Radiology,* **185**, 149–55.

Peterson, M.S., Baron, R.L. and Murakami, T. (1996) Hepatic malignancies: usefulness of acquisition of multiple arterial and portal venous phase images at dynamic gadolinium-enhanced MR imaging. *Radiology,* **201**, 337–45.

Rapaccini, G.L., Pompili, M., Catarelli, E. *et al.* (1994) Ultrasound-guided fine-needle biopsy of hepatocellular carcinoma: comparison between smear cytology and microhistology. *American Journal of Gastroenterology,* **89**, 898–902.

Reimer, P., Rummeny, E.J., Wissing, M. *et al.* (1996) Hepatic MR imaging: comparison of RARE derived sequences with conventional sequences for detection and characterization of focal liver lesions. *Abdominal Imaging,* **21**, 427–32.

Reuter, S.T., Redman, H.C. and Siders, D.B. (1970) The spectrum of angiographic findings in hepatoma. *Radiology,* **94**, 89–94.

Santis, M.D., Romagnoli, R., Cristani, A. *et al.* (1992) MRI of small HCC: comparison with US, CT, DSA and lipiodol CT. *Journal of Computer Assisted Tomography,* **16**, 189–97.

Seldinger, S.L. (1953) Catheter replacement of needle in percutaneous arteriorgraphy: a new technique. *Acta Radiologica,* **39**, 368.

Sheu, J.C., Sung, J.L., Yu, J.Y. *et al.* (1984) Ultrasonography of small hepatic tumors using high-resolution linear-array real-time instrument. *Radiology,* **150**, 797–802.

Slater, G.J., Saini, S., Mayo-Smith, W.W. *et al.* (1996) Mn-DPDP enhanced MR imaging of the liver: analysis of pulse sequence performance. *Clinical Radiology,* **51**, 484–6.

Soyer, P. (1993) Segmental anatomy of the liver: utility of a nomenclature accepted worldwide. *American Journal of Roentgenology,* **161**, 572–3.

Soyer, P., Bluemke, D.A., Sitzmann, J.V. *et al.* (1995) Hepatocellular carcinoma: findings on spiral CT during arterial portography. *Abdominal Imaging,* **20**, 541–6.

Soyer, P., Elias, D., Zeitown, G. *et al.* (1993) Surgical treatment of hepatic metastases: impact of intraoperative sonography. *American Journal of Roentgenology,* **160**, 511–14.

Stevens, W.R., Gulino, S.P., Batts, K.P. *et al.* (1996) Mosaic pattern of hepatocellular carcinoma: histologic basis for a characteristic CT appearance. *Journal of Computer Assisted Tomography,* **20**, 337–42.

Stevens, W.R., Johnson, C.D., Stephens, D.H. *et al.* (1994) CT findings in hepatocellular carcinoma: correlation of tumor characteristics with causative factors, tumor size, and histologic tumour grade. *Radiology,* **191**, 531–7.

Suto, Y., Tanigawa, N., Iwamiya, T. *et al.* (1994) The potential use of I-123 IMP scintigraphy for pelvic bone metastases in hepatocellular carcinoma. A comparison with Ga-67 scintigraphy. *Clinical Nuclear Medicine,* **19**, 302–6.

Takayasu, K., Moriyama, N., Muramatsu, Y. *et al.* (1990) The diagnosis of small hepatocellular carcinomas: efficacy of various imaging procedures in 100 patients. *American Journal Roentgenology,* **155**, 49–54.

Tanaka, J., Kitamra, T., Fujita, M. *et al.* (1992) Small HCC: differentiation from adenomatous hyperplastic nodule with color Doppler flow imaging. *Radiology,* **182**, 161–5.

Tanaka, S., Kitamura, T., Ohishi, A. *et al.* (1986) Diagnostic accuracy of ultrasonography for hepatocellular carcinoma. *Cancer,* **58**, 344–7.

Tano, S., Ueno, N., Tomiyama, T. *et al.* (1997) Possibility of differentiating small hyperechoic liver tumours using contrast-enhanced colour Doppler ultrasonography: a preliminary study. *Clinical Radiology,* **52**, 41–5.

Torizuka, T., Tamaki, N., Inokuma, T. *et al.* (1994) Value of fluorine-18-FDG-PET to monitor hepatocellular carcinoma after interventional therapy. *Journal of Nuclear Medicine,* **35**, 1965–9.

Torizuka, T., Tamaki, N., Inokuma, T. *et al.* (1995) *In vivo* assessment of glucose metabolism in hepatocellular carcinoma with FDG-PET. *Journal of Nuclear Medicine,* **36**, 1811–17.

Urban, B.A., Fishman, E.K., Kuhlman, J.E. *et al.* (1993) Detection of focal hepatic lesions with spiral CT: comparison of 4- and 8-mm interscan spacing. *American Journal of Roentgenology,* **160**, 783–5.

Veltri, A., Capello, S., Faissola, B. *et al.* (1994) Dynamic contrast-enhanced ultrasound with carbon dioxide microbubbles as adjunct to arteriography of liver tumours. *Cardiovascular and Interventional Radiology,* **17**, 133–7.

Vogl, T.J., Kummel, S., Hammerstingl, R. *et al.* (1996) Liver tumours: comparison of MR imaging with Gd-EOB-DTPA and Gd-DTPA. *Radiology*, **200**, 59–67.

Walkey, M.M. (1991) Dynamic hepatic CT: how many years will it take until we learn? *Radiology*, **181**, 17–24.

Yamashita, Y., Matsukawa, T., Arakawa, A. *et al.* (1995) US-guided liver biopsy: predicting the effect of interventional treatment of hepatocellular carcinoma. *Radiology*, **196**, 799–804.

Yu, S.C.H., Metreweli, C., Lau, W.Y. *et al.* (1997) Safety of percutaneous biopsy of hepatocellular carcinoma with an 18 gauge automated needle – the importance of liver parenchymal tract. *Clinical Radiology*, **52**, 907–11.

Yumoto, Y., Jinno, K., Tokuyama, K. *et al.* (1985) Hepatocellular carcinoma detected by iodized oil. *Radiology*, **154**, 19–24.

FINE NEEDLE ASPIRATION CYTOLOGY DIAGNOSIS OF PRIMARY LIVER CANCER

A.R. Chang

5.1 INTRODUCTION

In current medical practice, fine needle aspiration (FNA) cytology implies the use of a 22-gauge or smaller diameter needle to obtain a sample for cytological evaluation. The FNA technique is not as useful for parenchymatous liver diseases such as cirrhosis and hepatitis. For these conditions it is important to assess changes in liver architecture and this is best achieved with a core needle biopsy for histological examination. However, FNA is ideal for mass lesions which include primary and metastatic carcinoma. In malignant disease of the liver meticulous evaluation of cells in an adequate FNA sample will allow a diagnosis to be made. This chapter will concentrate on the cytological diagnosis of primary liver carcinoma or hepatocellular carcinoma (HCC).

The use of cytology to obtain a cellular diagnosis predates the use of histology as it was not possible to produce satisfactory tissue sections for microscopic examination prior to the advent of wax embedding and the microtome. The first recorded use of needle puncture for diagnosis was by an Arabian doctor in the 11th century to diagnose different types of goitre (Anderson and Webb, 1987) but further advances had to wait until the microscope was invented in the 16th century. In the 19th century, pathologists employed scrapings, imprints and aspirates for microscopic diagnosis. According to Webb (1974, 1975) the first recorded use of needle aspiration biopsy was by Kun in 1841. In 1853, both Sir James Paget and, independently, Erichsen used needle aspiration to diagnose breast diseases. However, in 1869 Klebs devised the method of embedding tissues in wax so that thin sections could be cut and stained, and following this the use of cytology for diagnosis declined (Trott, 1996).

Some desultory interest in cytology persisted in the 1920s with scrapings from freshly excised surgical specimens being used to obtain a rapid diagnosis (Dudgeon and Patrick, 1927). In the 1930s, Martin, a head and neck surgeon, and Ellis, a laboratory technologist, and with crucial input from Fred Stewart, a pathologist, reported on the use of needle aspiration for securing a diagnosis in many tumors at the Memorial Hospital for Cancer and Allied Diseases, New York. This group used 18-gauge needles to obtain biopsies from patients (Frable, 1994; DeMay, 1996). The modern practice of FNA cytology using 21–23-gauge needles originated in Scandinavia in the 1950s and 1960s. The technique was initiated by a group of physicians who were primarily hematologists and included Söderström (1966) and Dahlgren and Nordenström

Hepatocellular Carcinoma: Diagnosis, investigation and management. Edited by Anthony S.-Y. Leong, Choong-Tsek Liew, Joseph W.Y. Lau and Philip J. Johnson. Published in 1999 by Arnold, London. ISBN 0 340 74096 5.

(1966). This method of FNA was further advanced in the 1970s by cytopathologist Josef Zajicek, who described the use of FNA to diagnose lesions in various body sites (Zajicek 1974, 1979). The first use of needle biopsy to obtain a diagnosis of liver disease was attributed to Lucatello in 1895 (Theise and Cohen, 1989) but the extensive use of FNA for hepatic diagnosis did not occur until after Lundquist published his landmark paper in 1971 (Lundquist, 1971). In his paper, Lundquist, who had trained with Söderström, reported on his experience with over 2600 liver FNAs.

5.2   COOPERATION OF PATHOLOGIST AND RADIOLOGIST

FNA cytology has wide application for securing a diagnosis in many superficial and deep-seated structures. For superficial lesions which can be easily palpated, no guidance is necessary, but for successful FNA of deep-seated lesions the sampling needle needs to be accurately placed with the aid of imaging techniques, e.g. fluoroscopy, ultrasound and computed tomography (CT). Typically, a 150- or 200-mm-long 22-gauge Chiba® or similar type of needle is used for liver FNA. Prior to insertion of the needle, the puncture site is infiltrated with local anesthetic and a small skin nick aids insertion of the needle. The latter is carefully guided into the lesion with imaging. Like FNA carried out at other sites, the needle is rapidly moved back and forth in a cutting action as suction is applied with a syringe.

Having a pathologist in attendance to prepare smears and also to provide instant microscopic evaluation will ensure specimen adequacy. The aspirate is immediately smeared onto glass slides, wet fixed by immersing in 95% ethyl alcohol and then stained by a modified hematoxylin and eosin (H&E) method or air dried smears are stained by Dif Qick®. If the former stain is used, slides are ready for examination in < 4 min, while for the latter stain the process is even more rapid.

The cellular content can be assessed and, if possible, a provisional diagnosis proffered. If there is insufficient material for diagnosis in the initial aspirate, the radiologist can perform a further FNA, unless there are clinical reasons for not repeating the procedure. Any slides which are not immediately stained can be set aside for standard H&E, Papanicolaou or special stains to detect specific cellular components. To ensure all aspirated material are available for diagnosis each needle is also rinsed out with a 25% saline–alcohol solution. In the laboratory, cells can be retrieved from the solution with one of the following methods: Cytospin®, Millipore® filter or agar cell block sections.

If the initial microscopic examination indicates an infection, appropriate material is sent for microbiological studies while other ancillary tests which include electronmicroscopy and immunocytochemistry are also possible. Good co-operation between pathologist and radiologist will ensure optimal FNA results.

5.3   COMPLICATIONS

The complication rate for liver FNA is exceedingly low when there is good clinical judgment, patient selection and if painstaking care is exercised at the time of aspiration. Reported rates of complications for transabdominal FNA range from 0.05 to 0.008% (Niemann *et al.*, 1996). Liver FNA should not be carried out on patients with a bleeding diathesis or suspected hydatid disease. In the latter condition an anaphylactic reaction is possible and may be life-threatening. Thus, the patient's clotting profile and relevant investigations should be done prior to the procedure.

In general, complications are related to three factors: aspirator experience, technique and needle size. Most serious complications following needle biopsy of the liver are associated with the use of large-gauge needles. With needles which are 22-gauge, the risk of complications is negligible. In a comprehensive review of the literature,

Powers (1996) found few documented cases of serious complication following liver FNA. Two cases of subcutaneous needle track tumor seeding were recorded (Onodera *et al.*, 1987; McGrath *et al.*, 1991) and a fatal case of bleeding involved a 22-gauge needle which penetrated a small artery (Martinez-Noguera *et al.*, 1991). A further death was due to carcinoid crisis which followed FNA of a metastatic carcinoid tumor (Bissonnette *et al.*, 1990).

Viral hepatitis and HIV are not uncommon infections and the outcome from accidental needle inoculation can be grave. Physicians who do not exercise caution when performing FNA can easily sustain needle stick injuries and such accidents are said to be more common than patients having complications from an FNA procedure (DeMay, 1996). Thus, it goes without saying that a high standard of practice will help to minimize the chance of needle stick accidents.

5.4 FNA APPEARANCE OF CELLS FOUND IN THE NORMAL LIVER

5.4.1 NORMAL HEPATOCYTES

In FNA samples hepatocytes (Fig. 5.1) are usually found in monolayered clusters and chords although a small number of cells may lie dispersed. The cells are polygonal shaped and have distinct cytoplasmic borders and abundant cytoplasm. The latter is finely granular and has an eosinophilic color when H&E is used. If Papanicolaoau, May–Grunwald Giemsa or Diff-Quik® stains are used the cytoplasm is a light blue. The cytoplasmic granularity is due to the presence of many micro-organelles including lysozomes, smooth and rough endoplasmic reticulum, and mitochondria (DeMay, 1996). The nuclear/cytoplasmic ratio is low. Other cytoplasmic findings include fat vacuoles and lipofucsin pigment and the latter is more

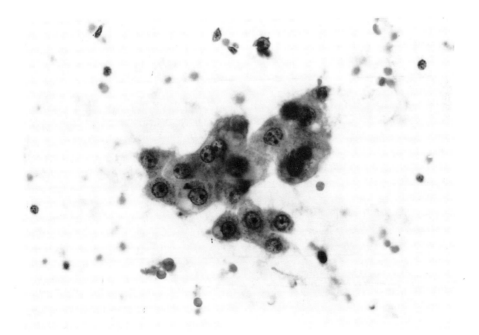

Fig. 5.1 Normal hepatocytes with one or two centrally placed nuclei, small nucleolus and distinct cell borders. The cytoplasm is granular and several cells have small cytoplasmic fat vacuoles. Papanicolaou stain, ×600.

abundant in older individuals. Hepatocytes have a round and bland nucleus which is centrally located. The chromatin is finely granular and the nucleolus is indistinct but may be more prominent. Depending on the age of the individual, nuclear size may vary a little and binucleate cells are not uncommon in older subjects. If there is a delay in fixing smears, naked hepatocyte nuclei may result and to the unwary these can mimic a small cell carcinoma (Tao, 1997). Thus many of the FNA findings are not unlike those found in tissue sections.

5.4.2   BILE DUCT EPITHELIAL CELLS

Bile duct cells (Fig. 5.2) are usually found only in small numbers in a FNA sample. The cells are cuboidal or columnar in shape and have a monolayer arrangement. If seen *en-face*, a honeycomb pattern is apparent. The nucleus is round and a little larger than an erythrocyte and the nucleolus is inconspicuous.

5.4.3   KUPFFER CELLS

These are phagocytic cells and have oval or elongated nuclei and small amounts of cytoplasm. In aspirated material they are often seen clinging to hepatocytes. Those with ingested debris have an oval- or bean-shaped nucleus which is eccentrically located.

5.4.4   OTHER CELLS

These include sinusoidal endothelial cells and connective tissue elements. The former are elongated to spindle shaped and have scanty cytoplasm, and in FNA specimens they are seen to line groups of hepatocytes.

5.5   FINDINGS IN HEPATOCELLULAR CARCINOMA

Using criteria derived from both FNA and histological findings, cytologically HCC can be classified into three categories: (1) well-differentiated cell, (2) pleomorphic large cell

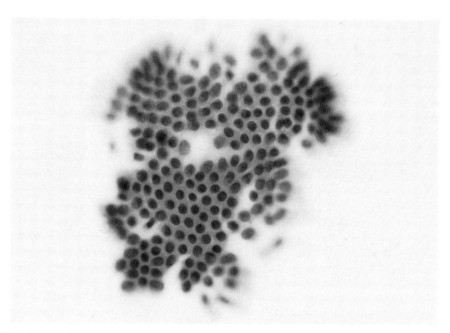

Fig. 5.2   Bile duct epithelial cells are in a monolayer and have a honeycomb arrangement. The nuclei are round or oval shaped. Papanicolaou stain, ×500.

and (3) poorly differentiated cell types (Tao, 1997). Histologically, most HCCs can be categorized into well-differentiated and poorly differentiated tumors.

5.5.1 WELL-DIFFERENTIATED HCC

The most important cytological criteria (Cohen *et al.*, 1991) for distinguishing a well-differentiated HCC from benign proliferative liver lesions such as adenoma and focal nodular hyperplasia are:

- nuclear cytoplasmic ratio;
- tumor cells forming cords or trabeculae; and
- single lying or disaggregated abnormal bare cell nuclei.

Aspirates are typically very cellular and the tumor cells are in trabeculae, papillae, clusters and balls (Fig. 5.3). The cells are smaller than normal hepatocytes and have comparatively uniform round centrally located nuclei which

have a fine chromatin pattern. The majority of cells have increased N/C ratio when compared with hepatocytes seen in other lesions. A helpful feature is the presence of thick cords and papillae which are often surfaced by flattened sinusoidal endothelial cells which can be seen in H&E- or Papanicolaou-stained smears (Fig. 5.4). The nature of these endothelial cells can be confirmed by imunocytochemical stains for markers such as Factor VIII related protein, CD31 or CD34 (Fig. 5.5). However, with meticulous examination immunostaining is not necessary for their delineation. A trabecular pattern can also be found in cirrhotic livers but the cell plates are thinner and have fewer cells.

Other less discriminating diagnostic features which can be helpful are the presence of intracytoplasmic bile which stains a khaki green and intranuclear cytoplasmic inclusions. Finding abnormal bare and enlarged nuclei (Fig. 5.6) which have a coarse chromatin pattern and prominent nucleoli is a further

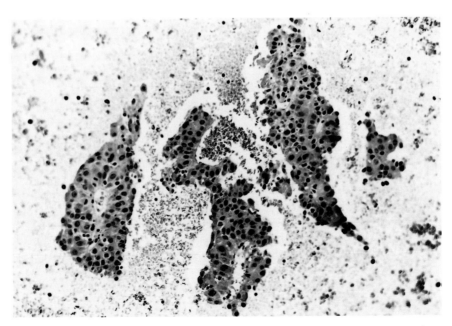

Fig. 5.3   Well-differentiated HCC with cells in a distinctive trabecular arrangement. Note the variation in nuclear size which is evident even at this magnification. H&E, ×100.

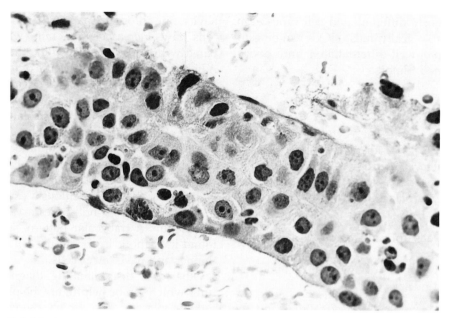

Fig. 5.4 Cell block section showing sinusoidal endothelial cells present on the surface of a thick trabeculum in a well-differentiated HCC. H&E, ×600.

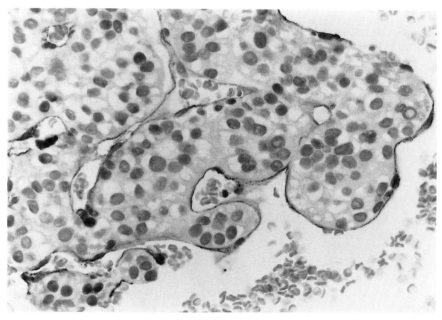

Fig. 5.5 CD34 immunohistochemical stain verifies the endothelial cells lining the tumor cell trabeculae. ×500.

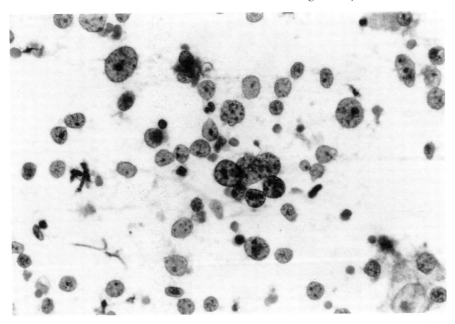

Fig. 5.6   Well-differentiated HCC with a group of bare nuclei displaying variation in nuclear size and granular chromatin and prominent nucleoli. Papanicolaou stain, ×600.

clue for HCC and such cells are not seen in benign lesions (Pedio *et al.*, 1988).

A few well-differentiated HCCs may have extremely prominent cytoplasmic vacuolation and these lesions have been designated the clear cell variant. The cell cytoplasm in this form of HCC contain glycogen which is readily demonstrated by a periodic acid Schiff (PAS) stain. A honeycomb arrangement of tumor cells can also be found (Tao, 1997). Intracytoplasmic lipid vacuoles and hyaline globules which are PAS diastase-positive may also be found. However, hyaline globules are not pathognomonic for HCC and they can be found in numerous other tumors including lung, ovary, breast and adrenals (DeMay, 1996). An uncommon sclerosing variant of well-differentiated HCC has also been described and in FNA samples two types of cells are found: cells which resemble hepatocytes and have a round to oval shaped nuclei and abundant granular cytoplasm and a second

population made up of ductal-like cells (Tao, 1997). In one series of 111 cases of HCC, 62 were well-differentiated HCC and in this category, three were of the clear cell type and two cases were sclerosing HCC (Tao, 1997). Multinucleated cells and mitoses are not a feature in well-differentiated HCC.

5.5.2   PLEOMORPHIC LARGE CELL HCC

The aspirates contain large bizarre cells with abundant cytoplasm and an eccentrically located nucleus and a conspicuous solitary nucleolus (Fig. 5.7). Multinucleated cells are also frequently found (Fig. 5.8) but cells which form a trabecular pattern and are lined by endothelial cells are absent. In general, the cells are in small loosely cohesive clusters or are dispersed. In both the mononuclear and multinucleated tumor cells, intracytoplasmic bile may be conspicuous.

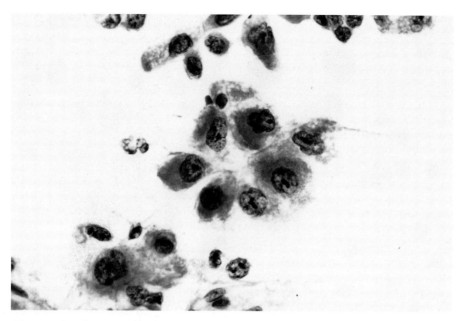

Fig. 5.7 Pleomorphic large cell HCC composed of dispersed tumor cells with eccentrically placed hyperchromatic nucleus, conspicuous nucleoli and ample cytoplasm. H&E, ×500.

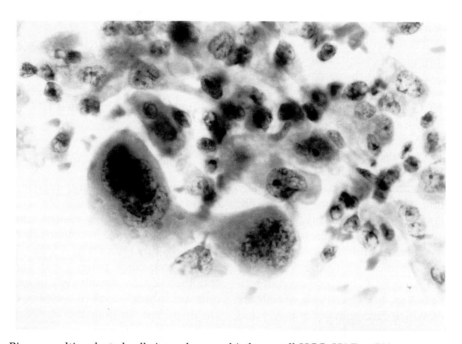

Fig. 5.8 Bizarre multinucleated cells in a pleomorphic large cell HCC. H&E, ×500.

The pleomorphic cells which have been described are also seen in the so-called fibrolamellar variant of HCC. In aspirates of this uncommon form of HCC fibrous stromal fragments may be seen (Suen *et al.*, 1985) but the fibrous component can be sparse or totally absent (Tao, 1997). Tumor cells with multiple intranuclear cytoplasmic invaginations and intracytoplasmic hyaline globules and well-delineated pale bodies are further useful findings which can aid diagnosis. However, without the presence of parallel rows of fibrocytes a dogmatic FNA diagnosis of this uncommon tumor is not possible. Fibrolamellar HCC is found in young adults and there is an equal incidence in both sexes. In addition, fibrolamellar HCC is not associated with cirrhosis, HBV infection or alcoholism. Individuals with this tumor may have no elevated α-fetoprotein and clinically there may be non-specific abdominal pain and/or a palpable abdominal mass. Radiological features of a central vascular scar in the tumor are charac-

teristic of fibrolamellar HCC but may mimic focal nodular hyperplasia. This tumor has a better prognosis than conventional types of HCC (Ng, 1996) after resection. Thus, an accurate diagnosis is important and confirmation with histology may be necessary.

5.5.3 POORLY DIFFERENTIATED HCC

There should be little difficulty in reaching a cytological diagnosis with this HCC. In FNA specimens many dyshesive cells are present and cellular pleomorphism is a key feature. The cells are bizarre and have large round-to-oval-shaped nuclei and prominent nucleoli (Fig. 5.9). Cytoplasm is sparse giving rise to a very high N/C ratio. Some cells are binucleated but it is rare to find multinucleation which is common in pleomorphic HCC. In addition, intranuclear cytoplasmic inclusions (Fig. 5.10), and intracytoplasmic hyaline globules with a peripheral lucid zone (Fig. 5.11) which are positive may be found (Tao, 1997).

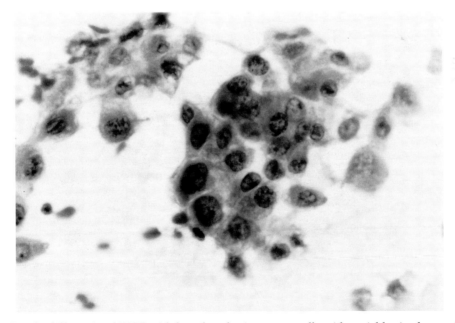

Fig. 5.9 Poorly differentiated HCC with loosely cohesive tumor cells with variable sized, round to oval nuclei, which are mainly centrally located. Some cells are binucleated and nucleoli are conspicuous. H&E, ×500.

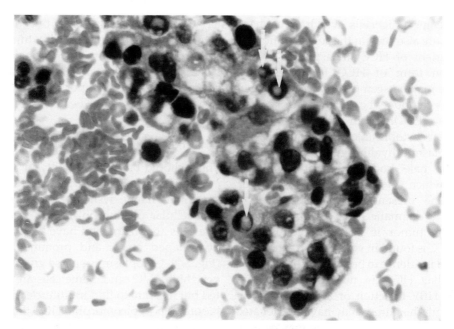

Fig. 5.10 Cell block section of a poorly differentiated HCC with several tumor cells with intranuclear vacuoles (arrows). H&E, ×500.

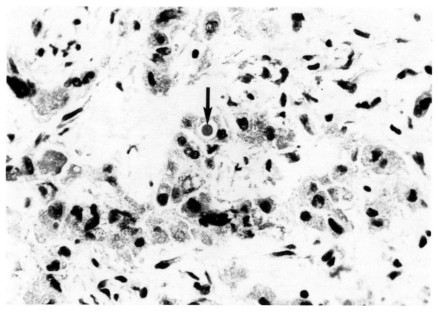

Fig. 5.11 Cell block section of a poorly differentiated HCC with one tumor cell with a distinctive cytoplasmic hyaline globule with a lucid zone (arrow). H&E, ×500.

Table 5.1 Main cytological differences of the three types of HCC

	Well-differentiated	Pleomorphic large cell	Poorly differentiated
Cellular grouping	papillae/trabeculae	loss of cohesion single cells	mostly dispersed cells
Sinusoidal endothelial cells	frequent on surface of cell fragments	nil	infrequent
N/C ratio	increased	low	high
Nucleus	small/round/oval/central	irregular shape and size/eccentric	large/round/oval
Nucleolus	small/indistinct	prominent	prominent
Multinucleation	rare	common	uncommon
Cytoplasm	reduced	plentiful	uncommon
Bile	common	frequent	uncommon

5.6 ANCILLARY STUDIES

Immuncytochemical stains for both AFP and hepatitis-B surface antigen when present will give a strong positive reaction, but unfortunately many HCCs may be non-reactive. However, metastatic tumors to the liver are negative. Thus these two antigens may be useful in some situations when the diagnosis of HCC is not clear cut and metastatic disease needs to be excluded (Bedrossian *et al.*, 1989; Waters and Armstrong, 1996).

Many lesions, including metastatic cancers and cholangiocarcinoma, are positive for CEA and hence CEA positivity *per se* does not confirm a diagnosis. However, CEA may assist in the diagnosis of HCC when a canaliculi pattern is demonstrated (Fig. 5.12) and this may be useful for separating HCC from other tumors (Wong and Yazdi,

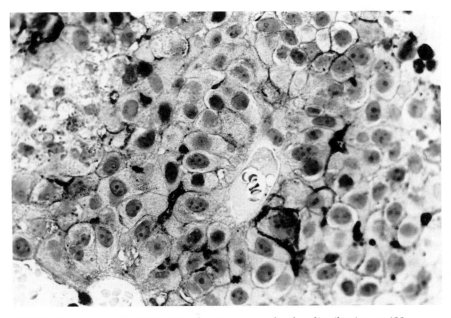

Fig. 5.12 Cell block section with CEA stain showing a canalicular distribution. ×600.

1990; Carrozza *et al.*, 1991; Wolber *et al.*, 1991)

Factor VIII, CD31 or CD34 have already been mentioned and in well-differentiated HCC can be useful in demonstrating the endothelial sinusoidal cells which are found on the surface of tumor cells forming trabeculae. Despite being a very useful ancillary procedure in certain cases, immunostaining cannot be relied upon to clinch a diagnosis of HCC and the pathologist will have to fall back on the cytological criteria previously described.

5.7   CONCLUDING REMARKS

Percutaneous FNA cytology is a safe, rapid and accurate method for the investigation of HCC. A key to successful FNA is having a cytopathologist in attendance to ensure specimen adequacy by the immediate assessment of the specimen and to guarantee that the aspirated material is handled optimally. Cases which require further sampling can be quickly identified. The number of unsatisfactory and false-negative FNA are therefore reduced and the complication rate is minimized by decreasing the number of liver punctures. In the drive to ensure that medical care is more cost-effective, FNA of the liver should be more widely used as it may replace more costly and difficult procedures for obtaining a diagnosis of HCC.

REFERENCES

Anderson, J.B. and Webb, A.J. (1987) Fine-needle aspiration biopsy and the diagnosis of thyroid cancer. *British Journal of Surgery,* **74,** 292–6.

Bedrossian, C.W.M., Davila, R.M. and Merenda, G. (1989) Immunocytochemical evaluation of liver fine-needle aspirations. *Archives of Pathology and Laboratory Medicine,* **113,** 1225–30.

Bissonnette, R.T., Gibney, R.G., Berry, B.R. and Buckley, A.R. (1990) Fatal carcinoid crisis after percutaneous fine needle biopsy of hepatic metastasis: case report and literature review. *Radiology,* **174,** 751–2.

Carrozza, M.J., Calafati, S.A. and Edmonds, P. (1991) Immunocytochemical localization of polyclonal carcinoembryonic antigen in hepatocellular carcinoma. *Acta Cytologica,* **35,** 221–4.

Cohen, M.B., Haber, M.M., Ahn, D. and Bottles, K. (1991) Cytologic criteria to distinguish hepatocellular carcinoma from non-neoplastic liver. *American Journal of Clinical Pathology,* **95,** 125–30.

Dahlgren, S.E. and Nordenström, B. (1966) *Transthoracic Needle Biopsy,* Almqvist & Wiksell, Stockholm.

DeMay, R.M. (1996) *The Art and Science of Cytopathology,* vol. 2, American Society of Clinical Pathologists Press, Chicago.

Dudgeon, L.S. and Patrick, C.V. (1927) A new method for the rapid microscopical diagnosis of tumours. *British Journal of Surgery,* **15,** 250–61.

Frable, W.J. (1994) The history of fine needle aspiration biopsy: the American experience, in *Cytopathology Annual 1994* (eds W. Schmidt., T. Miller, R. Katz and P. Ashton), American Society of Clinical Pathologists Press, Chicago, pp. 91–9.

Lundqvist, A. (1971) Fine-needle aspiration biopsy of the liver: applications in clinical diagnosis and investigation. *Acta Medica Scandinavica,* **520 (Suppl.),** 1–28.

Martinez-Noguera, A., Donoso, L. and Coscojuela, P. (1991) Fatal bleeding after fine needle aspiration biopsy of a small hepatocellular carcinoma. *American Journal of Roentgenology,* **156,** 1114–15.

McGrath, F.P., Gibney, R.G., Rowley, V.A. and Scudmore, C.H. (1991) Case report; cutaneous seeding following fine needle biopsy of colonic liver metastases. *Clinical Radiology,* **43,** 130–1.

Ng, I.O.L. (1996) Liver tumours, in *Topics in Pathology for Hong Kong,* (eds F.C.S. Ho and P.C. Wu), Hong Kong University Press, pp. 101–13.

Niemann, T.H., Miller, T.R., Bottles, K. and Cohen, M.B. (1996) Fine needle aspiration biopsy of the liver, in *Cytopathology Annual 1996,* (eds W. Schmidt, R. Katz., T. Miller *et al.*), American Society of Clinical Pathologists Press, Chicago, pp. 159–73.

Onodera, H., Oikawa, M., Abe, M. *et al.* (1987) Cutaneous seeding of hepatocellular carcinoma after fine needle aspiration biopsy. *Journal of Ultrasound in Medicine,* **6,** 273–5.

Pedio, G., Landolt, U., Zobeli, L. and Gut, D. (1988) Fine needle aspiration of the liver. Significance of naked nuclei in the diagnosis of hepatocellular carcinoma. *Acta Cytologica,* **32,** 437–42.

Powers, C.N. (1996) Complications of fine needle aspiration biopsy: the reality behind the myths, in *Cytopathology Annual 1996*, (eds W. Schmidt., R. Katz., T. Miller *et al.*), American Society of Clinical Pathologists Press, Chicago, pp. 69–95.

Söderström, N. (1966) *Fine Needle Aspiration Biopsy*, Almqvist & Wiksell, Stockholm.

Suen, K.C., Magee, J.F., Halparin, L.S. *et al.* (1985) Fine needle aspiration cytology of fibrolamellar hepatocellular carcinoma. *Acta Cytologica*, **29**, 867–72.

Tao, L.C. (1997) Liver and pancreas, in *Comprehensive Cytology*, 2nd edn, (ed. M. Bibbo), W. B. Saunders, Philadelphia, pp. 827–63.

Theise, N. and Cohen, M.B. (1989) Classics in cytology. III: on puncture of the liver with diagnostic purpose. *Acta Cytologica*, **33**, 934–5.

Trott, P.A. (1996) Introduction, in *Breast Cytopathology. A Diagnostic Atlas* (ed. P.A. Trott), Chapman & Hall, London, pp. 2–11.

Waters, E.D. and Armstrong, J.A. (1996) Disorders of the liver, in *Diagnostic Cytopatholgy* (ed. W. Gray), Churchill Livingstone, Edinburgh, pp. 353–401.

Webb, A.J. (1974) Through a glass darkly (the development of needle aspiration biopsy). *Bristol Medico-Chirurgical Journal*, **89**, 59–68.

Webb, A.J. (1975) Cytological study of mammary disease. *Annals of the Royal College of Surgeons of England*, **56**, 181–91.

Wolber, R.A., Greene, C.A. and Dupuis, B.A. (1991) Polyclonal carcinoembryonic antigen staining in the cytologic differential diagnosis of primary and metastatic hepatic malignancy. *Acta Cytologica*, **35**, 215–20.

Wong, M.A. and Yazdi, H.M.(1990) Hepatocellular carcinoma versus carcinoma metastatic to the liver: value of stains for carcinoembryonic antigen and aphthylamidase in fine needle aspiration biopsy material. *Acta Cytologica*, **34**, 192–6.

Zajicek, J. (1974) *Aspiration Biopsy Cytology. Part 1. Cytology of Supra-diaphragmatic Organs.* Monographs in clinical cytology, vol. 4., S. Karger, Basel.

Zajicek, J. (1979) *Aspiration Biopsy Cytology. Part 2. Cytology of Infra-diaphragmatic Organs.* Monographs in clinical cytology, vol. 7., S. Karger, Basel.

PATHOLOGY OF HEPATOCELLULAR CARCINOMA

6

C.-T. Liew and A.S.-Y. Leong

6.1 INTRODUCTION

The liver is predominantly composed of hepatocytes and bile duct cells, which together give rise to almost all the primary malignant tumors of the liver. Over 95% of such tumors are hepatocellular carcinoma (HCC). Cholangiocarcinoma is the next most common primary malignant tumor and others, such as hepatoblastoma, embryonal sarcoma, malignant hemangioendothelioma, angiosarcoma and carcinoid tumor, are rare.

In Hong Kong, HCC ranks as the second and fourth most frequent cause of death from cancer in males and females respectively, and it is estimated that the hepatitis B virus (HBV) carrier rate is >30 per 100 000 population (Leung et al., 1992; Hong Kong Cancer Registry, 1993). Over 350 cases of HCC are diagnosed annually at the 1350-bed Prince of Wales Hospital, Shatin, Hong Kong, and only 60–80 of these cases are deemed resectable. Of the patients who die from liver cancer, 85% are chronically infected with HBV and >85% have liver cirrhosis. Chronic hepatitis C infection and aflatoxin do not appear to be important risk factors in Hong Kong and <7.3% of patients with HCC in have chronic hepatitis C infection (Leung et al., 1992).

6.2 MORPHOLOGY

6.2.1 GROSS APPEARANCE

Various classifications of the gross appearance of HCC have been proposed. Eggel classified HCC into diffuse, nodular and massive types (year). Nakashima et al. (1974) emphasized the differences in growth pattern and subdivided the tumors into diffuse, fine nodular diffuse, oligonodular, confluent massive, multinodular, solitary massive, encapsulated and massive nodular types. The classification into diffuse, multicentric, inductive, expanding, meganodular and sclerosing types proposed by Peters (1976) attempted to group HCC into different subsets that may have similar etiologic and pathogenetic processes. He further emphasized the importance of the following features: (1) relation of tumor to non-tumor liver; (2) the pattern of growth within the tumor (relationship of tumor to tumor); and (3) the stromal reaction (relationship of tumor to stroma). Kojiro and Nakashima (1987) classified advanced HCC according to the difference in the growth pattern with consideration of capsule, cirrhosis and portal vein tumor thrombosis. Recently, the Liver Cancer Study Group of Japan (1992) proposed a subclassification of nodular HCCs into four

6

Hepatocellular Carcinoma: Diagnosis, investigation and management. Edited by Anthony S.-Y. Leong, Choong-Tsek Liew, Joseph W.Y. Lau and Philip J. Johnson. Published in 1999 by Arnold, London. ISBN 0 340 74096 5.

types that allowed adaptation to relatively small HCCs. These were single nodular, single nodular with perinodular tumor growth, multinodular and confluent multinodular types. This subclassification system is only widely accepted in Japan but not elsewhere.

We describe the gross appearance of HCC as follows:

1. Massive, in which a solitary mass replaces most of one or both lobes of the liver with small satellite nodules in the surrounding liver (Fig. 6.1*a*).
2. Multi-nodular, comprising sharply demarcated, somewhat rounded nodules scattered throughout the liver (Fig. 6.1*b*).
3. Diffuse, in which numerous small tumor nodules are present throughout the liver. These tumor nodules are difficult to distinguish from the backgound of cirrhotic nodules (Fig. 6.1*c*).
4. Pedunculated, which is a subcapsular tumor often in the undersurface of the right lobe near the anterior edge; the location has suggested an origin from an accessory lobe (Fig. 6.1*d*).
5. Fibrolamellar, which is a well-circumscribed tumor of brown coloration and with a central scar.

For each type, consideration is given to the presence of encapsulation and cirrhosis in the surrounding liver. The presence of gross invasion of intrahepatic vessels and bile ducts is also noted. The nodular or massive type is the most common in our practice.

This method of classification is largely for descriptive convenience and does not reflect epidemiology, biology or prognosis other than fibrolamellar carcinoma. Pedunculated HCC may be the only variant of prognostic relevance, as such tumors tend to be more readily resected because of their peculiar exophytic nature and subcapsular location. Furthermore, they show little invasion into the liver and are not usually associated with cirrhosis. Encapsulation of solitary nodules also imparts a better prognosis, as such lesions are often associated with a lower incidence of liver invasion, vascular permeation and formation of daughter or microsatellite tumor nodules.

6.2.2   MICROSCOPIC

The histologic appearance of HCCs is highly variable between different tumors and within the same tumor, especially in larger tumor nodules. In a series of 6391 cases of primary liver cancer, 4317 (67.5%) were found to be HCCs (Carriaga and Henson, 1995). These tumors displayed a wide range of histologic patterns ranging from the classical trabecular carcinomas to undifferentiated carcinomas. Although clear cell and fibrolamellar carcinomas are uncommon, these are the more frequently described histologic variants of HCCs.

Adequate tissue sampling will reveal the full spectrum of the histologic appearances of the tumor. Most HCCs conform to a fairly monotonous pattern; however, the appearances may sometimes be quite variable and difficult to distinguish from cholangiocarcinoma and metastatic carcinoma. The identification of HCC is based on the resemblance of the tumor cells to normal hepatocytes both in its cytologic appearance as well as the plate-like pattern of growth. These features can usually be found in some part of the tumor with adequate sampling.

The World Health Organization (WHO) classification of HCC is probably one of the more commonly used classifications although there are minor modifications used by individual pathologists. In this classification, HCC is divided into five subtypes: trabecular plate-like type (sinusoidal), pseudoglandular type (acinar or adenoid), compact solid, scirrhous type and fibrolamellar carcinoma (Ishak *et al.*, 1994).

The trabecular or plate-like type is composed of well-formed trabeculae of five-to-eight cell layers thick (microtrabecular) (Fig. 6.2*a*) and it is sheathed by flattened endothelial cells of intervening sinusoidal blood

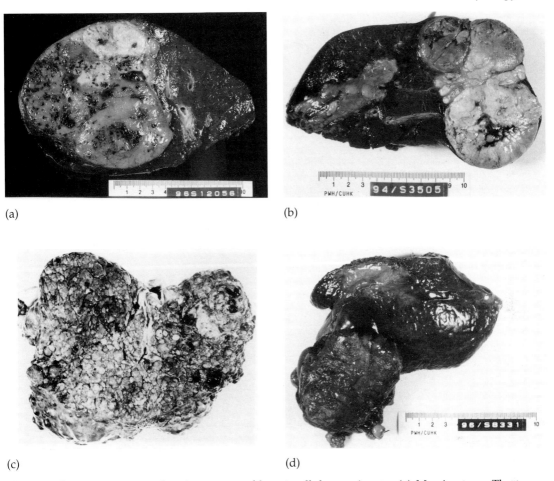

(a)

(b)

(c)

(d)

Fig. 6.1 Gross appearance of various types of hepatocellular carcinoma. (a) Massive type. The tumor replaces most of the resected left lobe of liver and has a bulging cut surface with areas of necrosis and hemorrhage. No obvious capsule is evident. (b) Multinodular tumor with several large nodules in the posterior part of the left lobe of liver, one of which shows distinct encapsulation. In addition, several smaller nodules are present in the anterior aspect of the lobe. These appear to be confluent and are not encapsulated. Note the presence of smaller detached nodules at the anterior edge of the lobe. (c) Diffuse variant with almost the entire liver replaced by multiple small nodules of tumor, many of which are necrotic. (d) A pedunculated tumor hangs from the anterior edge of the liver. There is an area of fibrosis in the base of the tumor pedicle and the liver is cirrhotic.

spaces. While often described as cord-like in appearance, they actually represent plates of cells of several layers thick. Occasionally, the less differentiated trabeculae are more than eight cell layers thick (macrotrabecular) (Fig. 6.2*b*). Sometimes cavernous blood filled spaces may be present in this type of HCC.

The pseudoglandular or acinar type is formed of trabeculae with intervening acinar-like spaces. These spaces are not true glands but represent dilated canaliculi and may contain bile or a dense eosinophilic material representing the breakdown products of inflammatory debris and exudate (Fig. 6.3).

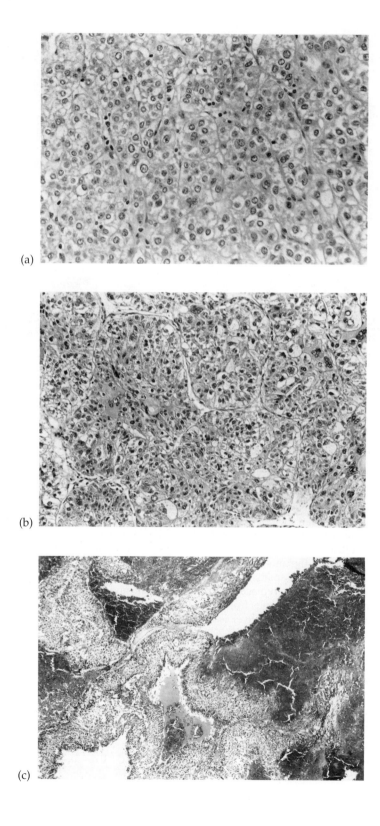

(a)

(b)

(c)

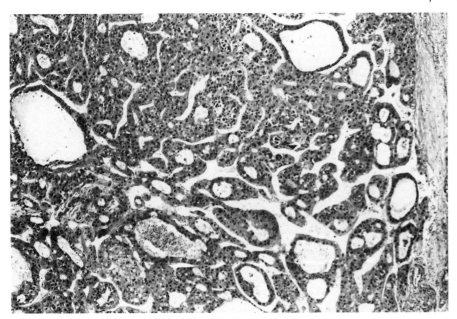

Fig. 6.3 Pseudoglandular or acinar variant of hepatocellular carcinoma in which acinar-like spaces are present in addition to the cords of tumor cells. These spaces represent dilated bile canaliculi, which may contain necrotic debris as seen in the lower half of the field, or bile or fibrin.

While occasionally staining with PAS-diastase, the colloid-like material is not mucin but fibrin. The trabecular and the pseudoglandular types are the most common histologic types seen in moderately to well differentiated HCCs.

The compact type of HCC is more often seen in moderately-to-poorly differentiated HCCs. In this variant, trabeculae are still present but they are poorly formed and often in disarray. The tumor appears to be composed of mostly solid sheets of cells with the blood spaces rendered inconspicuous by compression (Fig. 6.4).

Scirrhous HCC is uncommon and shows prominent desmoplasia with fibrous septa dissecting nests or groups of malignant cells. Although this variant is more often reported following irradiation or chemotherapy and infarction, it may also be seen in the absence of these factors (Fig. 6.5).

The fibrolamellar variant of HCC is distinctive because it is found in a younger age group, has better prognosis and usually occurs in non-cirrhotic livers. The tumor often has a distinctive gross appearance being well circumscribed with a rich brown color and central fibrosis. In addition to the unidirectional type

Fig. 6.2 Trabecular or plate-like pattern of hepatocellular carcinoma. In (a) the well-differentiated tumor cells are arranged in a compact trabecular pattern of three to five cells thick. Flattened endothelial cells lining compressed sinusoids are recognizable. In (b) the trabeculae are thicker and often formed of more than eight cell layers. This is a higher-grade tumor that shows a greater degree of nuclear pleomorphism. Sinusoidal clefts with lining endothelial cell ensheath the trabeculae. (c) Cavernous blood-filled spaces are present in this tumor.

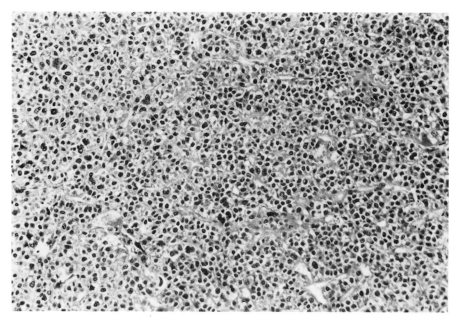

Fig. 6.4 Compact pattern of hepatocellular carcinoma of moderate differentiation. Trabeculae are poorly formed and difficult to recognize.

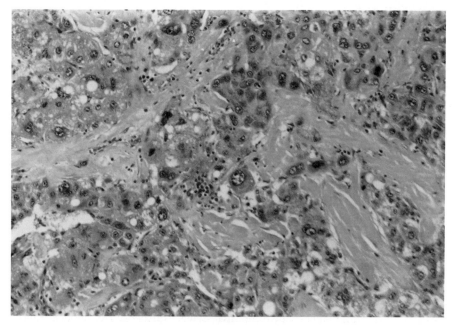

Fig. 6.5 Schirrous variant of hepatocellular carcinoma in which thick fibrous septae transect cords and nests of poorly differentiated tumor cells. Scattered inflammatory cells are present in the septae.

of fibrous septum, most of the malignant cells in this variant have distinctive cytoplasmic inclusions and display special ultrastructural features. This variant of HCC is discussed in greater detail in Chapter 13.

In addition to the histologic types, the WHO classification also includes cytological variants of the tumor. These are:

Hepatic or liver-like cell variant, which have polygonal cells and show vesicular nuclei with prominent nucleoli. The nuclear/cytoplasmic ratio and the degree of nuclear pleomorphism and hyperchromasia vary with the level of differentiation of the tumor. The cytoplasm is generally granular as in normal hepatocytes but it shows a greater degree of basophilia. Often it is this cytoplasmic basophilia which differentiates the cells of HCC from non-neoplastic cells (Fig. 6.6).

Pleomorphic cells, which are often large and contain multiple bizarre nuclei. These cells rarely form sheets or compact masses and usually comprise only a small portion of the tumor (Fig. 6.7).

Clear cells have an abundant, pale, finely granular or vacuolated cytoplasm as a result of abundant glycogen, fat or water (Fig. 6.8). The nuclei are centrally located. The clear cells can predominate in the tumor but they often retain their trabecular growth pattern. Rarely, they grow in solid sheets and require distinction from metastatic renal cell carcinoma and other metastatic clear cell tumors. Although there is a suggestion of better prognosis with this variant (Lai *et al.*, 1979), this claim has not been substantiated (Yang *et al.*, 1996).

Less common cytologic variants are the oncocyte-like cells seen in fibrolamellar HCC, spindle cell, giant cell and rhabdoid types. The oncocyte-like cells are moderately-to-well-differentiated and are fairly regular in size and shape. These cells have pink cytoplasm and small hyperchromatic nuclei. The spindle cell variant is reported to be more

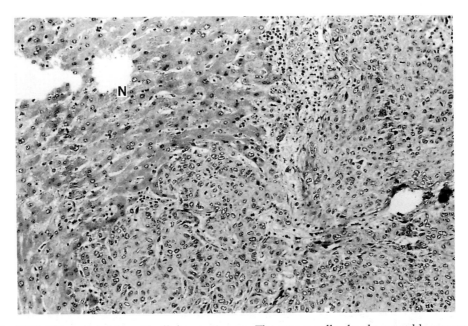

Fig. 6.6 Well-differentiated hepatocellular carcinoma. The tumor cells closely resemble non-neoplastic hepatocytes (N) and are differentiated by their smaller size, increased nuclear cytoplasmic ratio and cytoplasmic basophilia. This tumor shows an infiltrative pattern of growth with compression of the non-neoplastic liver.

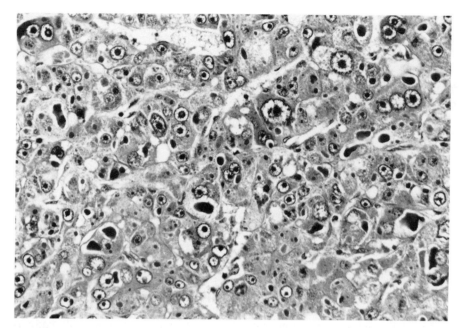

Fig. 6.7 Pleomorphic cells in a poorly differentiated hepatocellular carcinoma. The tumor cells have large vesicular nuclei with prominent central nucleoli and are arranged in compact sheets. Bile thrombi are also prominent in this field.

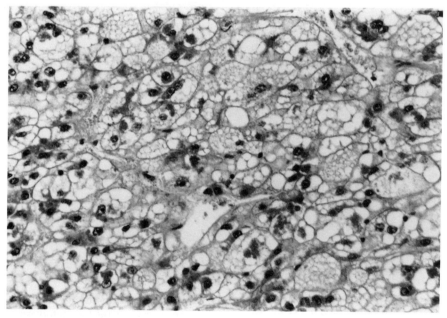

Fig. 6.8 Clear cells of a hepatocellular carcinoma. The cells have vacuolated cytoplasm as a result of abundant glycogen accumulation.

common in patients with a history of anti-cancer therapy which can result in phenotypic changes in HCC cells. Often the spindle cells show a transition from more conventional HCC, either of the trabecular or compact type, and immunostaining reveals the co-expression of cytokeratin and vimentin. Such tumors should be considered spindle cell carcinomas and not carcinosarcomas or mixed tumors.

Several types of cytoplasmic inclusions may be seen in the tumor cells of HCC. These include Mallory bodies that have been demonstrated to be masses of clumped intermediate filaments by electron microscopy (Nakanuma and Ohta, 1984). Pale cytoplasmic inclusions or bodies are frequently seen in fibrolamellar HCC. These stain positive with antifibrinogen antibodies and represent fibrillary structures within cystically dilated endoplasmic reticulum (Nakanuma and Ohta, 1984). Granular hyaline bodies of varying sizes may be seen in as many as 15% of HCCs and may be intracellular or extracellular in location. These granules are often weakly acidophilic and stain with the PAS stain. They stain orange to red with trichrome stains and can be shown immunohistochemically to be one of the liver products such as albumin, α-fetoprotein, α-1-antitrypsin, bile or ferritin. The presence of Mallory's hyaline and α-1-antitrypsin globules is not related to alcohol intake or deficiency of α-1-antitrypsin respectively. Although HBV infection with surface antigen (HBsAg) producing the characteristic ground glass cytoplasm in the tumor cells may occur, it is a very rare occurrence. The pale cytoplasmic bodies in the tumor cells of fibrolamellar HCC may be mistaken for ground glass hepatocytes but they do not stain for HbsAg.

6.2.2.1 Growth pattern

Most HCCs show a sinusoidal or a replacing growth pattern that is most evident at the periphery or the advancing edge of the tumor. The tumor cells grow in the sinusoids in an infiltrative fashion and compress the surrounding liver cell cords (Fig. 6.6). HCCs may also show a replacing growth pattern in which the tumor cells replace hepatocytes within the liver cell cords (Fig. 6.9). This method of infiltration is considered to be basic growth pattern in HCC and is the pattern frequently observed in small HCCs. A direct infiltrative method of extension into adjacent liver tissue may be seen less commonly.

6.2.2.2 Grading

There have been proposals to grade HCC, and the Edmondson and Steiner (1945) system is probably the most widely used. In this system, HCC is graded into four grades. Grade I HCC shows well-differentiated tumor cells usually arranged as thin trabeculae (Fig. 6.10a). This is the tumor grade most commonly seen in lesions <3 cm diameter and it can be difficult to differentiate from hepatocellular adenoma. Grade II HCC shows tumor cells which still resemble hepatocytes but have round but larger hyperchromatic nuclei and abundant eosinophilic cytoplasm (moderately differentiated) compared with grade I cells. These tumor cells are typically arranged in the classical trabecular pattern of three-to-five cell layers thick. Acinar and/or glandular patterns are also often seen (Fig. 6.10b). Grade III HCC shows tumor cells with larger, more pleomorphic and hyperchromatic nuclei (moderately-to-poorly differentiated) compared with grade II tumors. The tumor cells show an increased nuclear cytoplasmic ratio and are more compact and arranged in a vaguely trabecular pattern. Most tumors with multinucleated giant cells fall into this grade (Fig. 6.10c). Grade IV HCC shows poorly differentiated tumor cells with intensely hyperchromatic and pleomorphic nuclei with scanty cytoplasm. The tumor cells are usually arranged in sheets without a regular trabecular pattern. Occasionally, spindle-shaped tumor cells are seen. Grade IV tumors may be difficult to distinguish from other metastatic

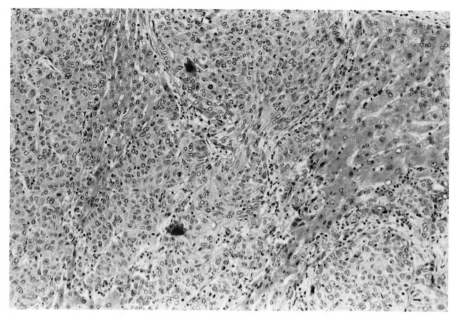

Fig. 6.9   The well-differentiated tumor shows a replacement pattern of growth with replacement of the normal cords of hepatocytes by tumor cells, which show increased nuclear cytoplasmic ratio and cytoplasmic basophilia.

carcinomas (Fig. 6.10*d*). While this grading system is reproducible, the two extremes of the spectrum can be difficult to recognize and the great variability of pleomorphism within the same tumor makes accurate grading a problem.

Despite the several classifications of HCC according to gross or microscopic parameters and the attempts at grading, few pathologic parameters have proven to be really useful in predicting the recurrence or prognosis of HCC. Besides providing prognostic information, the purpose of tumor grading is to provide a correlation with biological data such as laboratory parameters and tumor markers. However, the grading of HCC has had a very small impact on prognosis and it is probably not of significance. Furthermore, despite significant differences in the clinical presentation of HBV- and HCV-associated HCC, studies from Japan have failed to demonstrate clear differences in the pathology

of the tumors in these two groups (Shiratori *et al.*, 1995; Takenaka *et al.*, 1995).

Recently, a thorough analysis of 20 pathologic features in 278 resected tumors in Hong Kong found that capsule formation and heavy intratumoral chronic inflammatory cell infiltrate were independent favorable factors related to tumor recurrence (Ng *et al.*, 1994). Negative resection margins and heavy intratumoral chronic inflammatory infiltrate were independent favorable factors correlating with postoperative survival. The authors disputed claims of other studies, which suggested that recurrence and survival were related to the size of the tumor, a finding that was not substantiated in their study. Tumors >5 cm were associated with a higher tumor recurrence rate by univariate analysis, but this was not an independent prognostic factor by multivariate analysis. Furthermore, there was no difference in survival rates between patients with large and small tumors. This

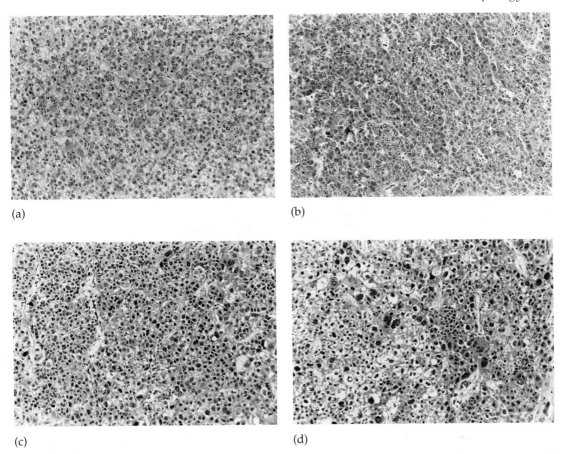

(a)

(b)

(c)

(d)

Fig. 6.10 Edmonson's grading system for hepatocellular carcinoma. (a) Grade 1 with well-differentiated tumor cells arranged in a trabecular pattern. The trabeculae are thicker than normal and there is mild disarray with a slightly increased nuclear–cytoplasmic ratio allowing the diagnosis of hepatocellular carcinoma. A reticulin stain is helpful in assessing the trabecular pattern. (b) Grade II tumor of cells clearly recognizable as hepatocytocytes but showing a greater degree of pleomorphism and thicker trabecular compared with grade I tumors. Small areas with a pseudoglandular pattern may be found in such tumors. (c) Grade III tumor. The degree of nuclear pleomorphism is greater and the cells are compact with only vaguely discernable trabeculae. (d) Hyperchromasia and pleomorphism are marked in grade IV hepatocellular carcinoma and the tumor cells occur in sheets. Occasional spindled forms may be seen.

finding contradicts Japanese findings (Nishi-mori *et al.*, 1994).

6.2.2.3 Small (early) HCC

Small (early) HCC is a more recent concept and when first introduced referred to tumors ≤5 cm diameter; however, currently, small HCCs are defined as tumors ≤2 cm diameter.

The definition of such tumors continues to change as smaller and smaller lesions are being diagnosed with increasingly sensitive imaging techniques. Small HCCs are reported to have better 5-year survival rates than other types of HCCs. Small HCCs can be further divided into two groups, namely, those with distinct and indistinct nodules (Fig. 6.11). The distinct nodule type usually shows clear demarcation and circumscription by a thin fibrous capsule. The indistinct nodule tumor is usually difficult to discern grossly in a macronodular cirrhotic liver because the tumor nodule blends in with the macronodular regenerative nodules. The tumor is usually paler or light yellow in color while the non-tumor nodules are usually tan or bile-stained (bile staining is enhanced by oxidation or fixation in formalin).

The most striking characteristic of small HCCs is that they are often composed of well-differentiated tumor cells resembling normal hepatocytes (Nakashima *et al.*, 1995). Cellularity is increased and the tumor cells are often compact and arranged in a vaguely trabecular

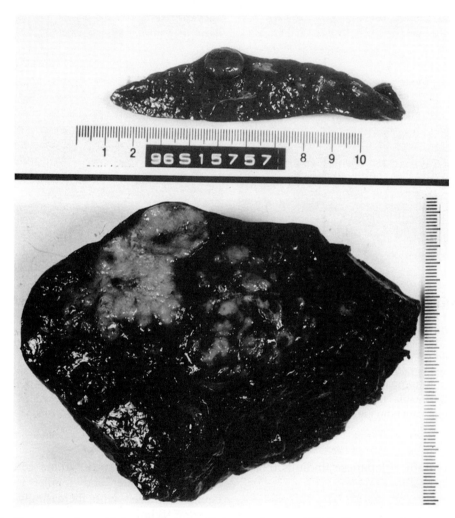

Fig. 6.11 Examples of so-called small hepatocellular carcinomas (HCC). The tumor in the upper frame was 15 mm in diameter and had a bulging cut surface. It was not encapsulated and arose in a bile-stained cirrhotic liver. The latter is not obvious here because of the strong bile staining. The second tumor does not fit the current definition of small HCC as it measured 40 mm. However, it shows a small tumor with irregular outlines and small nodules <5 mm in diameter in the adjacent parenchyma. It was not encapsulated and the pale tan color contrasted against the bile-stained cirrhotic liver.

pattern, frequently with pseudoglandular or acinar structures. The cytoplasm displays increased staining affinity and can be either eosinophilic or basophilic; the nuclei being round and mildly hyperchromatic, with increased nuclear/cytoplasmic ratio. Fatty change is frequent. Often there is a component of the tumor, which is less well differentiated, and this is invariably surrounded by the well-differentiated component, the areas of well-differentiated tumor diminishing in size as the tumor enlarges. If encapsulated, capsular invasion is unusual. If the capsule is absent, the neoplastic cells may blend in with the surrounding hepatocytes making microscopic delineation of the tumor nodule difficult.

The distinction of small HCC from border-line macroregenerative nodular hyperplasia is difficult. The later condition is discussed in detail in Chapter 7.

6.3 NATURAL HISTORY AND SPREAD

At the Prince of Wales Hospital, during 1993–96, >82% of resected livers with HCC had associated macronodular cirrhosis, 5% had mixed cirrhosis, 2% had micronodular and 4% had moderate to severe portal fibrosis (unpublished data). Only 7% had no evidence of fibrosis or cirrhosis. When the tumor was not resectable, the majority of patients, if symptomatic, died in 3–6 months.

The pattern of metastasis of hepatocellular carcinoma is monotonously similar and occurs at a relatively late stage of the disease. More than 70% show extrahepatic metastases, a feature more common in non-cirrhotic than cirrhotic livers. It was reported that nearly twice as many patients dying with HCC occurring in a cirrhotic liver were free of metastases compared with those patients with carcinomas in non-cirrhotic livers (Peters, 1976). It was speculated that the reason for such a difference was probably because the patient with HCC and cirrhosis developed hepatic failure and died sooner before metas-tases developed. An incidence of metastasis of 74.2 and 58.4% was reported in non-cirrhotic

and cirrhotic respectively in Japan (Kojiro, 1997).

Hematogenous and lymph node metastases are the most common routes for dissemination of the tumor cells. Kojiro (1997) reported hematogenous metastases in 50.8%, while lymph node metastases occur in 25.5% of HCCs. The most common site of spread is the lung, occurring in >40% of tumors in one series (Craig *et al.*, 1989). Nearly equal in frequency is involvement of the portal vein with retrograde extension into the extra-hepatic portion of that vessel. The next most common metastatic site is the periportal lymph nodes that accounted for 43% in non-cirrhotic and 16.5% in cirrhotic livers (Peters, 1976). Other sites of metastases are the adrenal gland, gastrointestinal tract, bone, spleen, serosal surfaces, gallbladder, heart and kidney. Lymph node metastasis was reported in 25.5% of 660 consecutive autopsy cases (Watanabe *et al.*, 1994); the hepatic hilar, peripancreatic, perigastric and periaortic being favored.

HCC has a tendency to extend into adjacent branches of the portal vein to result in multiple intrahepatic secondaries; rarely spreading to involve gastric and esophageal veins producing varices, sometimes account-ing for variceal hemorrhage in the absence of cirrhosis. HCC also extends into the hepatic venous system to involve the hepatic vein radicals with access to the right heart and lungs via the inferior vena cava. The pro-pensity for local intravascular invasion and spread is a major factor in the development of spontaneous tumor rupture, which results from widespread thrombotic occlusion, infarc-tion or hemorrhage seen in about 10% of our cases. HCC also infiltrates the intrahepatic bile ducts with extension into the common bile duct, both of which may be observed macroscopically. Obstruction and hemorrhage can produce obstructive jaundice. Other sites of metastases include the bones and lymph nodes of the porta hepatis. Decompensation of liver function is often the cause of death even before metastatic disease is extensive.

6.4 COMBINED HEPATOCELLULAR CARCINOMA AND CHOLANGIOCARCINOMA

Combined HCC and cholangiocarcinoma (CC) is rare and is defined as a tumor composed of both elements of HCC and CC (Allen and Lisa, 1949; Goodman *et al.*, 1985; Taguchi *et al.*, 1996) (Fig. 6.12). The components of the combined tumor may occur separately (double cancers), be adjacent to each other or mixed as one tumor mass (combined), or be intimately mixed (mixed) (Allen and Lisa, 1949). Another study separated combined tumors into 'collision' tumors, 'transitional' tumors and cases of fibrolamellar HCCs with a mucus-secreting component (Goodman *et al.*, 1985). The explanation for such combined tumors is based on the theory that hepatocytes and biliary epithelial cells originate from the same pleuripotent progenitor cell (Aterman, 1992). While clinically combined HCC-CC is similar to HCC, the presence of bile duct differentiation appears to impart a poorer prognosis (Wu *et al.*, 1996).

6.5 LIVER CARCINOMA IN CHILDREN

Lack *et al.* (1982) reported that HCC accounted for 20% of all primary hepatic tumors treated or seen at the Children's Hospital Medical Center in Boston, Masssachussetts and HCC is the third most common childhood hepatic tumor following hepatoblastoma and vascular tumors. The commonest disorders related to childhood HCC are biliary atresia, chronic hepatitis B infection, glycogen storage disease type I, hereditary tyrosinemia, and familial cholestasis.

6.5.1 HEPATOBLASTOMA

Hepatoblastoma is the most common tumor to arise in childhood; rare adult cases have been reported. Hepatoblastoma is a malignant tumor that arises in embryonic rests of fetal hepatocytes. It presents usually as a single large mass and its macroscopic appearance is determined by the presence or absence of mesenchymal components, often showing

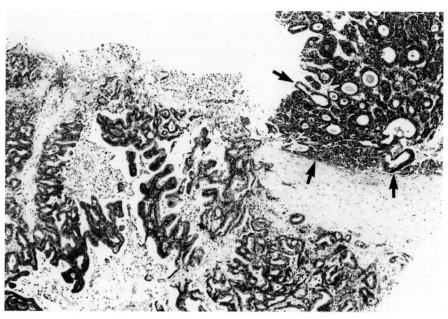

Fig. 6.12 Combined hepatocellular carcinoma (HCC) and cholangiocarcinoma. The HCC (arrows) displays an acinar pattern and the cholangiocarcinoma is clearly mucin-secreting and has a complex glandular pattern.

necrosis, cystic change and hemorrhage. Vascularity is prominent and a thin capsule may be present. The association of liver cirrhosis is not common.

The tumor can be epithelial or mixed with both epithelial and mesenchymal components. Rarely, they may be of the anaplastic small cell, macrotrabecular, teratoid or mucoid variants (Ishak and Glunz, 1967; Weinberg and Finegold, 1983; Dehner and Manivel, 1988). The epithelial variant shows two kinds of cells, namely, fetal and embryonal. The fetal-type cells resemble hepatocytes of the fetus and are arranged in irregular two cell-thick plates with bile canaliculi and sinusoids. The polygonal cells have round-to-oval nuclei and single nucleoli. Hematopoiesis is frequently seen in the fetal type of hepatoblastoma. The embryonic-type cells are small, elongated or spindled shaped with basophilic cytoplasm and a high nuclear/cytoplasmic ratio. They grow in a compact or trabecular pattern and often form rosettes, cords or ribbons. Extramedullary hematopoiesis is not found in this type of tumor. Transition between the two types of tissue is often present. A separate anaplastic type of hepatoblastoma with a poorer prognosis has been recognized (Kasai and Watanabe, 1970). These tumors are composed of small anaplastic cells that are poorly cohesive and difficult to distinguish from neuroblastomas and other small round cell tumors of childhood.

The mixed type of hepatoblastoma is composed of both epithelial and mesenchymal elements, the latter includes connective tissues such as osteoid, chondroid and undifferentiated spindle cells.

6.5.2 CHILDHOOD HCC

Landing (1976) argued that the data of many previous studies was confused by the failure to distinguish epithelial hepatoblastoma from true HCC. He suggested that helpful criteria to distinguish the two tumors included the presence of typical broad cord-like trabecular pattern in HCC and the presence of both a

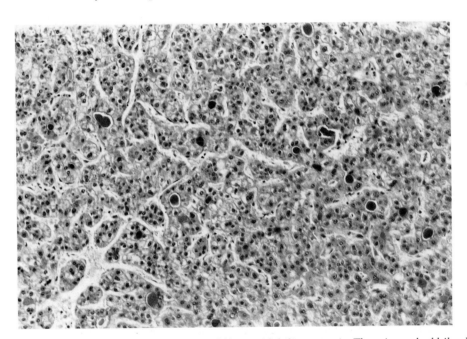

Fig. 6.13 Hepatocellular carcinoma in a 3-year-old boy with biliary atresia. There is marked bile plugging in this moderately differentiated tumor with a conventional trabecular pattern.

larger HCC and a smaller embryonic cell epithelial component in epithelial hepatoblastoma. In our experience with primary liver tumors in childhood, hepatoblastoma has been the commonest tumor. Of six cases of HCCs in patients <21 years of age, five were related to chronic viral B infection and the other was a small HCC (<2 cm) in a 3-year-old boy with biliary atresia (Fig. 6.13). All six patients had liver cirrhosis. The microscopic appearances of childhood HCC are not significantly different to that seen in adult patients with the exception that they are generally well-differentiated tumors.

REFERENCES

Allen, R.A. and Lisa, J.L. (1949) Combined liver cell and bile duct carcinoma. *American Journal of Pathology*, **25**, 647–55.

Aterman, K. (1992) The stem cells of the liver: a selective review. *Journal of Cancer Research and Clinical Oncology*, **118**, 87–115.

Carriaga, M.T. and Henson, D.E. (1995) Liver, gallbladder, extrahepatic bile ducts and pancreas. *Cancer*, **75 (1 Suppl.)**, 171–90.

Craig, J., Peters, R.L. and Edmondson, H.A. (1989) *Atlas of Tumor Pathology*, Second Series, Fascicle 26. *Tumors of the Liver and Intrahepatic Bile Ducts*. Armed Forces Institute of Pathology, Washington, pp. 123–38.

Dehner, L.P. and Manivel, J.C. (1988) Hepatoblastoma: an analysis of the relationship between morphologic subtypes and prognosis. *American Journal of Pediatric Hematology and Oncology*, **10**, 301–7.

Edmondson, H.A. and Steiner, P.E. (1945) Primary carcinoma of the liver. A study of 100 cases among 48,900 necropsies. *Cancer*, **7**, 462–563.

Goodman, Z.D., Ishak, K.G., Langloss, J.M. *et al.* (1985) Combined hepatocellular-cholangiocellular carcinoma. *Cancer*, **55**, 124–35.

Hong Kong Cancer Registry (1993) Annual Report 1993, Hospital Authority, Hong Kong.

Ishak, K.G., Anthony, P.P. and Sobin, L.H. (1994) *Histological Typing of Tumors of the Liver*, 2nd edn. WHO International Histological Classification of Tumours, Springer, Berlin, p. 20.

Ishak, K.G. and Glunz, P.R. (1967) Hepatoblastoma and hepatocarcinoma in infancy and childhood. Report of 47 cases. *Cancer*, **20**, 396–422.

Kasai, M. and Watanabe, I. (1970) Histologic classification of liver cell carcinoma in infancy and childhood: clinical evaluation. *Cancer*, **25**, 551–60.

Kojiro, M. and Nakashima, T. (1987) Pathology of hepatocellular carcinoma, in *Neoplasms of the Liver*, (eds K. Okuda and K.G. Ishak), Springer, Berlin, pp. 81–104.

Kojiro, M. (1997) Pathology of hepatocellular carcinoma, in *Liver Cancer*, (eds K. Okuda and E. Tabor), Churchill Livingstone, New York, pp. 165–87.

Lack, E.E., Neave, C. and Vawter, C.G. (1982) Hepatoblastoma. A clinical and pathologic study of 54 cases. *American Journal of Surgical Pathology*, **6**, 693–705.

Lai, C.L., Wu, P.C., Lam, K.C. and Lok, A.S.F. (1979) Histologic prognostic indicators in hepatocellular carcinoma. *Cancer*, **44**, 1677–83.

Landing, B.H. (1976) Tumors of the liver in childhood, in *Hepatocellular Carcinoma*, (eds K. Okuda and R.L. Peters) Wiley, New York, pp 205–26.

Leung, N.W.Y., Tam, J.S., Lai, J.Y. *et al.* (1992) Does hepatitis C virus infection contribute to hepatocellular carcinoma in Hong Kong? *Cancer*, **70**, 40–4.

Liver Cancer Study Group of Japan (1992) *The General Rules for the Clinical and Pathological Study of Primary Liver Cancer*, 3rd edn, Kanechara Shuppan, Tokyo, pp. 14–26.

Nakanuma, Y. and Ohta, G. (1984) Is Mallory body formation a preneoplastic change? A study of 181 cases of liver bearing hepatocellular carcinoma and 82 cases of cirrhosis. *Cancer*, **55**, 2400–4.

Nakashima, O., Sugihara, S. and Kage, M. (1995) Pathomorphologic characteristics of small hepatocellular carcinoma: a special reference to small hepatocellular carcinoma with indistinct margins. *Hepatology*, **22**, 101–5.

Nakashima, T., Kojiro, M., Sakamoto, K. *et al.* (1974) Studies of primary liver carcinoma. I. Proposal of a new gross anatomical classification of primary liver cell carcinoma. *Acta Hepatologica Japanica*, **15**, 279–91.

Ng, I.O.L., Lai, E.C.S., Fan, S.T. *et al.* (1994) Prognostic significance of proliferating cell nuclear antigen expression in hepatocellular carcinoma. *Cancer*, **73**, 2268–74.

Nishimori, H., Tsukishiro, T., Nambu, S. *et al.* (1994) Analysis of proliferating cell nuclear antigen-positive cells in hepatocellular carcinoma: comparison with clinical findings. *Journal of Gastroenterology and Hepatology*, **9**, 425–32.

Peters, R.L. (1976) Pathology of hepatocellular carcinoma, in *Hepatocellular Carcinoma*, (eds K. Okuda and R.L. Peters), Wiley, New York, pp. 107–69.

Shiratori, Y., Shina, S., Imamura *et al.* (1995) Characteristic difference of hepatocellular carcinoma between hepatitis B- and C-viral infection in Japan. *Hepatology*, **22**, 1027–33.

Taguchi, J., Nakashima, O., Tanaka, M. *et al.* (1996) A clinicopathological study on combined hepatocellular and cholangiocarcinoma. *Journal of Gastroenterology and Hepatology*, **11**, 758–64.

Takenaka, K., Yamamoto, K., Taketomi, A. *et al.* (1995) A comparison of the surgical results in patients with hepatitis B versus hepatitis C-related hepatocellular carcinoma. *Hepatology*, **22**, 20–4.

Watanabe, J., Nakashima, O. and Kojiro, M. (1994) Clinicopathologic study on lymph node metastasis of hepatocellular carcinoma: a retrospective study of 660 consecutive autopsy cases. *Japanese Journal of Clinical Oncology*, **24**, 37–41.

Weinberg, A.G. and Finegold, M.J. (1983) Primary hepatocellular tumors of childhood. *Human Pathology*, **14**, 512–37.

Wu, P.C., Fang, J.W., Lau, V.K. *et al.* (1996) Classification of hepatocellular carcinoma according to hepatocellular and biliary differentiation markers. Clinical and biological implications. *American Journal of Pathology*, **149**, 1167–75.

Yang, S.H., Watanabe, J., Nakashima, O. and Kokuro, M. (1996) Clinicopathologic study on clear cell hepatocellular carcinoma. *Pathology International*, **46**, 503–9.

A.S.-Y. Leong and C.-T. Liew

7.1 INTRODUCTION

Numerous investigative modalities for hepatocellular carcinoma (HCC) are available but none has been as useful and accurate as histologic examination. A combination of clinical, radiological and biochemical information can produce a high diagnostic yield. However, rare cases of metastatic carcinoma in the liver are known to produce elevated levels of α-fetoprotein (Alpert *et al.*, 1971), whereas slightly over 20% of patients with HCC do not exhibit raised levels of α-fetoprotein (unpublished data), inconsistencies which contribute to the inaccuracy of clinical modalities of diagnosis. Thus, even in highly specialized centers, liver biopsy examination is highly desirable in all cases where HCC is clinically suspected.

Needle biopsy of the liver is contraindicated in certain situations. First, when there is a high risk of bleeding because of severely compromised blood coagulation. Strict observation of this precaution significantly reduces the risk of hemorrhage. There were only two fatalities from hemorrhage after biopsy during a 6-year period at the Liver Unit of the University of Southern California in the USA (Reynolds, 1976). Similarly, at the Prince of Wales Hospital where >1500 consecutive liver biopsies were performed for the diagnosis of

HCC over a 6-year period, there were only three cases of post-biopsy hemorrhage and none had a fatal outcome. Second, it has been suggested that if partial hepatectomy is planned in a patient with a liver mass associated with raised α-fetoprotein, it is probably best to delay biopsy until the time of surgery to avoid intraperitoneal dissemination of the tumor. However, the risk of needle tract dissemination is probably very small.

At the Prince of Wales Hospital, all liver biopsies for the diagnosis of HCC are performed under ultrasound guidance. If the tumor is vascular, smaller gauge biopsy needles or even FNA needles are used (Yu *et al.*, 1997).

7.2 PROBLEMS ASSOCIATED WITH NEEDLE BIOPSIES

The diagnosis of medical liver diseases normally requires a core of liver tissue >1 cm in length and containing at least four to five portal triads. However, the diagnosis of HCC often does not require a large core of tissue. Usually, a fragmented biopsy or only a few clusters of tumor cells are sufficient for a confident diagnosis if the classical trabecular pattern of HCC is identifiable. Paradoxically, grades I and II HCC require less tissue compared with grades III and IV HCC,

Hepatocellular Carcinoma: Diagnosis, investigation and management. Edited by Anthony S.-Y. Leong, Choong-Tsek Liew, Joseph W.Y. Lau and Philip J. Johnson. Published in 1999 by Arnold, London. ISBN 0 340 74096 5.

because the poorly differentiated tumors have a less well-defined trabecular pattern. The amount of tissue required for the histologic diagnosis of HCC therefore can range from a few tumor cell clusters to a long core of tissue. Although fragmentation may be encountered in needle biopsies of HCC, it often does not pose a diagnostic problem.

Adequacy of sampling is a problem in 'blind' needle biopsies as they may not be representative of the tumor mass. Ultrasound-guided biopsies provide the highest diagnostic yield by ensuring that the needle is directed into the lesion of interest. A minor drawback of obtaining tissue in this manner is the absence in the sample of normal or non-lesional tissue for comparison, unless a second core is obtained.

The pathology of HCC is detailed in the preceding chapter and this chapter discusses the differential diagnoses and ancillary investigations which help separate the histologic mimics of HCC.

7.3 DIFFERENTIAL DIAGNOSES

The differential diagnosis of HCC in a needle biopsy specimen includes both benign and malignant tumor masses.

The benign group comprises benign nodular proliferations of hepatocytes including macroregenerative nodules, borderline macroregenerative hyperplasia, adenoma, focal nodular hyperplasia, nodular regenerative hyperplasia, mesenchymal hamartoma, and non-neoplastic tumor-like proliferations such as inflammatory pseudotumor and focal (solitary) necrotic nodules. Other benign tumor masses including lipoma, angiomyolipoma, focal fatty change, cavernous hemangioma, epithelioid hemangioendothelioma and juvenile hemangioendothelioma make up the differential diagnosis clinically but they are readily identified histologically and do not pose a diagnostic problem.

The malignant group of tumors that may mimic HCC comprises cholangiocarcinoma, hepatoblastoma, carcinoid and metastatic carcinoma. Other malignant tumors that make up the clinical differential diagnosis but do not generally pose a problem in histologic identification include embryonal sarcoma, embryonal rhabdomyosarcoma, epithelioid leiomyosarcoma, angiosarcoma and malignant teratoma.

7.3.1 DIAGNOSIS OF HCC

The diagnosis of HCC on clinical grounds is still possible without histologic confirmation if the liver containing the space-occupying lesion is also cirrhotic as discerned by imaging and there is associated elevation of serum α-fetoprotein. Unlike resected specimens in which the tumor nodule is often clearly visible, the needle core is often fragmented and the diagnosis of HCC is dependent on the recognition of cytomorphologic and architectural features in the tumor that resemble normal liver. Normal liver lobules show the presence of portal triads and terminal hepatic veins. In regenerating nodules of cirrhotic livers and dysplastic nodules, the two-cell thick plates of liver cells generally display small nuclei with inconspicuous nucleoli. Fibrous bands circumscribe cirrhotic nodules and portal tract elements while absent within the nodules may be seen in the fibrous septae (Fig. 7.1a). Fragmentation may render the identification of fibrosis difficult as the thin fibrous bands often lie at the edge of the fragments and a reticulin or collagen stain is often helpful. The presence of chronic inflammatory cells in the fibrous bands is another helpful clue. HCC is composed of hepatocytes arranged in a plate-like growth pattern comprising cords or trabeculae of two or more cells thick, and intervening stroma with sinusoid-like blood spaces lined by a single layer of endothelial cells (Fig. 7.1b), a pattern revealed best by reticulin stains. While the neoplastic hepatocytes may closely resemble their normal counterparts in cytomorphology, they may also display a variation in the

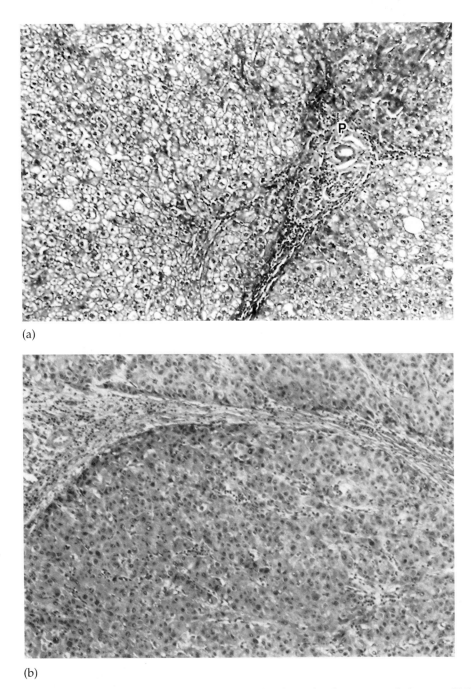

(a)

(b)

Fig. 7.1 (a) Cirrhotic nodules composed of thick trabeculae, loss of architecture and absence of bile ducts. Such nodules can be difficult to distinguish from hepatocellular carcinoma but the presence of intervening fibrous septae with portal tract elements and inflammatory cells (P) is a helpful discriminator. (b) In contrast, the cells of hepatocellular carcinoma display cytoplasmic basophilia and mild-to-moderate nuclear pleomorphism. The thick hepatocyte cords have discernable intervening sinusoids lined by flattened endothelial cells.

degree of differentiation and show a greater degree of cytoplasmic basophilia. Bile production, clear cell change, steatosis and various cytoplasmic inclusions such as eosinophilic hyaline, ground glass inclusions, pale bodies and eosinophilic globules may be present and the neoplastic cells may rarely show sarcomatoid transformation. The presence of architectural patterns such as pseudoglandular change, the features of the fibrolamellar and schirrous variants make the recognition of HCC easier. However, low-grade HCC may be difficult to distinguish from liver cell adenomas and other benign nodular proliferations. High-grade and anaplastic tumors may also be difficult to separate from other anaplastic tumors and may require ancillary investigations including immunohistochemistry and electron microscopy.

7.3.2 BENIGN NODULAR PROLIFERATIONS OF HEPATOCYTES

7.3.2.1 Dysplastic nodules (adenomatous hyperplasia, macroregenerative nodules) and borderline macroregenerative nodules (atypical regenerative nodules, 'nodule-within-nodule')

Liver cirrhosis, in particular, macronodular cirrhosis secondary to chronic hepatitis B infection, is the most common association of HCC. The regenerative nodules of macronodular cirrhosis can sometimes grow to a large size and present as a mass, mimicking a small HCC or metastatic tumor. These macroregenerative nodules have also been referred to as 'adenomatous hyperplasia', and the term 'dysplastic nodule' has been recently employed by a consensus group (Wanless *et al.*, 1995). There is no set size to these nodules which may measure >15 cm in diameter, but most reported cases have ranged from 2 to 3 cm (Crawford, 1990). Macroregenerative nodules occur in cirrhotic livers, particularly in the vicinity of HCC. Although most frequently described in the Japanese population,

macroregenerative nodules appear to have a comparable frequency in the West (Ferrell *et al.*, 1992). Macroscopically, such nodules are distinct from their surrounding tissue in terms of size, texture and color, being yellowish to greenish or bile-stained, sometimes of a lighter tan color than the surrounding cirrhotic liver. They have a bulging cut surface and may be surrounded by a fibrous rim with compression of the adjacent liver parenchyma. There are no internal septae or scars, and necrosis and hemorrhage are not present.

Such nodules, especially larger ones (Arakawa *et al.*, 1986), may show 'nodules within nodules', and varying degrees of atypia or 'early malignant' changes may be observed (Nakanuma *et al.*, 1990; Sakamoto *et al.*, 1991). Fatty change in such nodules is highly indicative of HCC transformation and has been used as a marker for the identification of HCC in laparoscopic examination of the liver (Kameda and Shinji, 1992). These nodules are considered to represent the early or small carcinomas identified by modern imaging techniques (Takayama *et al.*, 1990).

Microscopically, macroregenerative nodules may be difficult to distinguish from ordinary regenerative cirrhotic nodules. An apparent increase in the number of arteries without corresponding bile ducts, so-called 'unpaired arteries' is a clue that the lesion is a macroregenerative nodule. These nodules are divided into 'typical' and 'atypical' nodules. The typical nodules are composed of hepatocytes with no evidence of atypia and are often similar in appearance to the surrounding cirrhotic parenchyma. Atypical macroregenerative nodules are also known as 'borderline macroregenerative nodules'. They are composed of hepatocytes arranged in one-to-three-cell thick cords with areas of fatty change, cytoplasmic basophilia and foci of disordered growth in the form of pseudoacini and/or thickened trabeculae. Other features such as clear cell change, Mallory body clustering, iron resistance in an otherwise siderotic nodule and increased copper may be present (Thiese, 1997). There may be nuclear pleomorphism with increased nuclear cyto-plasmic ratio, nuclear crowding and enlarge-ment of nucleoli, besides increased cyto-plasmic basophilia (Eguchi *et al.*, 1992; Nakanuma *et al.*, 1990; Takayama *et al.*, 1990) (Fig. 7.2). Hepatocytes may be observed pro-liferating within the fibrous septae and portal tracts (Wada *et al.*, 1988; Nakanuma *et al.*, 1990).

The distinction of 'atypical' macroregener-ative nodules from small or early HCC is difficult. It is now accepted that macro-regenerative nodules are preneoplastic and may be the precursor lesion of HCC, or at least represent one mode of hepatocarcinogenesis. This contention is supported by the demon-stration of monoclonality of these nodules, and autopsy and liver explant studies have demonstrated a strong association with devel-opment of HCC in the adjacent liver. In addition, animal studies of hepatocarcinoge-nesis have demonstrated progression of 'bor-derline' lesions to overt HCC (Thiese, 1997). Furthermore, the finding of 'nodule in nodule' transformation in man adds further support to this contention. The subnodules display a pushing growth against the surrounding par-enchyma within the nodule and also show a more rapidly proliferative rate than the sur-rounding nodule (Thiese *et al.*, 1996).

The identification of small adenomas or HCC or 'nodule-in-nodule' has mostly been done with modern imaging techniques. Such transformed lesions show decreased Ga-67 uptake, and a negative colloid (Tc-99 m phy-tate) uptake and early uptake and subsequent retention of Tc-99 m PMT compared with normal liver. Macroregenerative nodules may accumulate iron and the development of iron-poor foci within these nodules corresponding to malignant transformation has been exploi-ted in magnetic resonance examinations for the detection of small HCCs (Mitchell *et al.*, 1991). Lipiodol retention is also fairly specific for HCC and can identify even lesions of

2 mm diameter; however, sensitivity is poor, being about 45% (Bhattacharya *et al.*, 1997). Macroregenerative nodules with cancerous foci tend to be significantly larger (15.8 +/− 2.2 mm) compared with those without (10.1 +/− 2.6 mm) (Eguchi *et al.*, 1992).

The microscopic features used to differ-entiate benign macroregenerative nodules from small HCC (see Chapter 6) include the architectural features of thickened cell plates, formation of trabeculae and loss of reticulin seen in HCC (Ferrell *et al.*, 1992). Nuclear crowding, pseudoacinar formation and increased cytoplasmic basophilia have also been employed although some of these fea-tures are also seen in 'typical' macroregener-ative nodules. By employing immunostaining, it has been demonstrated that normal livers, livers with chronic hepatitis, cirrhotic nodules and macroregenerative nodules display few or no arterial elements in the parenchyma and perisinusoidal cells are increased compared with HCC, allowing a method of distinguish-ing between these entities (Terada and Naka-numa, 1995). Staining for cytokeratin 19 to label biliary cells has been employed as an aid to distinguish small HCCs from borderline and cirrhotic nodules. Small HCCs and malignant foci in borderline macroregenerative nodules lacked cytokeratin 19-positive biliary cells, whereas benign nodules harbored a few intra-parenchymal ductules as well as peripheral reactive or proliferative ductules (Terada *et al.*, 1995). In an attempt to identify microscopic features in cirrhotic livers that are associated with concurrent HCC, Ojanguren *et al.* (1997) assessed the following: large cell dysplasia, small cell dysplasia, cytoplasmic basophilia, small microacinar structures, peripheral dis-tribution of nuclei, nuclear irregularities and thickened liver plates. They found that none was useful in discriminating between cirrhotic livers and HCC. On the other hand, cirrhotic nodules exhibiting three or fewer of these features were never associated with malig-nancy, whereas those with four or more alterations were often located in the vicinity of

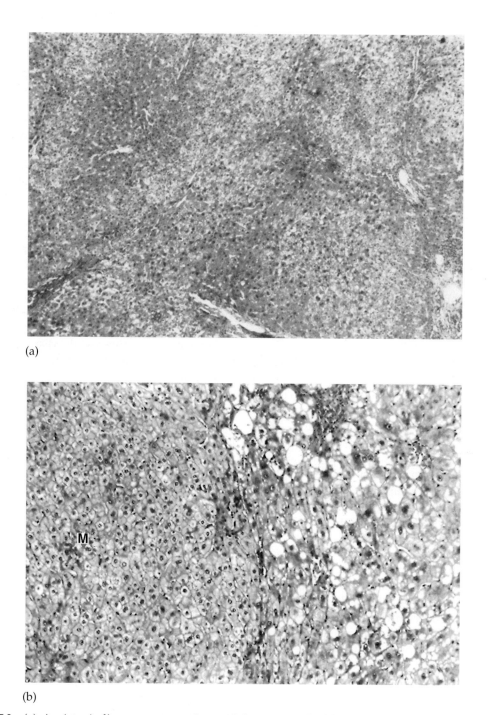

(a)

(b)

Fig. 7.2 (a) An 'atypical' macroregenerative nodule composed of hepatocytes arranged in cords of several cells thick and showing marked nuclear pleomorphism and cytoplasmic basophilia. Portal vessels and bile ducts are present in the nodule. (b) A 'typical' macroregenerative nodule (M) producing compression of adjacent hepatocytes. The nodule is composed of hepatocytes arranged as sheets of cells with mild nuclear pleomorphism and only slightly increased nuclear cytoplasmic ratio.

HCC. Acinar structures, thickened trabeculae, peripheral distribution of nuclei and nuclear irregularities seemed to be the most specific indicators of proximity to HCC.

In a study of 18 cases of adenomatous hyperplasia and 20 cases of so-called small HCCs, Yamamoto *et al.* (1996) found that there were significant differences between the two groups. These were differences in size (0.94 ± 0.36 and 1.69 ± 0.36 cm respectively; *p*<0.01), angiographic features and basement membrane immunohistochemistry of the sinusoids. The sinusoids of HCC acquire type IV collagen and laminin-staining reflecting their capillarization associated with the increased arterial blood flow that occurs with malignant transformation. These authors suggested that immunostaining for basal lamina components can help identify malignant change in adenomatous hyperplasia.

It is clear that the distinction of 'atypical' or 'borderline' macroregenerative nodules from early HCC is an area that requires further clarification. The definitions of diagnostic criteria require refinement (Ferrell *et al.*, 1993). Analyses of objective parameters including morphometry (Nagato *et al.*, 1991), proliferative indices (Thiese *et al.*, 1996) and image analysis (An *et al.*, 1997), together with careful correlation of histology and imaging findings will provide the foundation for such refinements.

7.3.2.2 Dysplasia

The term liver cell 'dysplasia' was first introduced by Anthony (1973) and refers to the presence of large, abnormal cells with bizarre, hyperchromatic and occasionally multiple nuclei. These cells occurred in clusters and sometimes occupied entire cirrhotic nodules. This form of dysplasia has come to be known as 'large cell dysplasia' (Fig. 7.3). While its occurrence is not disputed, the earlier suggestion that it represents an independent risk factor for the development of HCC has not been irrefutably proven. These findings require confirmation.

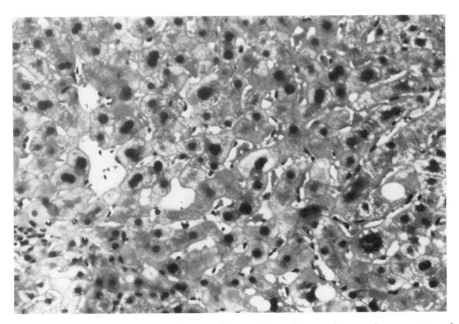

Fig. 7.3 Large cell dysplasia in a cirrhotic liver. Note the nuclear enlargement and marked pleomorphism.

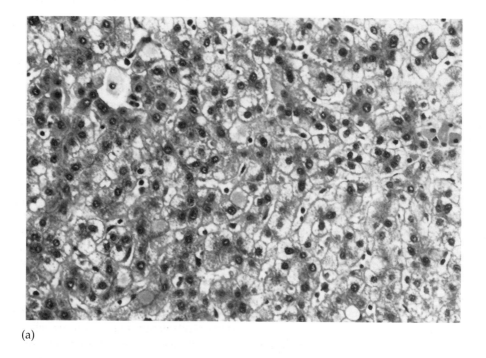

(a)

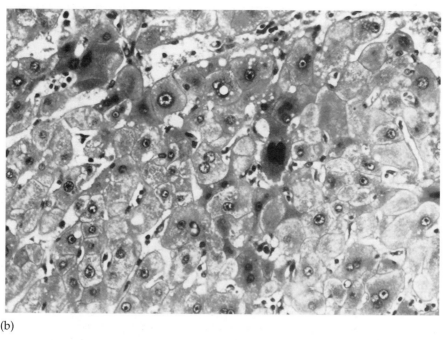

(b)

Fig. 7.4 'Small cell dysplasia' with ground glass hepatocytes (a) and a multinucleated cell (b). There is nuclear crowding and unlike the large cell variety, the nuclei are small and only mildly pleomorphic. The cytoplasm is slightly reduced resulting in an increased nuclear cytoplasmic ratio. Small cell dysplasia is difficult to distinguish from the changes in regenerative nodules of cirrhotic livers.

'Small cell dysplasia' is a more recent term first used by Watanabe *et al.* (1983) who found these cells in HCCs. These cells were observed in clusters and displayed nuclear crowding. The small nuclei and the relatively less than normal, often basophilic cytoplasm resulted in an increased nuclear-cytoplasmic ratio. In addition, there were cytologic abnormalities in the form of nuclear pleomorphism and sometimes multinucleation (Fig. 7.4). Watanabe *et al.* (1983) concluded that these cells were premalignant. While small cell dysplasia appears to be readily identified in HCCs in Japan and in the Asian population, it seems less common in the West and there is expressed uncertainty as to the distinction of the cytologic features of small cell dysplasia from those seen in regenerative changes (Thiese, 1997).

It should be noted that the diagnosis of 'dysplastic' nodules or 'adenomatous hyperplasia' does not require the presence of hepatocytes displaying the cytologic features of either large or small cell dysplastic changes (see above).

7.3.2.3 Hepatocellular adenoma

This benign tumor of hepatocytes is well recognized for its association with the use of oral contraceptive steroids as well as androgenic/anabolic steroids. True malignancy as a result of intake of such steroids is very rare. Progestogens do not appear to carry any risk and modern low dose oral contraceptives seem to carry a very much-reduced risk (Huggins and Zucker, 1987; Rosenberg, 1991; Nagorney, 1995). The most commonly incriminated androgens have been methyltestosterone, oxymetholone and norethandrolone. Other side effects of synthetic gonadal steroids include cholestatic jaundice, Budd–Chiari syndrome, sinusoidal dilatation and peliosis hepatis, and the latter associated with anabolic steroids. With the exception of peliosis hepatis, which can occur in adenomas due to androgenic steroids, these other side effects

are seldom seen in combination with adenoma. While other etiologic agents such as danazol, norethisterone, clomiphene, diabetes mellitus, glycogen storage disease type Ia and Klinefelter syndrome have been implicated, increasing number of cases do not seem to have an identifiable etiology. Glycogen storage disease types I and II have been associated with hepatocellular adenomas (Labrune *et al.*, 1997).

Patients with hepatocellular adenoma present mostly with acute abdominal pain, which is frequently due to intratumoral hemorrhage and less frequently, rupture into the peritoneum. Episodic abdominal pain may occur or the tumor may be asymptomatic at the time of discovery. Malignant transformation is rare (Foster and Berman, 1994).

Hepatocellular adenomas are usually solitary. Multiple adenomas are uncommon and rare instances of multiple adenomatosis have been reported (Le Bail *et al.*, 1992; Arsenault *et al.*, 1996). Macroscopically, the tumor mass may be as large as 30-cm diameter and 3000 g weight. Dilated vessels commonly traverse its bulging surface and it is clearly demarcated but not encapsulated. It has a soft friable consistency with areas of hemorrhage or necrosis (Fig. 7.5a). Focal scarring marks sites of previous hemorrhage and infarction. Microscopically, the tumor lacks a lobular architecture, bile ducts are completely absent and the liver plates are no more than two-to-three cells thick. The liver plates are separated by narrow, inconspicuous sinusoids lined by endothelium and Kupffer cells may be present in variable numbers (Fig. 7.5b). The hepatocytes do not display pleomorphism although they are generally larger than normal and their cytoplasm is pale or clear due to excess glycogen. Large tortuous arteries and dilated veins may be present and foci of hematopoiesis may be seen in adenomas occurring in children. Peliosis hepatis may be present in those tumors associated with anabolic steroid intake and occasionally α-1-antitrypsin globules and appearances simulating

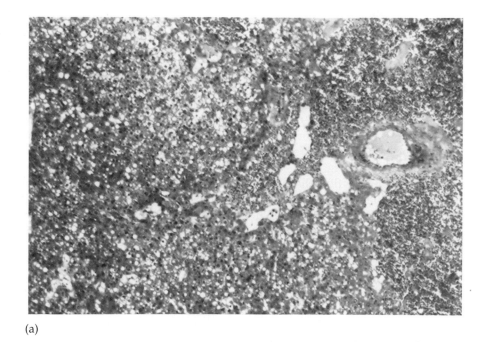

(a)

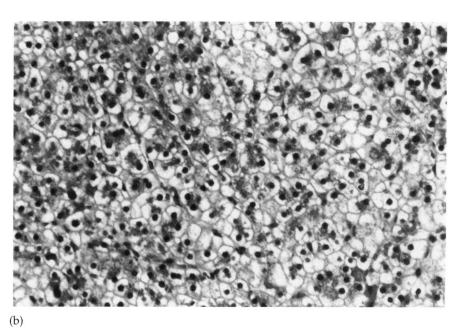

(b)

Fig. 7.5 (a) Prominent vascular channels in a hepatocellular adenoma. (b) Tumor composed of compact cords of hepatocytes of two-to-three cells thick. There is very mild pleomorphism and normal lobular architecture is lost with an absence of portal tracts and central veins throughout the adenoma.

alcoholic hepatitis with fatty change, neutrophils and giant cell granulomas may be present.

While not difficult to diagnose in the gross state, it can be difficult to separate hepatocellular adenoma from well-differentiated HCC in needle biopsies. The latter is diagnosed by the presence of thick liver plates of more than three cell layers, pseudoacinar formation, cytologic atypia, cytoplasmic basophilia, loss of the reticulin pattern, absence of Kupffer cells, stainable α-fetoprotein and vascular invasion. An appropriate clinical history is useful for the diagnosis of hepatocellular adenoma.

7.3.2.4 Focal nodular hyperplasia

Focal nodular hyperplasia (FNH) occurs most frequently in young women but it is also seen in both sexes and at all ages (Shortell and Schwartz, 1991; Reymond *et al.*, 1995). Its alleged association with oral contraceptive use is controversial and is thought to be a vascular malformation with arteriovenous anastomoses and local overgrowth of liver elements (Ndimbie *et al.*, 1990). This suggestion is supported by the lobulated outline of the lesion which appears to be associated with the vascular pattern in the fibrous scar, best displayed in a reticulin stain. FNH is usually asymptomatic and discovered incidentally as a solitary mass <5 cm in diameter with a prominent central fibrous scar. The cut surface bulges and it is of a brown-yellow color. Microscopically, it is composed of nodules of liver parenchyma separated by fibrous septae. The latter contain numerous bile ducts and variable numbers of lymphoid cells and thick walled vessels are seen in the central stellate scar (Fig. 7.6). The hepatocytes are arranged in liver plates of no more than three cell layers and may show variable amounts of glycogen or fat and other cytoplasmic inclusions such as Mallory's hyaline and bile.

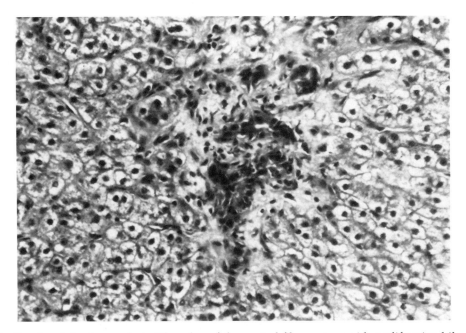

Fig. 7.6 Focal nodular hyperplasia. The edge of the central fibrous scar with proliferating bile ducts is clearly visible in the center of the field. The surrounding hepatocytes are normal appearing.

The distinction of FNH from hepatocellular adenoma in a needle biopsy specimen is often difficult and is sometimes not possible. Accurate diagnosis is dependent on tissue sampling. However, diagnosis is aided by the presence of prominent proliferating bile ductules in the fibrous septae and the radiological findings of a solitary lesion with a central vascular scar (Buetow *et al.*, 1996). The remaining liver is usually normal. Multifocal nodular hyperplasia has been described, sometimes associated with systemic vascular malformations and neoplasia of the brain (Wanless *et al.*, 1989).

7.3.2.5   Nodular regenerative hyperplasia

Nodular regenerative hyperplasia (NRH) is also known as non-cirrhotic nodulation, nodular transformation, partial nodular transformation and a variety of other names. NRH is now the generally accepted term. It is associated with a variety of diseases that seem to share the common feature of some sort of vascular or circulatory abnormality. These diseases include rheumatoid arthritis, Felty's syndrome, lupus erythematosus, scleroderma, polyarteritis nodosa, diabetes mellitus and hematolymphoid proliferative disorders. NRH has also been described following bone marrow and kidney transplantation. It has been suggested that NRH occurs as a result of tissue adaptation to heterogeneous distribution of hepatic blood from a variety of causes (Wanless, 1990). NRH is most often asymptomatic although it may be a cause of non-cirrhotic portal hypertension and, rarely, it has caused intraperitoneal hemorrhage.

Macroscopically, the liver shows multiple fine nodules of 0.1–1.0 cm. It is not associated with cirrhosis or fibrosis and the severity of nodulation may be variable, with accentuation near the porta hepatis. Microscopically, the nodules are composed of normal-appearing hepatocytes that are arranged in plates of two-to-three cell layers thick (Fig. 7.7a). Dysplastic cells may be present (Fig. 7.7b).

Lobular architecture is maintained with evenly distributed portal structures and no evidence of fibrosis. The expansive nature of these nodules is best demonstrated with reticulin stains. Obliterative vascular changes may be seen in all types of intrahepatic vessels. Diagnosis by needle biopsy is obviously difficult and the differential diagnoses are focal nodular hyperplasia and hepatocellular adenoma.

7.3.2.6   Mesenchymal hamartoma

Mesenchymal hamartoma is related to polycystic disease and congenital hepatic fibrosis. It occurs exclusively in young children (DeMaioribus *et al.*, 1990). The large multicystic lesion contains fluid or semi-solid gelatinous material. Microscopically, it shows a mixture of mesenchymal and epithelial elements. The mesenchymal component consists of loose connective tissue rich in acid mucopolysaccharides and dilated vessels, lymphatics and fluid-filled spaces. Prominent tortuous bile ducts and nodules of hepatocytes are present and distributed in a random fashion. Hematopoietic elements may be seen. The presence of the striking mesenchymal components readily distinguishes this lesion from focal nodular hyperplasia and hepatocellular (Stocker and Ishak, 1983).

Similarities have been drawn between the gross vascular and segmental anomalies, as well as the histologic features seen in mesenchymal hamartoma and torted accessory lobe of liver. These similarities have led to the suggestion that mesenchymal hamartoma may represent ischemic change in a sequestered lobe of liver (Lennington *et al.*, 1993).

7.3.3   NON-NEOPLASTIC TUMOR LIKE PROLIFERATIONS

7.3.3.1   Inflammatory pseudotumor

The inflammatory pseudotumor may be solitary or multiple and of variable size. It is

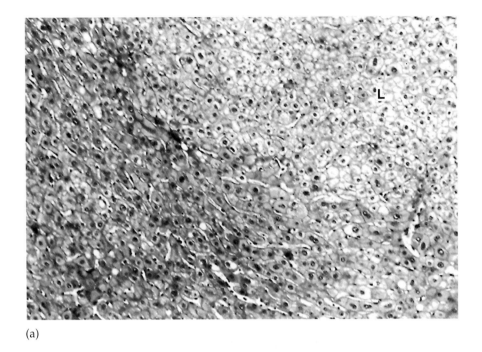

(a)

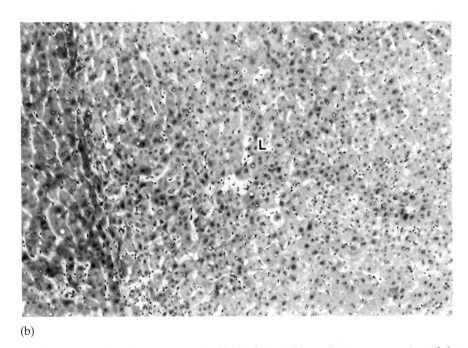

(b)

Fig. 7.7 Nodular regenerative hyperplasia. In (a) the lesion (L) produces compression of the adjacent liver tissue and shows greater cytoplasmic clearing but no atypia. There is no fibrousis or septum between the nodular expansion and adjacent liver tissue. In some nodules (L), mild-to-moderate degree of pleomorphism may be present (b).

usually associated with systemic symptoms and fever, and the patient may have similar lesions in other organs (Anthony, 1993). The histologic features are similar to those occurring in other sites such as the lung and soft tissue, and are composed of spindle shaped myofibroblasts mixed predominantly with lymphocytes, plasma cells, eosinophils and focal collections of foamy macrophages (Anthony, 1993; Noi *et al.*, 1994). Some acute inflammatory cells may also be present. The histologic features can sometimes resemble granulation tissue and thus suggest a healing and regeneration process. The proliferation of spindle-shaped myofibroblasts occasionally leads to the misdiagnosis of sarcoma. The differentiation of this tumor from HCC is usually not difficult.

More recently, two cases of 'inflammatory pseudotumor' of the liver have been shown to be proliferations of follicular dendritic reticulum cells associated with clonal Epstein–Barr virus (Selves *et al.*, 1996; Shek *et al.*, 1996).

7.3.3.2 Focal (solitary) necrotic nodule

The focal or solitary necrotic nodule is a rare benign lesion of unknown etiology. This lesion is clinically mistaken for a metastatic tumor (Alfieri *et al.*, 1997). Grossly, most of these nodules are small and well-demarcated by a thick capsule. They are filled with yellowish necrotic material and composed of acellular necrotic debris with no evidence of atypia. The wall is thick and occasionally shows granulation tissue similar to an abscess (Fig. 7.8). It has been suggested that these lesions represent the 'burnt-out phase' of a variety of benign conditions, in particular, hemangiomas (Berry, 1985; Sundaresan *et al.*, 1991). A parasitic origin such as from Clonorchis sinensis has also been suggested (Tsui *et al.*, 1992). While focal solitary necrotic nodules pose no difficulties in histologic recognition, they should be differentiated from infarcted HCC nodules following thrombosis after lipoidol injection. In the latter, a giant cell reaction is seen at or near

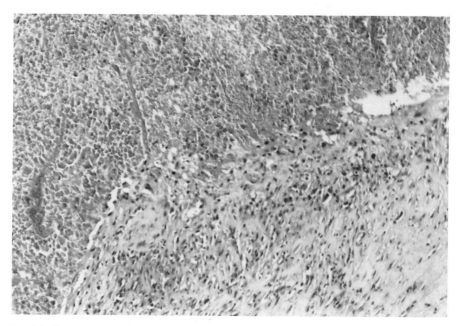

Fig. 7.8 Focal (solitary) necrotic nodule. The necrotic area is shown at top, and the fibrous wall in the lower half of the field contains inflammatory cells.

the capsule and a residual rim of tumor cells may be present.

7.4 MALIGNANT TUMORS

7.4.1 CHOLANGIOCARCINOMA

Cholangiocarcinomas arise within the liver, from the extrahepatic ducts or near the hilum (Klatskin tumor). Most cholangiocarcinomas are either well- or moderately differentiated adenocarcinomas and the major diagnostic difficulty is in distinguishing it from metastatic adenocarcinoma. In the absence of a source of primary tumor elsewhere, this distinction can be very difficult. Differentiation of cholangiocarcinoma and HCC is usually not a problem as the latter does not form true glands and rarely secretes mucin. Cholangiocarcinoma usually incites an abundant desmoplastic reaction, a feature uncommon in HCC (Nakajima *et al.*, 1988; Sugihara and Kojiro, 1988; Okuda *et al.*, 1993; Anthony, 1994). Immunostains are helpful in distinguishing it from HCC (see below).

7.4.1.1 Mixed HCC-cholangiocarcinoma (see Chapter 6)

Mixed or combined HCC-cholangiocarcinoma is composed of a mixture of both HCC and cholangiocarcinoma. These tumors are estimated to form about 2.5% of primary liver cancers (Okuda *et al.*, 1993). The two components of this tumor may be separate, adjacent to each other, or intimately mixed (Okuda *et al.*, 1993; Taguchi *et al.*, 1996). The recognition of this tumor in needle biopsies is dependent on the identification of characteristic HCC mixed or adjacent to an adenocarcinoma (with mucin production) (Fig. 7.9). In the absence of one component of the tumor, it is likely that the diagnosis will not be correctly made. There are no distinctive clinical features to allow identification. Biliary differentiation in HCC is associated with a poorer prognosis so that identification

of the cholangiocarcinoma component has prognostic relevance (Wu *et al.*, 1996).

7.4.1.2 Metastatic adenocarcinoma

The histologic distinction of metastatic adenocarcinoma from HCC is not a problem when the former is well differentiated. On the other hand, poorly differentiated metastatic carcinoma may occasionally pose a problem and identification of the cytomorphologic and architectural characteristics of HCC is required to separate them. Immunostains with a panel of antibodies can be helpful in this respect (see below). Microscopically, metastatic carcinomas frequently resemble their primary tumors and a strong desmoplastic reaction often accompanies metastases from pancreatic, breast and, less often, colonic and gastric carcinomas. Metastatic clear cell carcinoma of the kidney can mimic the clear cell variant of HCC. While clear cell change is common in HCC, it tends to be focal and adequate sampling will reveal the more diagnostic features of the tumor allowing its definitive identification.

7.4.1.3 Hepatoblastoma (see Chapter 6)

Hepatoblastoma is the commonest primary liver tumor in the pediatric age group and most frequently diagnosed before 5 years of age. It rarely occurs in adults. Hepatoblastoma arises from fetal or embryonal hepatocytes and it differentiates into epithelial and mixed epithelial and mesenchymal types (Anthony, 1994). The epithelial component may be of several types including squamous, glandular and macrotrabecular resembling adult liver. The tumor cells are generally of the fetal type, being about the size of normal hepatocytes and arranged into irregular plates with bile canaliculi and sinusoids. Embryonal-type cells are small, elongated or spindled, with hyperchromatic nuclei and scant cytoplasm. These cells may form rosettes, ribbons and cords. The anaplastic variant is difficult to

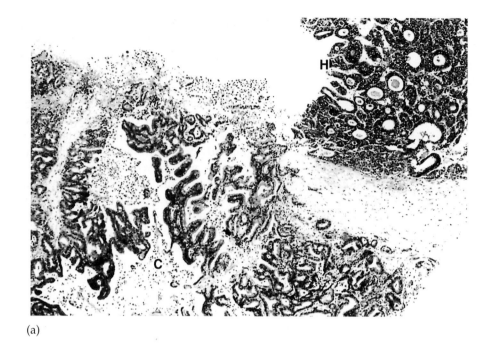

(a)

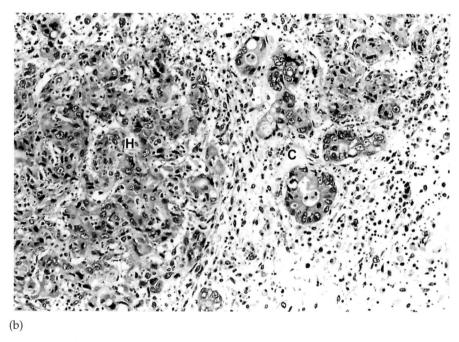

(b)

Fig. 7.9 Combined hepatocellular carcinoma (HCC) and cholangiocarcinoma. (a) The HCC (H) shows a pseudoglandular pattern while the cholangiocarcinoma (C) is characterized by a papillary growth pattern and mucin-secreting columnar cells. (b) Another example of this uncommon tumor in which the HCC (H) merges with the distinctly glandular cholangiocarcinoma (C).

distinguish from neuroblastoma and other small round cell tumors. This variant may display a mucoid stroma. The mesenchymal element is usually osteoid. Other elements such as striated muscle, cartilage and neural tissue are less common, their presence forming the teratoid variant. Hematopoiesis is usually present and cirrhosis is usually absent in the surrounding non-tumor liver tissue. This tumor is rarely mistaken for HCC.

7.4.1.4 Carcinoid

Primary hepatic or metastatic carcinoid tumors are uncommon (Krishnamurthy *et al.*, 1996; Mehta *et al.*, 1996). While the eosinophilic cytoplasm of carcinoid cells and the pseudoglandular and trabecular pattern can be mistaken for a HCC, the diagnosis can be readily confirmed with argyrophilic and argentaffin stains. Immunostaining of carcinoid tumors invariably reveals positivity for chromogranin, synaptophysin and neuron specific enolase (Leong and Gown, 1993). Electron microscopy frequently shows dense core granules characteristic of neuroendocrine tumors but this investigation is not necessary when histochemical or immunohistochemical stains are positive.

7.5 SPECIAL STAINS

Ancillary investigations are helpful in the distinction of HCC from its histologic mimics and are particularly useful in small biopsy samples. While histochemistry used to be the mainstay of such investigations, it is being superceded by immunohistochemistry. Electron microscopy remains a useful technique (Leong *et al.*, 1997), but, for a variety of reasons, is not popular as a diagnostic tool.

7.5.1 HISTOCHEMISTRY

Special stains such as periodic acid-Schiff (PAS) for glycogen and neutral mucosubstances, Gomori's or Masson's trichrome for collagen, Gordon and Sweet's stain for reticulin, Miller's stain for elastic fibers, Shikata's modified orcein stain for hepatitis B surface antigen and elastic fibers, Perl's Prussian blue reaction for ferric ions, rhodamine for copper deposits (Leong, 1996) and other histochemical stains remain the standard for the study of liver architecture and pathology but are not of great use in the identification of liver tumors.

The demonstration of bile production by the tumor cells is specific for HCC and can be done with the Fouchet's stain (Leong, 1996) but it is of low sensitivity, being positive in only 5–33% of HCCs (Anthony, 1973; MacSween, 1974; Cohen, 1976). The presence of PAS/diastase-positive mucosubstances in the tumor cells excludes the diagnosis of HCC but care should be taken not to mistake the PAS/diastase-positive material sometimes seen in the pseudoglandular spaces of HCC as this material represents fibrin and not mucin.

7.5.2 IMMUNOHISTOCHEMISTRY

Various immunohistochemical markers have been advocated for the identification of HCC and its distinction from cholangiocarcinoma (CC) and metastatic carcinoma. These markers include α-fetoprotein (AFP), α-1-antitrypsin, carcinoembryonic antigen (CEA) (Thung *et al.*, 1979, Hirohashi *et al.*, 1983; Imoto *et al.*, 1985; Ferrandez-Izquierdo and Llombart-Bosch, 1987; Hurlimann and Gardiol, 1991; Johnson *et al.*, 1992), factor XIIIa (Fucich *et al.*, 1994), ferritin (Johnson *et al.*, 1992), albumin (Papotti *et al.*, 1994) and cytokeratins 8, 18, 7 and 19 (Hurlimann and Gardiol, 1991; Maeda *et al.*, 1995; D'Errico *et al.*, 1996). However, their application has been met with varying success and none is specific (Geber *et al.*, 1983; Johnson *et al.*, 1992).

Eosinophilic cytoplasmic or intercellular globules that are PAS/diastase-positive may be observed in 10–15% of HCCs and represent AFP, α-1-antitrypsin or α-1-antichymotrypsin but these globules are not specific and may be seen in metastatic tumors from the ovary, testes or pancreas. AFP is also of low sensitivity, being found in no more than 50% of HCCs when immunostaining is performed (Thung *et al.*, 1979). A figure of 61.5% was obtained by Hurlimann and Gardiol (1991) who attributed the variation of positivity to the weak staining in many instances. Non-tumoral hepatocytes may also label for AFP (Hirohashi *et al.*, 1983).

The application of polyclonal antibodies to CEA produces a distinctive canalicular pattern (see Chapter 5, Fig. 5.12), which is specific for HCC compared with the diffuse cytoplasmic staining obtained for cholangiocarcinoma and metastatic carcinoma, but the incidence of positivity is very variable, ranging from 15–80% (Ferrandez-Izquierdo and Llombart-Bosch, 1987; Balaton *et al.*, 1988).

Two recent papers suggested that factor XIIIa, a blood proenzyme that plays a role in the blood coagulation may be a marker of hepatocytes and HCC (Hurlimann and Gardiol, 1991; Fucich *et al.*, 1994). However, a more recent study clearly showed that factor XIIIa is not expressed in HCCs and suggested that previous studies employed the antibodies to factor XIIIa at excessively high concentrations (Leong *et al.*, 1998).

Hep Par 1 (clone OCH 1E5) is a recently developed antibody specific for hepatocytes and their tumors (Wennerberg *et al.*, 1993). We have found this antibody to be the most sensitive and specific marker yet for neoplastic and non-neoplastic hepatocytes (Leong *et al.*, 1998). Hep Par 1 labeled 30 of 32 HCCs (Fig. 7.10) and all five cases of combined HCC-CC in our study. Previously, Wennerberg *et al.* (1993) found 37 of 38 HCCs to be positive and Wu *et al.* (1996) showed positivity for the antigen in 289 of 290 cases. Because of the marked heterogeneity of staining within individual tumors for the antigen, we recommend that Hep Par 1 be employed in conjunction with antibodies to cytokeratin 19 and 20 to provide the highest diagnostic yield. The latter cytokeratin isotypes are found in benign

and malignant bile duct epithelium (Fig. 7.11) and in carcinomas from the gastrointestinal tract respectively (Leong *et al.*, 1998). The addition of anti-CEA to the diagnostic panel of antibodies is useful.

Immunostaining for albumin is insensitive but recent studies suggest that *in situ* hybridization for albumin mRNA may be a useful marker for HCC, not being expressed in metastatic carcinomas, although it is occasionally seen in cholangiocarcinomas (D'Errico *et al.*, 1996). However, as with Hep Par 1, the expression is heterogeneous, and smaller samples show occasional false-negative results (Papotti *et al.*, 1994).

In general, hepatocytes lack basement membrane structures and laminin is not seen around normal hepatic cords; however, laminin was shown to be present in about 86% of HCCs (Yoshida *et al.*, 1996). The efficacy of this marker is yet to be proven as earlier studies found the frequency laminin expression to be much lower, particularly in poorly differentiated tumors (Grigoni *et al.*, 1987a, b). More recently, inhibin, a peptide hormone produced by ovarian granulosa cells, was employed as a marker of HCC. There was strong cytoplasmic staining of 17 of 19 cases of HCC whereas, six of 20 adenocarcinomas expressed the antigen. Staining in adenocarcinomas was weak and localized to the luminal surface of the tumor glands (McCluggage *et al.*, 1997).

7.6 CONCLUSIONS

While HCC can usually be readily distinguished from non-neoplastic and neoplastic proliferations of hepatocytes in resected specimens, this task may occasionally be difficult in needle core specimens. The advent of modern imaging techniques combined with isotopes has enabled the detection of small HCCs and malignant transformation in regenerative nodules, making available for microscopic examination ultrasound-guided core biopsy specimens of such lesions. Despite accumulating information, the refinement of diagnostic

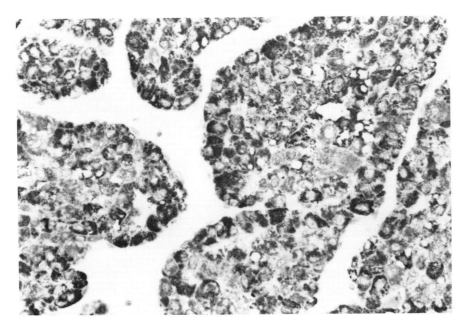

Fig. 7.10 Hep Par 1 antibody staining of hepatocellular carcinoma. The staining is granular and cytoplasmic but heterogenous within the tumor.

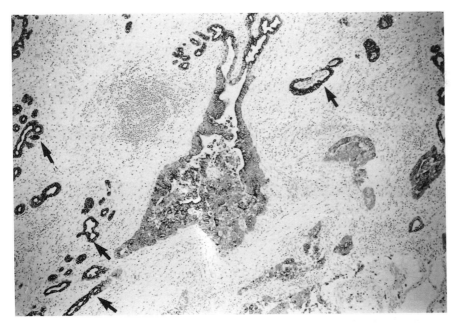

Fig. 7.11 Cholangiocarcinoma composed of well-formed glands showing positivity for cytokeratin 19. Benign bile ducts (arrows) in the vicinity also stain strongly positive. Hepatocytes do not label for this antigen.

criteria and the contributions of ancillary techniques such as immunohistochemistry, some of these lesions remain difficult to diagnose on morphological grounds alone, particularly in needle core biopsies. Accurate diagnosis requires clinical and radiological correlation as well as knowledge of other clinical data such as serum α-fetoprotein level and associated etiologic factors.

REFERENCES

Alfieri, S., Carriero, C., Doglietto, G.B. et al. (1997) Solitary necrotic nodule of the liver: diagnosis and treatment. *Hepatogastroenterology*, **44**, 1210–11.

Alpert, E., Pinn, V. and Isselbacher, K. (1971) Alpha-feto-protein in a patient with gastric carcinoma metastatic to the liver. *New England Journal of Medicine*, **285**, 1058–9.

An, C.S., Petrovic, L.M., Reyter, I. et al. (1997) The application of image analysis and neural network technology to the study of large cell liver dysplasia and hepatocellular carcinoma. *Hepatology*, **26**, 1224–31.

Anthony, P.P. (1973) Primary carcinoma of the liver: a study of 282 cases in Ugandan Africans. *Journal of Pathology*, **116**, 37–48.

Anthony, P.P. (1993) Inflammatory pseudotumor (plasma cell granuloma) of lung, liver and other organs. *Histopathology*, **23**, 501–3.

Anthony, P.P. (1994) Tumors and tumor-like lesions of the liver and biliary tract, in: *Pathology of the Liver*, 3rd edn (eds R.N.M. MacSween, P.J. Scheuer and A.D. Burt), Churchill Livingstone, London, pp. 635–711.

Arakawa, M., Sugihara, S., Kenmochi, K. et al. (1986) Small mass lesions in cirrhosis: transition from benign adenomatous hyperplasia to hepatocellular carcinoma? *Journal of Gastroenterology and Hepatology*, **1**, 3–14.

Arsenault, T.M., Johnson, C.D., Gorman, R. and Burgart, L.J. (1996) Hepatic adenomatosis. *Mayo Clinic Proceedings*, **71**, 478–80.

Balaton, A.J., Nehama-Sibony, M., Gotheil, C. et al. (1988) Distinction between hepatocellular carcinoma, cholangiocarcinoma, and metastatic carcinoma based on immunohistochemical staining for carcinoembryonic antigen and for cytokeratin 19 on paraffin sections. *Journal of Pathology*, **156**, 305–10.

Berry, C.L. (1985) Solitary 'necrotic nodule' of the liver: a probable pathogenesis. *Journal of Clinical Pathology*, **38**, 1278–80.

Bhattacharya, S., Dhillion, A.P., Rees, J. et al. (1997) Small hepatocellular carcinomas in cirrhotic explant livers: identification by macroscopic examination and lipiodol localization. *Hepatology*, **25**, 613–18.

Buetow, P.C., Pantongrag-Brown, L., Buck, J.L. et al. (1996) Focal nodular hyperplasia of the liver: radiologic-pathologic correlation. *Radiographics*, **16**, 369–88.

Cohen, C. (1976) Intracytoplasmic hyaline globules in hepatocellular carcinoma. *Cancer*, **37**, 1754–8.

Crawford, J.M. (1990) Pathologic assessment of liver cell dysplasia and benign liver tumors: differentiation from malignant tumors (review). *Seminars in Diagnostic Pathology*, **7**, 115–28.

D'Errico, A., Baccarini, P., Fiorentino, M. et al. (1996) Histogenesis of primary liver carcinomas: strengths and weaknesses of cytokeratin profile and albumin mRNA detection. *Human Pathology*, **27**, 599–604.

DeMaioribus, C.A., Lally, K.P., Sim, K. et al. (1990) Mesenchymal hamartoma of the liver. A 35 year review. *Archives of Surgery*, **125**, 598–600.

Eguchi, A., Nakashima, O., Okudaira, S. et al. (1992) Adenomatous hyperplasia in the vicinity of small hepatocellular carcinoma. *Hepatology*, **15**, 843–8.

Ferrandez-Izquierdo, A. and Llombart-Bosch, A. (1987) Immunohistochemical characterization of 130 cases of primary hepatic carcinomas. *Pathology, Research and Practice*, **182**, 783–91.

Ferrell, L., Wright, T., Lake, J. et al. (1992) Incidence and diagnostic features of macroregenerative nodules vs. small hepatocellular carcinoma in cirrhotic livers. *Hepatology*, **16**, 1372–81.

Ferrell, L.D., Crawford, J.M., Dhillon, A.P. et al. (1993) Proposal for standardized criteria for the diagnosis of benign, borderline, and malignant hepatocellular lesions arising in chronic advanced liver disease. *American Journal of surgical Pathology*, **17**, 1113–23.

Foster, J.H. and Berman, M.M. (1994) The malignant transformation of liver cell adenomas. *Archives of Surgery*, **129**, 712–17.

Fucich, L.F., Cheles, M.K., Thung, S.N. et al. (1994) Primary vs metastatic hepatic carcinoma. An immunohistochemical study of 34 cases. *Archives of Pathology and Laboratory Medicine*, **118**, 927–30.

Gerber, M.A., Thung, S.N., Shen, S. et al. (1983) Phenotypic characterization of hepatic proliferation: antigenic expression by proliferating epithelial cells in fetal liver, massive hepatic necrosis and nodular transformation of the liver. *American Journal of Pathology*, **110**, 70–4.

Grigoni, W.F., D'Errico, A., Biagini, G. *et al.* (1987a) Primary liver cell carcinoma. New insight for a more correct approach to its classification. *Acta Pathologica Japonica*, **37**, 929–40.

Grigoni, W.F., D'Errico, A., Mancini, A.M. *et al.* (1987b) Hepatocellular carcinoma: expression of basement membrane glycoproteins. An immunohistochemical approach. *Journal of Pathology*, **152**, 325–32.

Hirohashi, S., Shimosato, Y., Yoshinori, I. *et al.* (1983) Distribution of alpha-fetoprotein and immunoreactive carcinoembryonic antigen in human hepatocellular carcinoma and hepatoblastoma. *Japanese Journal of Clinical Oncology*, **13**, 37–44.

Huggins, G.R. and Zucker, P.K. (1987) Oral contraceptives and neoplasia: 1987 update. *Fertility and Sterility*, **47**, 733–61.

Hurlimann, J. and Gardiol, D. (1991) Immunohistochemistry in the differential diagnosis of liver carcinomas. *American Journal of Surgical Pathology*, **15**, 280–8.

Imoto, M., Nishimura, D., Fukuda, Y. *et al.* (1985) Immunohistochemical detection of alpha-fetoprotein, carcinoembryonic antigen, and ferritin in formalin-paraffin sections from hepatocellular carcinoma. *American Journal of Gastroenterology*, **80**, 902–6.

Johnson, D.E., Powers, C.N., Rupp, G. *et al.* (1992) Immunocytochemical staining of fine needle aspiration biopsies of the liver as a diagnostic tool for hepatocellular carcinoma. *Modern Pathology*, **5**, 117–23.

Kameda, Y. and Shinji, Y. (1992) Early detection of hepatocellular carcinoma by laparoscopy: yellow nodules as diagnostic indicators. *Gastrointestinal Endoscopy*, **38**, 554–9.

Kondo, F., Hirooka, N., Wada, K. and Kondo, Y. (1987) Morphological clues for the diagnosis of small hepatocellular carcinomas. *Virchow's Archives A Pathology Anatomy Histopathology*, **411**, 15–21.

Kondo, F., Wada, K., Nagato, Y. *et al.* (1989) Biopsy diagnosis of well-differentiated hepatocellular carcinoma based on new morphologic criteria. *Hepatology*, **9**, 751–5.

Krishnamurthy, S.C., Dutta, V., Pai, S.A. *et al.* (1996) Primary carcinoid tumor of the liver: report of four resected cases including one with gastrin production. *Journal of Surgical Oncology*, **62**, 218–21.

Labrune, P., Trioche, P., Duvaltier, I. *et al.* (1997) Hepatocellular adenomas in glycogen storage disease type I and III: a series of 43 patients and review of the literature. *Journal of Pediatric Gastroenterology*, **24**, 276–9.

Le Bail, H., Jouhanole, H., Deugnier, Y. *et al.* (1992) Liver adenomatosis in two patients on long-term oral contraceptives. *American Journal of Surgical Pathology*, **16**, 982–7.

Lennington, W.J., Gray, G.F. Jr and Page, D.L. (1993) Mesenchymal hamartoma of liver. A regional ischemic lesion of a sequestered lobe. *American Journal of Diseases of Childhood*, **147**, 193–6.

Leong, A.S.-Y. (1996) *Principles and Practice of Medical Laboratory Science*, vol. 1. *Basic Histotechnology*, Churchill Livingstone, London, pp. 59–78.

Leong, A.S.-Y. and Gown, A.M. (1993) Immunohistochemistry of 'solid tumors': poorly differentiated round cell and spindle cell tumors I, in *Applied Immunohistochemistry for the Surgical Pathologist*, (ed. A.S.-Y. Leong), Edward Arnold, London, pp. 23–72.

Leong, A.S.-Y. Wick, M.R. and Swanson, P.E. (1997) *Immunohistology and Electron Microscopy of Anaplastic and Pleomorphic Tumors*, Cambridge University Press, Cambridge, pp. 39–42.

Leong, A.S.-Y., Sormunen, R., Tsui, W.M.S. and Liew, C.T. (1998) Immunostaining of hepatocellular carcinoma, cholangiocarcinoma and metastatic adenocarcinoma. *Histopathology*, (in press).

MacSween, R.M.N. (1974) A clinicopathologic review of 100 cases of primary malignant tumors of the liver. *Journal of Clinical Pathology*, **27**, 669–82.

Maeda, T., Adachi, E., Kajiyama, K. *et al.* (1995) Combined hepatocellular and cholangiocarcinoma. Proposed criteria according to cytokeratin expression and analysis of clinicopathological features. *Human Pathology*, **26**, 950–64.

McCluggage, W.G., Maxwell, P., Patterson, A. and Sloan, J.M. (1997) Immunohistochemical staining of hepatocellular carcinoma with monoclonal antibody against inhibin. *Histopathology*, **30**, 518–22.

Mehta, D.C., Warner, R.R., Parnes, I. and Weiss, M. (1996) An 18-year follow-up of primary hepatic carcinoid with carcinoid syndrome. *Journal of Clinical Gastroenterology*, **23**, 60–2.

Mitchell, D.G., Rubin, R., Sieglman, E.S. *et al.* (1991) Hepatocellular carcinoma within siderotic regenerative nodules: appearance as a nodule within a nodule on MR images. *Radiology*, **178**, 101–3.

Nagato, Y., Kondo, F., Kondo, Y. *et al.* (1991) Histological and morphometrical indicators for a biopsy diagnosis of well-differentiated hepatocellular carcinoma. *Hepatology*, **14**, 473–8.

Nagorney, D.M. (1995) Benign hepatic tumors: focal nodular hyperplasia and hepatocellular adenoma. *World Journal of Surgery*, **19**, 13–18.

Nakajima, T., Kondo, Y., Miyazaki, M. and Okui, K. (1988) A histopathologic study of 102 cases of intrahepatic cholangiocarcinoma. *Human Pathology*, **19**, 1228–34.

Nakanuma, Y., Terada, T., Teraski, S. *et al.* (1990) 'Atypical adenomatous hyperplasia' in liver cirrhosis: low-grade hepatocellular carcinoma or borderline lesion? *Histopathology*, **17**, 27–35.

Ndimbie, O.K., Goodman, Z.D., Chase, R.L. *et al.* (1990) Hemangiomas with localized nodular proliferation of the liver. A suggestion on the pathogenesis of focal nodular hyperplasia. *American Journal of Surgical Pathology*, **14**, 142–50.

Noi, I., Loberant, N. and Cohen, I. (1994) Inflammatory pseudotumor of the liver. *Clinical Imaging*, **18**, 283–5.

Ojanguren, I., Castella, E., Ariza, A. *et al.* (1997) Liver cell atypias: a comparative study in cirrhosis with and without hepatocellular carcinoma. *Histopathology*, **30**, 106–12.

Okuda, K., Kojiro, M. and Okuda, H. (1993) Neoplasms of the liver, in *Diseases of the Liver*, 7th edn (eds L. Schiff and E.R. Schiff) J.B. Lippincott Philadelphia, pp. 1236–96.

Papotti, M., Pacchioni, D., Negro, F. *et al.* (1994) Albumin gene expression in liver tumors: Diagnostic interest in fine needle aspiration biopsies. *Modern Pathology*, **7**, 271–5.

Reymond, D., Plaschkes, J., Luthy, A.R. *et al.* (1995) Focal nodular hyperplasia of the liver in children: review of follow-up and outcome. *Journal of Pediatric Surgery*, **30**, 1590–93.

Reynolds, T.B. (1976) Diagnostic methods in hepatocellular carcinoma. In *Hepatocellular Carcinoma*, (eds K. Okuda and R.L. Peters) Wiley, New York, pp. 437–48.

Rosenberg, L. (1991) The risk of liver neoplasia in relation to combined oral contraceptive use. *Contraception*, **43**, 643–52.

Sakamoto, M., Hirohashi, S. and Shimosato, Y. (1991) Early stages of multistep hepatocarcinogenesis: adenomatous hyperplasia and early hepatocellular carcinoma. *Human Pathology*, **22**, 172–8.

Selves, J., Meggetto, F., Brousset, P. *et al.* (1996) Inflammatory pseudotumor of the liver. Evidence for follicular dendritic reticulum cell proliferation associated with clonal Epstein–Barr virus. *American Journal of Surgical Pathology*, **20**, 747–53.

Shek, T.W., Ho, F.C., Ng, I.O. *et al.* (1996) Follicular dendritic cell tumor of the liver. Evidence for an Epstein–Barr virus-related clonal proliferation of follicular dendritic cells. *American Journal of Surgical Pathology*, **20**, 313–24.

Shortell, C.K. and Schwartz, S.I. (1991) Hepatic adenoma and focal nodular hyperplasia. *Surgery, Gynecology and Obstetrics*, **173**, 426–31.

Stocker, J.T. and Ishak, K.G. (1983) Mesenchymal hamartoma of the liver: report of 30 cases and review of the literature. *Pediatric Pathology*, **1**, 245–67.

Sugihara, S. and Kojiro, M. (1988) Pathology of cholangiocarcinoma, in *Neoplasms of the Liver*, (eds K. Okuda and K.G. Ishak) Springer, Berlin, pp. 143–58.

Sundaresan, M., Lyons, B. and Akosa, A.B. (1991) 'Solitary' necrotic nodule of the liver: an aetiology affirmed. *Gut*, **32**, 1378–80.

Taguchi, J., Nakashima, O., Tanaka, M. *et al.* (1996) A clinicopathological study on combined hepatocellular and cholangiocarcinoma. *Journal of Gastroenterology and Hepatology*, **11**, 758–64.

Takayama, T., Makuuchi, M., Hirohashi, S. *et al.* (1990) Malignant transformation of adenomatous hyperplasia to hepatocellular carcinoma. *Lancet*, **336**, 1150–3.

Terada, T., Hoso, M. and Nakanuma, Y. (1995) Distribution of cytokeratin 19-positive biliary cells in cirrhotic nodules, hepatic borderline nodules (atypical adenomatous hyperplasia), and small hepatocellular carcinomas. *Modern Pathology*, **8**, 371–9.

Terada, T. and Nakanuma, Y. (1995) Arterial elements and perisinusoidal cells in borderline hepatocellular nodules and small hepatocellular carcinomas. *Histopathology*, **27**, 333–9.

Thiese, N.D. (1997) Precursor lesions of hepatocellular carcinoma, in: *Pathology of Liver Transplantation, Viral Hepatitis, and Tumors*, (eds W.M.S. Tsui, A.S.-Y. Leong, C.T. Liew and W.F. Ng), International Academy of Pathology Hong Kong Division, pp. 87–92.

Thiese, N.D., Marcelin, K., Goldfischer, M. *et al.* (1996) Low proliferative activity in macroregenerative nodules: evidence for an alternative hypothesis concerning human hepatocarcinogenesis. *Liver*, **16**, 134–9.

Thung, S.N., Gerber, M.A., Sarno, E. and Popper, H. (1979) Distribution of 5 antigens in hepatocellular carcinoma. *Laboratory Investigation*, **41**, 101–5.

Tsui, W.M., Yuen, R.W., Chow, L.T. and Tse, C.C. (1992) Solitary necrotic nodule of the liver: parasitic origin? *Journal of Clinical Pathology*, **45**, 975–8.

Wada, K., Kondo, F. and Kondo, Y. (1988) Large regenerative nodules and dysplastic nodules in cirrhotic livers: a histopathologic study. *Hepatology*, **8**, 1684–8.

Wanless, I.R. (1990) Micronodular transformation (nodular regenerative hyperplasia) of the liver: a report of 64 cases among 2500 autopsies and a new classification of benign hepatic nodules. *Hepatology*, **11**, 787–97.

Wanless, I.R., Albrecht, S., Bilbao, J. *et al.* (1989) Multiple focal nodular hyperplasia of the liver associated with vascular malformations of various organs and neoplasia of the brain: a new syndrome. *Modern Pathology*, **2**, 456–62.

Wanless, I., Callea, F., Craig, J. *et al.* (1995) (International Working Party). Terminology of nodular hepatocellular lesions. *Hepatology*, **22**, 983–93.

Watanabe, S., Okita, K., Harada, T. *et al.* (1983) Morphologic studies of the liver cell dysplasia. *Cancer*, **51**, 2197–2205.

Wennerberg, A.E., Nalesnik, M.A. and Coleman, W.B. (1993) Hepatocyte paraffin 1: A monoclonal antibody that reacts with hepatocytes and can be used for differential diagnosis of hepatic tumors. *American Journal of Pathology*, **143**, 1050–4.

Wu, P.-C., Fang, J.W.-S., Lau, V.K.-T. *et al.* (1996) Classification of hepatocellular carcinoma according to hepatocellular and biliary differentiation markers. Clinical and biological implications. *American Journal of Pathology*, **149**, 1167–75.

Yamamoto, T., Ikebe, T., Mikami, S. *et al.* (1996) Immunohistochemistry and angiography in adenomatous hyperplasia and small hepatocellular carcinomas. *Pathology International*, **46**, 364–71.

Yoshida, K., Tadaoka, Y. and Manabe, T. (1996) Expression of laminin in hepatocellular carcinoma: an adjunct for its histological diagnosis. *Japanese Journal of Clinical Oncology*, **26**, 70–76.

Yu, S.C.H., Metreweli, C., Lau, W.-Y. *et al.* (1997) Safety of percutaneous biopsy of hepatocellular carcinoma with an 18 gauge automated needle. *Clinical Radiology*, **52**, 907–11.

MOLECULAR ASPECTS

8

J.Y.-H. Chan, K.-W. Lo, H.-M. Li and C.-T. Liew

8.1 INTRODUCTION

Epidemiological and experimental evidences have shown that the etiology of hepatocellular carcinoma (HCC), like other kinds of cancer, is multifactorial and multistage. The risk factors for HCC may be divided into environmental factors including biological and chemical agents, and genetic factors (Fig. 8.1). The major biological agents are the hepatitis viruses including the hepatitis B virus (HBV) and hepatitis C virus (HCV), and parasites such as the liver fluke which contributes to parasitic hepatitis. Chemical agents that contribute to HCC are aflatoxin, nitrosamines, vinyl chloride, peroxisome proliferators and alcohol. Most of these agents either directly or indirectly induce mutations or alterations in DNA, or act as promoters which facilitate the proliferation of hepatocytes and the fixation of DNA lesions. In addition, genetic factors such as metabolic disorders, DNA repair defects and altered susceptibility genes may also contribute to the development of HCC. Differential susceptibility to the development of liver cancers varies considerably among different rodent species and strains, while in man, familial clustering of HCC have been described in Chinese and Alaskan natives (Alberts *et al.*, 1991; Shen *et al.*, 1991). The evolution of HCC may be divided into several stages: genomic/DNA damage (initiation); chronic liver injury (promotion) which produces inflammation, cirrhosis and cell death; regeneration (promotion); adenomatous hyperplasia/dysplasia (progression), and HCC. Specific genetic and epigenetic changes including the differential expression of genes have been identified for some of these stages. It is hoped that the molecular studies will be informative in dissecting the multifactorial etiology of HCC, and in setting priorities for the implementation of prevention and treatment.

8.2 MOLECULAR ANALYSIS OF HEPADNAVIRUSES INFECTION AND HCC

8.2.1 HBV AND HCV GENOMES

Hepadnaviruses including HBV and HCV are known to be associated with the development of liver neoplasia, accounting for >80% of human HCCs worldwide yet the molecular mechanism is still unclear (Brechot, 1994; Robinson, 1994; Hoppe-Seyler and Butz, 1995; Kasai *et al.*, 1996). The HBV genome is relatively small, consisting of a 3.2 kb circular DNA with single-stranded region of variable length in different molecules (Fig. 8.2). It contains four open reading frames (ORFs) in the complete strand of DNA (Brechot, 1994).

Hepatocellular Carcinoma: Diagnosis, investigation and management. Edited by Anthony S.-Y. Leong, Choong-Tsek Liew, Joseph W.Y. Lau and Philip J. Johnson. Published in 1999 by Arnold, London. ISBN 0 340 74096 5.

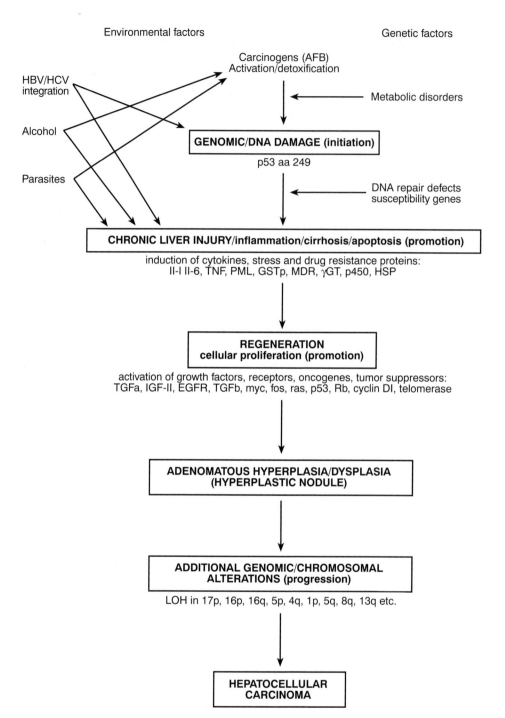

Fig. 8.1 Proposed sequence of carcinogenesis of human hepatocellular carcinoma. The environmental risk factors including HBV/HCV, chemical carcinogens such as aflatoxin B1, alcohol and parasites are listed. Genetic factors such as intrinsic levels of metabolizing enzymes, DNA repair defects and others are also shown.

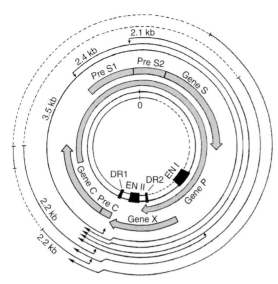

Fig. 8.2 Genetic map of the HBV DNA. The broad arrows represent the four open reading frames (ORFs) encoding the envelope (preS1, preS2 and S), capsid (preC and C), polymerase (P) and X proteins. The thin arrows indicate mRNA of the HBV. The direct repeats (DR1 and DR2) and the regulatory elements (enhancer I and II) are involved in replication and transcription.

The four ORFs are: (1) the envelope protein which encodes the hepatitis B surface antigen (HBsAg); (2) the core protein, which encodes the nucleocapsid core protein including the core antigen (HBcAg) and the e antigen (HBeAg) which is a truncated form of the major core protein; (3) the polymerase (P) protein which encodes the reverse transcriptase, DNA polymerase and RNAase H activities; and (4) the HBX protein which is a small polypeptide with the capability to trans-activate cellular genes. Moreover, two direct repeat sequences of 11 bp in length, namely DR1 and DR2, which are involved in viral DNA replication, are localized at the terminal ends on the DNA strands. In addition, the viral DNA contains four promoter elements for transcription, two enhancer elements designated enhancer 1 and 2, and a polyadenylation signal used by all major transcripts lie within the pre-C region.

On the other hand, the genome of HCV was identified in 1989 and shown to comprise of a positive-stranded RNA molecule of approximately 9500 nucleotides (Brechot, 1994). Sequence comparisons indicate that HCV is distantly related to both the animal pestiviruses and the human flaviviruses. The genome of HCV contains a single ORF which encodes a large polyprotein precursor of just over 3000 amino acids. The proteins encoded by HCV include the structural protein genes: RNA binding nucleocapsid C, and the envelope glycoprotein gene E1 and E2, followed by six genes that encode the presumed nonstructural proteins: NS2, a Zn metallo-proteinase, NS3, a serine protease/helicase, NS4a and NS4b with unknown function, NS5a, with possibly replicase function, and NS5b with RNA-dependant RNA polymerase homology. HCV has been found to be associated with non-A, non-B hepatitis and has been suggested to be the main cause of cryptogenic chronic hepatitis, cirrhosis and HCC. Although chronic HCV infection is considered a global disease and the number of carriers is estimated to be about 300 million, the numbers of HCV associated HCC are still much less than those associated with HBV.

8.2.2 INSERTIONAL MUTAGENESIS AND *CIS*-ACTIVATION OF CELLULAR GENES BY HBV DNA

HBV DNA has been found in approximately 85% of HCC and mostly occurs as the integrated form of viral DNA. It is believed that the integrated HBV DNA may play a role in the pathogenesis of HCC. However, the complete viral sequence is usually not found in the integrated DNA and the infected tissues do not contain the replicative form of viral DNA. In the woodchuck model of HCC, HBV-DNA is preferentially integrated in the *c-myc* or *N-myc* regulatory or coding sequences (Robinson, 1994), while in man, specific HBV insertion in cellular genes has been found only in single cases in genes such as *erb A*, *cyclin A*, and retinoic acid receptor. However, the viral DNA appears to contain preferred sites for integration, since >50% of the junctions are at or near the cohesive 5' ends of the direct repeat (DR) sequences. The sites of integration in the host DNA are random but a certain degree of preference has been found. The integration appears to occur mostly at repeated sequences such as Alu DNA, satellite III DNA, α-satellite, minisatellite or VNTR DNA. Most of the integrations are of multiple clonal type, each at a different cellular site. At the site of integration, alterations in the host chromosomal DNA have also been found. These alterations include: (1) microdeletion (approximately 10 bp) which is apparently a part of the illegitimate recombination process; (2) large deletion which occurs in some HCC and it appears to be formed by mechanism other than illegitimate recombination; (3) translocations, which involve host DNA from two different chromosomes joined to the viral sequence; (4) inverted repeats of viral and cellular DNA, which are identical or common sequences brought together during the recombination process; (5) amplification of cellular DNA; and (6) other alterations including allelic deletion and point mutation in host DNA. Although these genetic changes in the HCC DNA indicate that the viral genome can act as a factor for insertional mutagenesis, there has been no consensus on specific cellular genes being disrupted by the virus insertion.

8.2.3 TRANSACTIVATION OF CELLULAR GENES BY HBV DNA

HBV still appears to be a prime candidate for the initiation event in the multifactorial-multistep model of hepatocarcinogenesis. Since HBV does not contain a direct oncogene, and the virus apparently integrates randomly into the human genome, a common *cis*-acting effect on activating cellular genes appears to be unlikely. There is therefore great interest in identifying the role of the virus in the development of HCC (Yen, 1996). Whether the proliferative stimuli created by chronic inflammation of the liver by HBV might be sufficient for HCC induction is still debatable. Moreover, recent publications indicate that HBV genes may act in *trans*-effect in activating critical cellular genes (Caselmann, 1995). The first is the *HBX* gene, which encodes the HBx protein (Yen, 1996). The HBx protein has been found to interact with the tumor suppressor p53 and with the repair protein excision repair cross complementation group 3 (ERCC3) (Harris, 1994; Greenblatt *et al.*, 1997). Recently, interaction between HBx and a cellular protein XAP-1 was also reported. XAP-1 is apparently the human homologue of the monkey UV-damaged DNA binding protein (UV-DDB) which is defective in some xeroderma pigmentosum group E patients. This suggests that important DNA repair process may be affected by HBV and that the resulting genetic instability may contribute to HCC development. In addition, HBX can abrogate p53-induced apoptosis, whereas the wild-type p53 could inhibit the function of the promoter of HBV core gene (Wang *et al.*, 1995). It is likely that the *HBX* gene may play some role in viral–cell interactions, but the oncogenicity of *HBX* is still unclear. Although one report indicated that HBX has an oncogenic potential in transgenic mice (Kim *et al.*, 1991), opposite findings have been reported (Lee *et al.*, 1995). Moreover, the *HBX* gene had no effect on the malignant transformation of normal cells, and only partially transformed cells such as NIH-3T3, or cells immortalized by SV40 T antigen were affected (Yen, 1996). As not all HBV-associated HCCs contain activated *HBX* gene, the role of HBx in hepatocarcinogenesis remains unclear.

The second HBV-transactivator is the truncated middle surface (*preS2/S*) gene (Caselmann, 1995). The 3' truncations of the HBV middle surface gene (*MHBs^t*) were found in some HCC-DNA, and in co-transfection experiments, this truncated gene was demonstrated to have transactivation function. The truncated region is defined as 'TransActivator On' domain (TAO), and the aberrant protein was found to be localized to the endoplasmic reticulum of the cells. The truncated *preS2/S* gene can utilize transcriptional factors such as NF-kB and AP1 for transactivation. In addition, the target genes for the transactivation were found to include the proto-oncogenes *c-myc*, *c-fos*, and the inflammation-associated cytokine *Il-6*. The activation of these proto-oncogenes or critical cellular genes may be the basis of cellular transformation and oncogenesis in HCC.

In a majority of HBV-associated HCCs from Asia and elsewhere, novel mutations at or around the TAO region of the *preS2/S* gene were found (Brechot, 1994; Zhong, 1997). Moreover, a large number of the HCC displayed mutations at codons 124–47 of the surface antigen *S* gene, defined as 'a loop', which is known to cause immunoescape for the virus against the host defense mechanism. The frequent occurrence of mutations around the transactivator domain of the *preS2/S* gene in the HCCs of this endemic region indicate that these molecular defects may be causally related to the development of HCC from HBV carriers. In addition, a high proportion of HBV from chronic active hepatitis and HCC contained aberrant sequences for the *preS1* and the *preC/C* region of the HBV (Brechot, 1994). Since both the *preS1* and the *preC/C* regions of the HBV are associated with the immunodeterminants, these mutations may play important roles in the immuno-escape for the virus against the host defense mechanisms.

8.3 INTERACTIONS BETWEEN CHEMICAL CARCINOGENS, HBV AND CELLULAR GENES

Another major risk factor for HCC is the hepatocarcinogen aflatoxin. Aflatoxins are mycotoxins generated by the fungi *Aspergillus flavus* and related strains (Brechot, 1994). The carcinogens are generated because of the improper storage of crops including peanuts, corn and rice, which occur most frequently in underdeveloped nations. Under hot and humid conditions, the molds grow favorably. To assess the extent of exposure to aflatoxin, antibodies against aflatoxin B1 (AFB), the most potent moiety of the compounds, have been generated. In addition, the measurement of minute amounts of DNA adducts in body fluids and tissues was made possible by innovative techniques such as the [^{32}P]-post-labeling technique and the immunodetection of protein and DNA adducts. For individuals who are at risk for both HBV infection and exposure to aflatoxin, such as those living in Qidong Province of China and sub-Saharan Africa, the relative risk was found to be significantly higher (Wogan, 1992). Moreover, in reviewing the mutation spectrum of p53 gene in HCC from endemic regions for the fungus, high frequency of mutations were found in codon 249 (50% or eight of 16; of which seven were G to T, and one G to C transversions) which are apparently specific for AFB–DNA interactions (Harris, 1994). However, the gene was found to be less involved in the non AFB$_1$-associated cases (20–25%). A variety of mutations were found in different sites of the *p53* gene in this non AFB$_1$-associated HCCs. Moreover, it is also reported that the *p53* mutation is rare in the HBV-associated HCC. The HBV-encoded X antigen (HBxAg) has recently been suggested to be bound to the wild-type *p53* and inactivating it. The low frequency of p53 mutation in these cases implies that *p53* inactivation may occur predominantly by complex formation with HBxAg (Greenblatt *et al.*, 1997). In HBV transgenic mice, treatment with several chemical carcinogens including AFB resulted in an earlier appearance and higher incidence of HCC, suggesting an interaction between HBV and chemical hepatocarcinogens. In addition, two isoforms of the cytochrome p450 (2a and 3a) which are involved in the activation of AFB, were progressively induced in hepatocytes of HBV transgenic mice. Similarly, the p450–2A6 and 3A4, both of which are involved in AFB activation in man, are also induced in cirrhotic liver and HBV hepatitis. This is consistent with the notion that HBV-infected cells are more susceptible to AFB by increasing the enzymes for activating carcinogens. It is also known that the expressions of genes for drug metabolism, including the phase I and II enzymes, are altered during hepatocarcinogenesis. Enhanced expression of multiple drug resistance (*mdr*) genes was previously reported in human and rodent HCC (Teeter *et al.*, 1991, 1993). In addition, GSH-*S*-transferase π (GSTπ), γ-glutammyl transferase (γGT), ornithine decarboxylase (ODC) are known to be induced during hepatocarcinogenesis and in HCC. Abnormal cytoplasmic localization of the O^6-alkyl-guanine DNA transferase in HBV induced cirrhotic liver has been reported (Lee *et al.*, 1996). The increased expression of these drug-metabolizing proteins is apparently a programmed cascade of events during hepatocarcinogenesis, but they may also play a role in the natural selection of malignant clones and may account for the intrinsic drug resistance of HCC.

8.4 ALTERATIONS OF PROTO-ONCOGENES, TUMOR SUPPRESSOR GENES AND GENES ASSOCIATED WITH PROLIFERATION AND INFLAMMATION

The third etiological factor for HCC is cirrhosis and chronic inflammation of the liver. There is an associated liver cirrhosis in 70–90% of Oriental HCC patients. The overall rate of HCC developing in patients with hepatic cirrhosis is about 2–5% annually. In addition, other risk factors for HCC such as HBV and HCV infection, and alcohol consumption all cause liver cirrhosis. However, the role of cirrhosis is believed to be at the promotion or progression phase of the carcinogenic process. One notion for the involvement of cirrhosis in HCC development is that cell damage and programed cell death in cirrhotic liver induce signals for liver regen-

eration. The proliferative stimuli can then act as a promoter for carcinogenesis in pre-initiated hepatocytes. The subsequent rounds of replication act to fix the DNA lesions as mutations. In addition, chronic inflammation of the liver may induce the expression of many growth factors, cytokines, stress proteins and hormones which directly or indirectly promote the clonal expansion of preneoplastic cells (Fausto, 1991). The growth factors for hepatocytes that have been documented previously are: (1) direct mitogens such as hepatocyte growth factor (HGF), epidermal growth factor (EGF), transforming growth factor α (TGF-α) acidic fibroblast growth factor (aFGF) and hepatocyte stimulatory substance (HSS); (2) indirect or co-mitogens including insulin, glucagon, norepinephrine, vasopressin, angiotensin II, vasoactive intestinal peptide (VIP); and (3) inhibitors such as the transforming growth factor β (TGF-β), interleukin 1, interleukin 6 and leukemia inhibitory factor (LIF). Enhanced expression of growth-related proto-oncogenes including *c-fos*, *c-jun*, *c-myc*, *c-H-ras*, *c-met* and *MAGE-1* have been reported (D'Errico *et al.*, 1996; Yamashita, 1996). In addition increased mRNA and proteins for growth factors, receptors and molecules for the signal transduction pathways such as TGF-α (Fig. 8.3), IGF-II, EGFR (*erbB*) have been reported earlier in human and in experimental rodent HCCs (Yamaguchi *et al.*, 1995). The increased expressions of many of these growth-related genes are apparently not specific for HCC, since many of these changes have been observed in cirrhotic and regenerating livers. However, studies on amplification and over-expression of the *cyclin D1* gene which is located at 11q13 demonstrated that such alterations occurred in the HCC in patients at advanced stage (11–13%) (Zhang *et al.*, 1993; Nishida *et al.*, 1994). The authors suggested that these changes may be associated with the aggressive behavior of tumors. It is believed that amplification and over-expression of the *cyclin D1* gene result in the deregulation of the cell

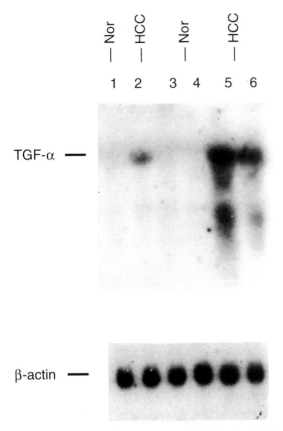

Nor | HCC | Nor | HCC

1   2   3   4   5   6

TGF-α —

β-actin —

Fig. 8.3 Increased expression of TGF-α in HCC. Equal amounts of total RNA (10 μg) isolated from HCC and normal liver tissues were analyzed by Northern blotting with 1% agarose-formaldehyde gel electrophoresis. After transferring to a nylon membrane filter, the samples were hybridized to a [32P]-labeled TGF-α probe, and the membrane was exposed to X-ray autoradiography. After washing off the labeled probe, the filter was rehybridized to the control of β-actin cDNA. The results showed that >5–10-fold increase in expression of TGFα mRNA was found in HCC as compared with normal liver tissues.

cycle. Moreover, amplification of the *c-myc* gene was also detected in 50% of HCC by differential PCR. These findings correlated with over-expression of the *c-myc* gene found in many HCCs (Saegusa *et al.*, 1993; Tabor, 1994). In addition, transgenic mice harboring the *c-myc* and *TGF-α* transgenes were found to

develop HCC, indicating that *c-myc* and *TGF-α* play a role in HCC development. Similarly, altered or decreased expression of tumor suppressor genes such as *Rb*, *p53* and *PML* have been documented (Zhang *et al.*, 1994; Terris *et al.*, 1995). Whether these alterations may reflect the increases in cellular proliferation or the appearance of the transformed or malignant phenotypes of those neoplasias is still unknown. Nevertheless, these alterations are part of the programed cascades of growth signals leading to the development of HCC (Mehta, 1995). Other alterations include the membrane proteins such as annexin I and adhesion molecules which may play a role in the loss of contact inhibition and disrupted intercellular communications (Masaki *et al.*, 1996). Recently, it was reported that the PML-RAR-α protein induces hepatic neoplastic lesions in transgenic mice (David *et al.*, 1997) indicating that this fusion gene deregulates hepatocyte proliferation and is involved in hepatocarcinogenesis *in vivo*. It is interesting to note that mutations of the *ras* genes are frequently found in many cancer types. The *ras* family genes (*Ha-*, *Ki-* and *N-ras*) are activated by point mutation at codons 12, 13 and 61. Although these mutations have been reported in considerable numbers of HCC from rodents, yet they are infrequent in human HCC (0–20%) (Tada *et al.*, 1990; Challen *et al.*, 1992), and their role remains obscure.

8.5 GENOMIC INSTABILITY AND CHROMOSOMAL ALTERATIONS IN HCC

Cancer is believed to arise from cells that have undergone genetic alterations and clonal expansion. These genetic alterations include activation of proto-oncogenes, inactivation of the tumor suppressor genes, and reactivation of the telomerase activity. As the altered hyperplastic foci of hepatocytes progress to the intermediate stage, namely that of adenomatous dysplasia (dysplastic/hyperplastic nodules), and then into HCC, additional genetic changes, expressed as chromosomal aberrations, are observed. The identification of specific genetic changes that drive the neoplastic process has led to a better understanding of the process of cancer progression and has provided useful markers for early detection and prognosis, and they will be discussed in the following sections. The accumulation of somatic genetic changes in the HCC cells have been investigated with a number of techniques, including cytogenetic, molecular genetic, and, recently, molecular cytogenetic methods.

8.5.1   ALLELOTYPING

A widely used strategy to search for the allelic alterations in the genome is through loss of heterozygosity (LOH) analysis at polymorphic markers mapped to specific chromsomal regions. By PCR-based microsatellite polymorphism analysis, specifically deleted regions which contain tumor suppressor genes involved in the tumorigenesis of HCC can be identified. Allelotypes of HCC have been completed by several groups. A comprehensive study by Boige *et al.* (1997), examined 275 microsatellite loci across the entire genome in 48 HCCs. The frequently deleted chromosome regions were: 8p (60%), 17p (48%), 1p (44%), 4q (42%), 16p (40%), 16q (39%), 6q (35%), 9p (30%) and 13q (29%). Nagai *et al.* (1997) studied allelic loss in 120 HCCs and found significantly elevated LOH in loci on 1p, 4q, 6q, 8p, 13q and 16p. In contrast, allelotype studies by our group in 45 HBV-associated HCCs from Chinese patients in Hong Kong showed a different pattern of deletion. The highest frequency of LOH was found in chromosome 16q (80%), while other regions frequently affected by deletion included: 17p (71%), 13q (67%), 8p (60%), 4q (60%), 16p (60%), 9p (56%), 1p and 1q (50% each) (unpublished data; Fig. 8.4). The reason for the difference in the patterns of LOH is not known, but may be related to the different

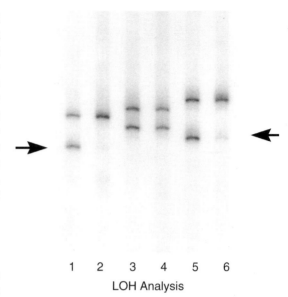

1   2   3   4   5   6
LOH Analysis

Fig. 8.4 Loss of heterozygocity in HCC. Labeled primers for chromosome 17 (D17S695) were used to amplify DNA from HCC and adjacent non-tumor tissue by PCR. The PCR-products were then fractionated by urea-polyacrylamide gel electrophoresis. Lanes 1 and 2 are the non-tumor (N) and tumor (T) tissues from one patient with HCC respectively. Lanes 3 and 4, and 5 and 6 are the corresponding N and T samples from two other HCC patients. The arrows indicate tumor samples with loss of heterozygocity. The results show that the first and the third samples of HCC contained LOH at chromosome 17 while the second HCC showed a normal pattern.

etiological factors involved in specific populations from different geographic regions.

8.5.2   COMPARATIVE GENOMIC HYBRIDIZATION ANALYSIS

The classical methods of cytogenetic analysis are generally not applicable in HCC, since most solid tumors including HCC produce very limited numbers of mitotic figures. Only few karyotypings have been reported and no consistant abnormalities have been found (Simon *et al.*, 1990, 1991; Bardi *et al.*, 1993; Chen *et al.*, 1996). However, with the new developed comparative genomic hybrid-ization (CGH) analysis which hybridizes dif-ferentially labeled DNA from tumor and normal tissues to mitotic figures of normal cells, non-random genomic changes have been demonstrated (Marchio *et al.*, 1997). In 50 primary HBV-related HCC, chromosome los-ses were frequently found in the regions of 4q (70%), 8p (65%), 16q(54%), 17p (51%), 13q and 6q (37% each). Deletions observed in these regions agree well with the findings of allelo-typing and LOH studies described earlier, and indicated that inactivation of the tumor sup-pressors on these regions may contribute to the HCC tumorigenesis. On the other hand, frequent gains were found to occur in the chromosome regions of 8q (60%), 1q (58%), 6p (33%) and 17q (33%) respectively. This study has also revealed several amplified regions including 11q12, 12p11, 14q12, and 19q13.1 in some of the cases, suggesting that there could be oncogene(s) residing on these chromosome regions. A recent CGH study in Hong Kong indicates that DNA losses were frequently seen in chromosomes 4, 10q, 11q, 14q, 17p, 18q and X while consistent chromosomal gains were found in 1q21–22, 6p, 8q, 17q and 20 (Wong *et al.*, unpublished data).

8.5.3   CHROMOSOME 16Q AND E-CADHERIN

In CGH and allelotyping studies, frequent deletion of several chromosomal regions including chromosome 16q, 17p, 8p, 13q, 4q and 1p were observed. Despite the large number of potential tumor suppressor gene (TSG) loci that have been identified, only few specific genes have been conclusively impli-cated in the development of HCC. Loss of chromosome 16q appears to be one of the most common genetic defects in HCC. A high frequency of 16q deletion has been documented in both LOH and CGH studies. LOH of 16q has been found in up to 80% of HCCs from Hong Kong patients. A com-monly deleted region, 16q22–23, has been reported suggesting the presence of a tumor

suppressor gene in this region (Yeh *et al.*, 1996). One of the candidate targets is the E-cadherin gene, which is located on 16q22.1. Although no mutations or gross structural alterations of this gene have been reported in HCC, loss of E-cadherin expression has been observed (Shimoyama and Hirohashi, 1991). Recently, *de novo* methylation of the 5'CpG island of the E-cadherin gene has been found in 46% of liver tissue showing chronic hep-atitis or cirrhosis and in 67% of HCCs ana-lysed (Kanai *et al.*, 1997). Moreover, it was also demonstrated that such epigenetic change correlated significantly with reduced E-cardherin expression. The silencing of the E-cadherin gene may lead to the loss of intercellular adhesiveness which may con-tribute to unrestrained cell growth. It is suspected that the inactivation of this gene by deletion or hypermethylation of the pro-moter region may play an important role in the development of HCC.

8.5.4   CHROMOSOME 17P AND *P53*

Deletion at 17p and alterations of the *p53* gene at 17p13 are common genetic changes repor-ted in human cancers. The tumor suppressor gene *p53* encodes a 53 kD nuclear phospho-protein that acts as a transcription factor. The major functions of the gene are the blockage of the progression of the cell cycle in response to DNA damage, and the mediation of DNA repair or apoptosis. In HCC, a high percentage of LOH at 17p was identified (48–71%) (Boige *et al.*, 1997). This finding strongly suggests that the *p53* gene is the target gene involved during the development of HCC. As men-tioned previously it was hypothesized that *p53* mutations were common in the HCCs associated with aflatoxin B exposure (about 50%) and a consistent mutation at codon 249 was observed in these tumors (Harris, 1994). On the other hand, the discrepancy between the consistant high frequencies of LOH at 17p and low frequencies of *p53* deletion in some of the HCC reported indicated that there may be other deleted tumor suppressor gene(s) on 17p in HCC.

8.5.5   CHROMOSOME 13Q AND *RB* AND *BRCA2*

Chromosome 13q is often found to be deleted in HCC by both LOH and CGH analysis (37–67%) (Boige *et al.*, 1997; Marchio *et al.*, 1997). Detailed deletion mapping have identified two distinct common deletion regions which appear to contain the tumor suppressor genes, *Rb* (13q14) and *BRCA2* (13q12). These genes have been suggested to be the candidate targets for the HCC tumorigenesis. The status of the *Rb* gene in HCC has been investigated previously and alterations of the gene seems to be rare in this cancer (Zhang *et al.*, 1994). For *BRCA2*, mutations were found in three of the 60 HCCs examined (Katagiri *et al.*, 1996). It is possible that other genes on this region may contribute to the development of this cancer or the *Rb* or *BRCA2* genes are inactivated by epigenetic changes such as aberrant methylation.

8.5.6   CHROMOSOME 8P AND THE PLATLET DERIVED GROWTH FACTOR (PDGF) RECEPTOR β-LIKE TUMOR SUPPRESSOR

Both LOH and CGH analysis (Boige *et al.*, 1997; Machio *et al.*, 1997) indicate that chromosome 8p loss is also a common abnormality (60–5%). Becker *et al.* (1996) have found that LOH at 8p was present in up to 85% of HBV-positive HCCs from China. The loci with the highest frequency of LOH have been observed in 8p21 and 8p23. The study of Emi *et al.* (1993) showed a 8-cM commonly deleted region at 8p21.3-p22 on deletion mapping of 142 HCCs. This region contains a putative tumor suppressor gene, PDGF-receptor β-like tumor suppressor, which has been shown to be mutated in two HCCs (Fujiwara *et al.*, 1994, 1995). However, the involvement of this gene in HCC needs further examination and no

other candidate tumor suppressor genes have been reported in this region.

8.5.7   CHROMOSOME 9P AND *P16*

Although reports of chromosome 9 loss are uncommon in HCC, recent data demonstrated LOH at 9p21 occurs frequently in HCC (54–63%) (Biden *et al.*, 1997). A homozygous deletion region at 9p21 has also been identified in some of our cases from Hong Kong (Liew *et al.*, unpublished data). This region includes the tumor suppressor genes *p16* and *p15*. It is suspected that these genes may be inactivated in HCC. Both *p16* and *p15* genes encode the negative regulator proteins for cell cycle progression. These proteins bind to cyclin-dependent protein kinases, CDK-4 and CDK-6, and prevent the CDKs from forming an active complex with the cyclin D protein. Inhibition of the catalytic activity of the CDK/cyclin D complex will prevent the phosphorylation of the Rb protein, and subsequently inhibits the cell cycle progression from G_1 to S phase. The alteration of the *p16* gene has been examined by several groups (Hui *et al.*, 1996; Kita *et al.*, 1996; Biden *et al.*, 1997; Chaubert *et al.*, 1997), and it was noted that mutations and homozygous deletion of the *p16* gene were infrequent in HCC. However, Chaubert *et al.*, (1997) have demonstrated *de novo* methylation of the 5'CpG island of the *p16* gene in 48% of HCCs examined. These findings indicate that alterations of the *p16* gene may be involved in the genesis of HCC, although it is not directly related to the LOH observed in 9p. On the other hand, the relationship of the *p15* gene in HCC is still not known.

8.5.8   OTHER CHROMOSOMAL ALTERATIONS

Several other losses of chromosomal regions that are not associated with known tumor suppressor genes have been found in HCC. For example, chromosome 4q has been reported to undergo LOH in 50–77% of HCC, while this region is less involved in other cancers (Zhang *et al.*, 1994; Yeh *et al.*, 1996). The commonly deleted region was localized between 4q12 and 4q23. Deletion of chromosome 1p was found to occur frequently in early- and well-differentiated HCC (Kuroki *et al.*, 1995), and this abnormality is clustered at the distal part of chromosome 1p, with a common deleted region at either 1p35–36 or 1p34–36 (Kuroki *et al.*, 1995). Amplification of chromosome 8q has been found in 44% of HCC examined by Southern blotting of the polymorphic markers on this region (Fujiwara *et al.*, 1993), a finding later confirmed by CGH analysis (Marchio *et al.*, 1997). The earlier study defined the amplification region to be distal to 8q24 where the proto-oncogene *c-myc* resides.

8.5.9 REACTIVATION OF TELOMERASE ACTIVITY IN HCC

Progressive shortening of telomeres with age is known to occur in normal somatic cells in culture and *in vivo*. Thus, the maintenance of telomere length and the expression of the enzyme activity is assumed to be an obligatory step(s) in the progression of tumor cells (Fig. 8.5). Reactivation of telomerase activity and shortening of the length of terminal restriction fragment (TRF) have been reported in a majority of human and rodent HCCs (Tahara *et al.*, 1995; Kojima *et al.*, 1997; Miura *et al.*, 1997). Our study of Chinese patients from Hong Kong showed that >80% of HCC analyzed contained telomerase activity (Liew *et al.*, unpublished data). However, there was no significant correlation between telomerase activity and clinical-pathological features of HCC. Nevertheless, it was suggested that telomerase may be a useful diagnostic discriminant for HCC regardless of tumor size.

Moreover, detection of new genes associated with HCC were also reported. Using the innovative technique of differential display of mRNA in HCC and normal tissues, a mitochondria proteolipid like gene (MPL) that was repressed in HCC has been identified (Wu *et al.*, 1995)

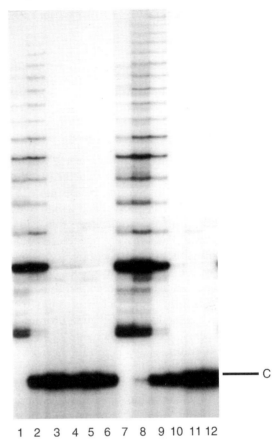

1 2 3 4 5 6 7 8 9 10 11 12

— C

Fig. 8.5 Increased telomerase activity in HCC. Increasing dilutions of cell extracts from HCC and adjacent non-tumor tissues were incubated with reaction mixture containing [^{32}P]-labeled primers for the telomeric repeat amplification protocol (TRAP) assay (Oncor Lab) for telomerase activity. After the reaction, the samples were analyzed by polyacrylamide-urea gel-electrophoresis and the gel was exposed to X-ray autoradiography. Lanes 1–3 are 1×, 10× and 100× dilution of 1 μg/μl of cell extract from a sample of HCC respectively; while lanes 4–6 are 1×, 10× and 100× dilution of 1 μg/μl of cell extract from the adjacent non-tumor tissues. Similarly, lanes 7–9 are 1×, 10× and 100× dilution of 1 μg/μl of cell extract from a different sample of HCC respectively, while lanes 10–12 are the corresponding samples from the adjacent non-tumor tissue. The results show that HCCs contain increased activity of telomerase as compared to the control non-tumor tissues which is apparently a diagnostic determinant for HCC.

8.6 GENE TRANSFER AND GENE THERAPY IN HCC

Gene transfer and gene therapy are two major innovative treatment approaches currently pursued by many investigators. Several reports utilizing restriction of tumoricidal gene therapy to selected HCC cells have recently been documented (Zern and Kresina, 1997). The 5′ flanking sequence of the α-fetal protein (*AFP*) gene was constructed as the promoter for the thymidine kinase gene of herpes simplex virus (HSV-TK), which was then cloned in an adenovirus vector. AFP-producing cells (HuH7) were specifically killed after transduction of the HSV-TK gene followed by the administration of the anti-viral TK drug ganciclovir (Kaneko and Tsukamoto, 1995). Another approach was to link the wild-type *p53* gene to the *AFP* gene promoter in a retrovirus vector to achieve selective growth inhibition of AFP-producing cells. Introduction of this gene into AFP-positive HCC cells resulted in inhibition of clonal growth and increased the sensitivity of these cells to cisplatin. Thus, restoring wild-type *p53* expression in HCC in combination with chemotherapy can be considered as a strategy for the treatment of HCC (Xu *et al.*, 1996). However, retrovirus vectors suffer from the drawback of low frequency of gene transfer, and the need of hepatocyte proliferation to allow the vector to replicate. Thus, another novel method is first to transduce hepatocytes with adenovirus that transiently express the urokinase gene, resulting in a high rate of asynchronous liver regeneration (Lieber *et al.*, 1995). This approach resulted in a 10-fold increase in the efficiency of subsequent transfection with retrovirus. Other methods of improving gene transfer in liver include the liposome-encapsulated DNA-mediated gene transfer with intravenous injection, and the use of the MoMLV LTR encapsulated in multilamellar liposomes of egg phosphatidylcholine. Chloroquine and colchicine pretreatment increase the levels of plasmid DNA in liver. Although adenovirus-based vectors are capable of transducing a high percentage of cells, the effects are transient and usually last no more than a few weeks (Kaneko *et al.*, 1995). Other difficulties include the low rates of penetration of these vectors in solid tumors. Nevertheless, new discoveries in molecular genetics and the significant potential of utilizing these findings to treat HCC, together with improved vectors and vehicles that are targeted to HCC cells and membranes, will make molecular therapy of HCC possible in the foreseeable future.

In conclusion, recent molecular studies have revealed a great deal about the role of proto-oncogenes, tumor suppressor genes and hepadnavirus in the development of HCC. The diagnosis and therapy of neoplastic diseases using the techniques of molecular biology is just beginning. The first rays of light on what promises to be a glorious period in the history of medicine are on the horizon.

REFERENCES

Alberts, S.R., Lanier, A.P., McMahon, B.J. *et al.* (1991) Clustering of hepatocellular carcinoma in Alaska native families. *Genetic Epidemiology*, **8**, 127–19.

Bardi, G., Pandis, N., Fenger, C. *et al.* (1993) Deletion of 1p36 as a primary chromosomal aberration in intestinal tumorigenesis. *Cancer Research*, **53**, 1895–8.

Becker, S.A., Zhou, Y.Z. and Slagle, B.L. (1996) Frequent loss of chromosome in hepatitis B virus-positive hepatocellular carcinomas from China. *Cancer Research*, **56**, 5092–7.

Biden, K., Young, J., Buttenshaw, R. *et al.* (1997) Frequency of mutation and deletion of the tumor suppressor gene CDKN4A (MST1/p16) in hepatocellulat carcinoma from an Australian population. *Hepatology*, **25**, 593–7.

Boige, V., Laurent-Puig, P., Fouchet, P. *et al.* (1997) Concerted nonsyntenic allelic losses in hyperploid hepatocellular carcinoma as determined by a high-resoulation allelotype. *Cancer Research*, **57**, 1986–90.

Brechot, C. (ed) (1994) *Primary Liver Cancer: Etiological and Progression Factors*, CRC Press, Boca Raton.

Caselmann, W.H. (1995) Transactivation of cellular gene expression by hepatitis B viral proteins: a possible molecular mechanism of hepatocarcinogenesis. *Journal of Hepatology*, **22 (Suppl. 1)**, 34–7.

Challen, C., Guo, K., Collier, J.D. *et al.* (1992) Infrequent point mutations in codons 12 and 61 of ras oncogenes in human hepatocellular carcinoma. *Journal of Hepatology*, **14**, 342–6.

Chaubert, P., Gayer, R., Zimmermann, A. *et al.* (1997) Germ-line mutation of the *p16INK4(MST1)* gene occur in a subset of patients with hepatocellular carcinoma. *Hepatology*, **25**, 1376–81.

Chen, H.L., Chen, Y.C. and Chen, D.S. (1996) Chromosome 1p aberrations are frequent in human HCC. *Cancer Genetic Cytogenetic*, **86**, 102–6.

David, G., Terris, B., Marchio, A. *et al.* (1997) The acute promyelocytic leukemia PML-RARα protein induces hepatic preneoplastic and neoplastic lesions in transgenic mice. *Oncogene*, **14**, 1547–54.

D'Errico, A., Fiorentino, M., Ponzetto, A. *et al.* (1996) Liver hepatocyte growth factor does not always correlate with hepatocellular proliferation in human liver lesions: its specific receptor c-met does. *Hepatology*, **24**, 60–4.

Emi, M., Fujiwara, Y., Ohata, H. *et al.* (1993) Allelic loss at chromosome band 8p21.3-p22 is associated with progression of hepatocellular carcinoma. *Genes, Chromosomes and Cancer*, **7**, 152–7.

Fausto, N. (1991) Growth factors in liver development, regeneration and carcinogenesis. *Progress in Growth Factor Research*, **3**, 219.

Fujiwara, Y., Monden, M., Mori, T. *et al.* (1993) Frequent multiplication of the long arm of chromosome 8 in hepatocellular carcinoma. *Cancer Research*, **53**, 857–60.

Fujiwara, Y., Ohata, H., Emi, M. *et al.* (1994) A 3-Mb physical map of the chromosome region 8p21.3-p22, including a 100-kb region commonly deleted in human hepatocellular carcinoma, colorectal cancer, and non-small cell lung cancer. *Genes, Chromosomes and Cancer*, **10**, 7–14.

Fujiwara, Y., Ohata, H., Kuroki, T. *et al.* (1995) Isolation of a candidate tumor suppressor gene on chromosome 8p21.3-p22 that is homologous to an extracellular domain of PDGF receptor β gene. *Oncogene*, **10**, 891–5.

Greenblatt, M.S., Feitelson, M.A., Zhu, M. *et al.* (1997) Integreity of p53 in hepatitis Bx antigen-positive and -negative hepatocellular carcinomas. *Cancer Research*, **57**, 426–32.

Harris, C.C. (1994) Solving the viral-chemical puzzle of human liver carcinogenesis. *Cancer Epidemiology Biomarkers and Prevention*, **3**, 1–2.

Hoppe-Seyler, F. and Butz, K. (1995) Molecular mechanisms of virus-induced carcinogenesis: the interaction of viral factors with cellular tumor suppressor proteins. *Journal of Molecular Medicine*, **73**, 529–38.

Hui, AM., Sakamoto, M., Kanai, Y. *et al.* (1996) Inactivation of p16INK in hepatocellular carcinoma. *Hepatology*, **24**, 575–9.

Kanai, Y., Ushuma, S., Hui, A.M. *et al.* (1997) The E-cadherin gene is silenced by CpG methylation in human hepatocellular carcinomas. *International Journal of Cancer*, **71**, 355–9.

Kaneko, S., Hallenbeck, P., Kotani T. *et al.* (1995) Adenovirus mediated gene therapy of HCC using cancer-specific gene expression. *Cancer Research*, **55**, 5283–7.

Kaneko, Y. and Tsukamoto, A. (1995) Gene therapy of hepatoma: bystander effects and non-apoptotic cell death induced by thymidine kinase and ganciclovir. *Cancer Letters*, **96**, 105–10.

Kasai, Y., Takeda, S. and Takagi, H. (1996) Pathogenesis of hepatocellular carcinoma: a review from the viewpoint of molecular analysis. *Seminars on Surgical Oncology*, **12**, 155–9.

Katagiri, T., Nakamura Y. and Yoshio, M. (1996) Mutation in the *BRCA2* Gene in hepatocellular carcinomas. *Cancer Research*, **56**, 4575–7.

Kim, C.M., Koike, K., Saito, I. *et al.* (1991) *HBx* gene of hepatitis B virus induces liver cancer in transgenic mice. *Nature*, **351**, 317–20.

Kita, R., Nishida, N., Fukuda, Y. *et al.* (1996) Infrequent alterations of the p16 INK4A gene in liver cancer. *International Journal of Cancer*, **67**, 176–80.

Kojima, H., Yokosuka, O., Imazeki, F. *et al.* (1997) Telomerase activity and telomere length in hepatocellular carcinoma and chronic liver disease. *Gastroenterology*, **112**, 493–550.

Kuroki, T., Fujiwara, Y., Nakamori, S. *et al.* (1995) Evidence for the presence of two-suppressor genes for hepatocellular carcinoma on chromosome 13q. *British Journal of Cancer*, **72**, 383–5.

Lee, S.M., Portmann, B.C. and Margison, G.P. (1996) Abnormal intracellular distribution of O^6AG-DNA alkyltransferase in hepatitis B cirrhotic human liver: a potential cofactor in the development of HCC. *Hepatology*, **24**, 987–90.

Lee, T.H., Finegold, M.J., Shen, R.F. *et al.* (1995) Hepatitis B virus tansactivator X protein is not tumorigenic in transgenic mice. *Journal of Virology*, **69**, 1107–14.

Lieber, A., VranckenPeeters, M.-J.T.F.D., Meuse, L. *et al.* (1995) Adenovirus-mediated urokinase gene transfer induces liver regeneration and allows for efficient retrovirus transduction of hepatocytes *in vivo. Proceedings of the National Academy of Sciences, USA,* **92,** 6210–14.

Marchio, A., Meddeb, M., Pineaui, P. *et al.* (1997) Recurrent chromosomal abnormalities in HCC detected by comparative genomic hybridization (CGH). *Genes, Chromosomes and Cancer,* **18,** 59–65.

Masaki, R., Tokuda, M., Ohnishi, M. *et al.* (1996) Enhanced expression of the protein kinase substrate Annexin I in human HCC. *Hepatology,* **24,** 72–81.

Mehta, R. (1995) The potential for the use of cell proliferation and oncogene expression as intermediate markers during liver carcinogenesis. *Cancer Letters,* **93,** 85–102.

Miura, N., Horikawa, I., Nishimoto, A *et al.* (1997) Progressive telomere shortening and telomerase reactivation during hepatocellular carcinogenesis. *Cancer Genetics and Cytogenetics,* **93,** 56–62.

Nagai, H., Pineau, P., Tiollais, P. *et al.* (1997) Comprehensive allelotyping of human hepatocellular carcinoma. *Oncogene,* **14,** 2927–33.

Nishida, N., Fukuda, Y., Komeda, T. *et al.* (1994) Amplification and overexpression of the cyclin D1 gene in aggressive human hepatocellular carcinoma. *Cancer Research,* **54,** 3107–10.

Robinson, W.S. (1994) Molecular events in the pathogenesis of hepadnavirus-associated hepatocellular carcinoma. *Annual Review of Medicine,* **45,** 297–323.

Saegusa, M., Takano, Y., Kishimoto, H. *et al.* (1993) Comparative analysis of p53 and c-myc expression and cell proliferation in human hepatocellular carcinomas-an enhanced immunohischemical approach. *Journal of Cancer Research and Clinical Oncology,* **119,** 737–44.

Shen, F.M., Lee, M.K., Gong, H.M. *et al.* (1991) Complex segregation analysis of primary hepatocellular carcinoma in Chinese families: interaction of inherited susceptibility and hepatitis B viral infection. *American Journal of Human Genetics,* **49,** 88.

Shimoyama, Y. and Hirohashi, S. (1991) Cadherin intercellular adhesion molecule in hepatocellular carcinoma: loss of E-cadherin expression in an undifferentiated carcinoma. *Cancer Letters,* **57,** 131–5.

Simon, D., Knowles, B.B. and Weith, A. (1991) Abnormalities of chromosome 1 and loss of heterozygosity on 1p in primary hepatomas. *Oncogenes,* **6,** 765–70.

Simon, D., Munoz, S.J., Maddrey, W.C. and Knowles, B.B. (1990) Chromosomal rearrangements in a primary hepatocellular carcinoma. *Cancer Genetics and Cytogenetics,* **45,** 255–60.

Tabor, E. (1994) Tumor suppressor genes, growth factor genes, and oncogenes in hepatitis B virus-associated hepatocellular carcinoma. *Journal of Medical Virology,* **42,** 357–65.

Tada, M., Omata, M. and Ohto, M. (1990) Analysis of *ras* gene mutations in human hepatic malignant tumors by polymerase chain reaction and direct sequencing. *Cancer Research,* **50,** 1121–4.

Tahara, H., Nakanishi, T., Kitamoto, M. *et al.* (1995) Telomerase activity in human liver tissues: comparison between chronic liver disease and hepatocellular carcinomas. *Cancer Research,* **55,** 2734–56.

Teeter, L.D., Chan, J.Y.H. and Kuo, M.T. (1991) Coordinate activation of multidrug-resistance (P-glycoprotein) genes *mdr2* and *mdr3* during mouse liver regeneration. *Molecular Carcinogenesis,* **4,** 358–61.

Teeter, L.D., Estes, M., Chan, J.Y.H. *et al.* (1993) Activation of distinct multidrug resistance (P-glycoprotein) genes during rat liver regeneration and hepatocarcinogenesis. *Molecular Carcinogenesis,* **8,** 67–73.

Terris, B., Baldin, V., Dubios, S. *et al.* (1995) PML nuclear bodies are general targets for inflammation and cell proliferation. *Cancer Research,* **55,** 1590–7.

Wang, X.W., Gibson, M.K., Vermeulen, W. *et al.* (1995) Abrogation or p53-induced apoptosis by the hepatitis B virus X gene. *Cancer Research,* **55,** 6012–16.

Wogan, G.N. (1992) Aflatoxins as risk factors for hepatocellular carcinoma in humans. *Cancer Research,* **52 (Suppl.),** 2114.

Wu, G.S., Kar, S. and Carr B.I. (1995) Identification of a human hepatocellular carcinoma-associated tumor suppressor gene by differential display polymerase chain reaction. *Life Science,* **57,** 1077–85.

Xu, G.W., Sun, Z.T., Forrester, K. *et al.* (1996) Tissue specific growth suppression and chemosensitivity promotion mediated transfer of the wild-type *p53* gene. *Hepatology,* **24,** 1264–8.

Yamaguchi, K., Carr B.I. and Nalesnik M.A. (1995) Concomitant and isolated expression of TGF-α and EGF-R in human hepatoma cells supports the hypothesis of autocrine, paracrine, and endocrine growth of human hepatoma. *Journal of Surgical Oncology*, **58**, 240–5.

Yamashita, N. (1996) High frequency of *MAGE-1* gene expression in HCC. *Hepatology*, **24**, 1437–40

Yeh, H.Y., Chen, P.J., Lai, M.Y. and Chen, D.S. (1996) Allelic loss on chromosome 4q and 16q in hepatocellular carcinoma: association with elevated α-fetoprotein production. *Gastroenterology*, **110**, 184–92.

Yen, T.S.B. (1996) Hepadnaviral X protein: review of recent progress. *Journal of Biomedical Science*, **3**, 20–3.

Zern, M.A. and Kresina, T.F. (1997) Hepatic drug delivery and gene therapy. *Hepatology*, **25**, 484–91.

Zhang, X., Xu, H.J., Murakami, Y. *et al.* (1994) Deletions of chromosome 13q, mutations in retinoblastoma 1, and retinoblastoma protein state in human hepatocellular carcinoma. *Cancer Research*, **54**, 4177–82.

Zhang, Y.J., Jiang, W., Chen, C.J. *et al.* (1993) Amplification and over-expression of cyclin D1 in human hepatocellular carcinoma. *Biochemical and Biophysical Research Communications*, **196**, 1010–16.

Zhong, S. (1997) Novel mutations in the hepatitis B virus genome in human HCC, PhD thesis, Chinese University of Hong Kong.

9

SURGICAL MANAGEMENT (INCLUDING LIVER TRANSPLANTATION)

J.W.Y. Lau and C.K. Leow

Of the many therapeutic options available for treating hepatocellular carcinoma (HCC), surgery, that is liver resection or liver transplantation, is the only treatment which has the potential to cure. Recent improvements in preoperative diagnosis and perioperative management of these patients have made liver resection safe. As most HCC develops in a cirrhotic liver, the specific risks associated with operating on a cirrhotic patient, with diminished functional liver reserve and impaired hepatic regenerative capability, make the perioperative management and surgery difficult and challenging.

9.1 SURGICAL ANATOMY OF THE LIVER

A detailed and accurate knowledge of the anatomy of the liver is vital and application of this knowledge to surgery on the liver has led to a rapid development in the art of precise operations.

As early as 1898, Cantlie noted 'The present anatomical division of the liver into right and left lobes is unscientific and consequently untrue and untenable'. On gross inspection, the liver appears divided anteriorly into two lobes, right and left, by the line of insertion of the falciform ligament. The right lobe, as defined by this anatomical division, is approximately six times the size of the left and includes the caudate lobe posteriorly and quadrate lobe inferiorly. Cantlie found that the physiological (or functional) right and left lobes were of equal size and divided by a plane of symmetry, often considered as the Rex–Cantlie line, passing through the bed of the gallbladder and the notch of the inferior vena cava (Cantlie, 1898). Fifty-five years later, Healey and Schroy, after examining the intrahepatic biliary architecture, proposed that the liver be divided into five segments: anterior, posterior, medial, lateral and caudate (Healey and Schroy 1953), and advocated a segmental approach to hepatic anatomy. The modern segmental nomenclature of the anatomy of the liver hinged on the published works of Couinaud (1954), who presents the French nomenclature based on the venous anatomy of the liver, and the Anglo-Saxon nomenclature of Healey and Schroy (1953) and Goldsmith and Woodburne (1957) which is based on the biliary structures (Figs 9.1–.3).

Healey and Schroy divided the liver into right and left lobes according to the primary division of the bile ducts, i.e. right and left hepatic ducts. The secondary biliary division further divides the right and left lobes of the liver into *segments*. On the right, the right segmental fissure divides the right lobe into anterior and posterior segments while the left segmental fissure divides the left lobe into

Hepatocellular Carcinoma: Diagnosis, investigation and management. Edited by Anthony S.-Y. Leong, Choong-Tsek Liew, Joseph W.Y. Lau and Philip J. Johnson. Published in 1999 by Arnold, London. ISBN 0 340 74096 5.

148   *Surgical management*

medial and lateral segments. The tertiary biliary divisions further divide the segments into equal superior and inferior parts called *areas*. The nomenclature of Goldsmith and Woodburne differs from that of Healey and Schroy in that the *areas* of Healey and Schroy are termed *subsegments*. Couinaud's nomenclature is based on the interdigitating fingers of the portal and hepatic veins: four portal and three hepatic fingers. When the hepatic veins constitute the basis of division, the planes are called *portal* scissurae or *portal* fissures. The planes are called *hepatic* scissurae or *hepatic* fissures when the portal veins form the basis of division. In Couinaud's nomenclature, the main portal scissura divides the liver into right and left livers or hemilivers. The secondary division of the liver by the right and left portal scissurae further divides the right and left hemiliver into *sectors*. On the right, the right portal scissurae divides the hemiliver into the anterior and posterior sectors while the left portal scissurae divides the left hemiliver into the medial and lateral

sectors. The tertiary division of the liver, according to Couinaud, by the portal veins further divides the sectors into *segments*. As a result Couinaud's *segments* correspond to Healey and Schroy's *areas* and Goldsmith and Woodburne's *subsegments*. This gives rise to confusion as Healey and Schroy termed the secondary divisions segments while Couinaud called them sectors! Although the French nomenclature on the divisions of the liver is more widely used, the presence of two classifications sharing some common terms but referring to differing anatomical parts of the liver has given rise to confusion in the surgical literature.

Based on Couinaud's nomenclature, the main *portal* scissura, which corresponds to the Rex–Cantlie line, runs anteriorly from the middle of the gallbladder bed to the left edge of the inferior vena cava posteriorly. The middle hepatic vein follows this scissura. The right liver is divided into two sectors by the right portal scissura: anteromedial (or anterior) and posterolateral (or posterior). The

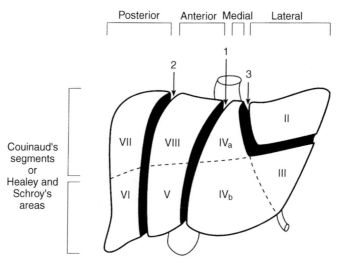

Fig. 9.1 Couinaud's, and Healey and Schroy's classification of liver divisions. The three portal scissurae of Couinaud are: main (1), right (2), and left (3). Healey and Schroy used the terms 'right and left segmental fissure' for dividing the right and left liver. Note the left segmental fissure extends to the umbilical fissure giving rise to the difference between Couinaud's, and Healey and Schroy's classification. Couinaud's lateral 'sector' consists of segment II only while Healey and Schroy's lateral 'segment' is made up of Couinaud's segments II and III.

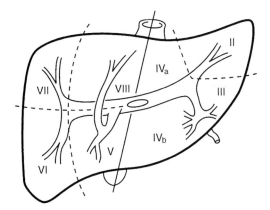

Fig. 9.2 Portal vein divisions and zones of supply according to Couinaud. The Rex-Cantlie line (solid line) divides the liver into 'hemilivers' with its primary division of right and left portal veins. The portal vein secondarily divides into anterior and posterior branches (on the right) and medial and lateral branches (on the left). These secondary divisions supply the anterior, posterior, medial and lateral 'sectors' of the liver. Further divisions of the secondary branches supply the eight 'segments', the caudate lobe (segment I) and the other seven segments (segments II–VIII).

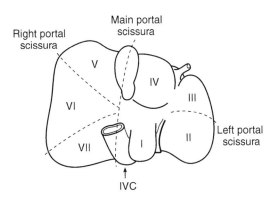

Fig. 9.3 Inferior view of the liver. IVC, inferior vena cava.

location of this scissura on the anterior surface of the right liver, according to Couinaud (1957), extends from the midpoint between the angle of the liver and the right side of the gallbladder bed to the confluence of the right hepatic vein and the inferior vena cava posteriorly. The right hepatic vein runs along this

scissura. The anterior sector of the right liver is further divided into segment V inferiorly and segment VIII superiorly by the anterior hepatic scissura (which contains the portal pedicle). Similarly, the posterior hepatic scissura divides the posterior sector into segment VI inferiorly and segment VII superiorly. The left portal scissura divides the left liver into the superior and posterior sectors. The scissura is located within the left liver posterior to the ligamentum teres and runs posteriorly to the confluence of the left hepatic vein and the inferior vena cava. The left hepatic vein lies within this scissura. The superior (called anterior or medial by some) sector is divided by the umbilical fissure into segment IV medially and segment III laterally. Segment II alone forms the posterior sector. Functionally, the caudate or Spigel lobe (segment I) is considered an autonomous segment.

9.2 CLASSIFICATION OF HEPATECTOMIES

The classification of the various types of liver resection in the literature can be confusing. This arose because of the confusing nomenclature based on the work of Couinaud (1957), Healey and Schroy (1953) and Goldsmith and Woodburne (1957). The more common major resections include right hepatectomy, left hepatectomy, right lobectomy (or right trisegmentectomy), left lobectomy (or left lateral segmentectomy) and extended left hepatectomy (or left hepatic trisegmentectomy). The confusion in terminology arose because the liver can be divided into right and left lobes based on anatomical markings, physiological divisions of the liver and the nomenclature accorded by Couinaud, Healey and Schroy, and Goldsmith and Woodburne (Fig. 9.4, Table 9.1). For example, the term trisegmentectomy was coined by Starzl *et al.* (1980, 1982) and the term right trisegmentectomy is commonly used in the literature. However, this operation, which involves the removal of Couinaud segments IV–VIII, has been called extended right lobectomy (Goldsmith and Woodburne,

HEPATECTOMY

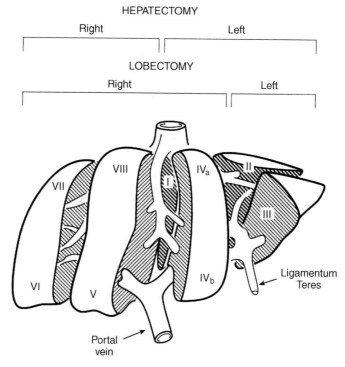

Fig. 9.4 Exploded view of the eight Couinaud's segments and the more common nomenclature of liver resections.

Table 9.1 Nomenclature of major liver resections.

Liver segments	*Couinaud (1957)*	*Goldsmith and Woodburne (1957)*
V, VI, VII, VIII	Right hepatectomy	Right hepatic lobectomy
II, III, IV	Left hepatectomy	Left hepatic lobectomy
IV, V, VI, VII, VIII +/− I	Right lobectomy (≡ right trisegmentectomy)	Extended right hepatic lobectomy
II, III	Left lobectomy	Left lateral segmentectomy
II, III, IV, V, VIII	Extended left hepatectomy (≡ left hepatic trisegmentectomy)	Extended left lobectomy

1957), right lobectomy (Bismuth, 1982) and right trisectorectomy (Scheele and Stangl, 1994) by others. Based on the nomenclature of Healey and Schroy, trisegmentectomy is correct and trisectorectomy is equally appropriate if Couinaud's classification is adopted! The confusing state of the nomenclature of hepatic resections and associated anatomic terms has been reviewed by Strasberg (1997) who proposed a more logical and less confusing way of naming hepatic structures and resections.

Isolated resection of one of the eight segments of the liver is called a segmentectomy: unisegmentectomy when one segment is removed, bisegmentectomy when two segments are removed and plurisegmentectomy when three or more segments are removed. Segmentectomies allow anatomical resection of liver lesions without sacrificing large amount of non-involved liver parenchyma. They are particularly useful in the removal of small central hepatomas, hepatomas situated at the periphery and for liver resections in cirrhotics (Bismuth *et al.*, 1982; Lau, in press). Theoretically segmentectomy I (excision of segment I/Spigel lobe) can be performed for isolated HCC situated in segment I but to gain access to this rather inaccessible segment, its resection is usually preceded by a left lobectomy (excision of segment II and III) (Ton, 1979; Bismuth *et al.*, 1982) or an excision of segment IV (Launois and Jamieson, 1993).

Uni- or bisegmentectomy performed on a normal liver is considered by many a minor resection and removing the entire lobe of the liver is a major resection. However, many factors determine what type of liver resection is a 'major' or 'minor'. Isolated resection of segment VIII is technically more difficult and challenging than resecting segments II and III and it can be associated with significantly more blood loss during liver transection. Performing a unisegmentectomy in a small, shrunken cirrhotic liver is a major undertaking as it is associated with a substantial risk of intra- and postoperative bleeding and the development of postoperative liver failure. Depending on the circumstances, what is a minor liver resection to one patient can be a major resection to another.

9.3 PREOPERATIVE INVESTIGATIONS

Preoperative investigations help to confirm or refute the diagnosis of hepatocellular carcinoma, to determine the extent of local disease and any evidence of distant spread, and to assess the general status of and operative risk to the patient. These investigations also form a baseline for subsequent management.

9.3.1 DIAGNOSIS

The true nature of the suspicious hepatic lesion in patients with a non-diagnostic α-fetal protein (AFP) level can be confirmed by percutaneous needle biopsy prior to resection. Hemorrhage and tumor rupture are possible complications of the biopsy procedure. We are concerned with the small but definite risk of tumor seeding in the biopsy needle tract, and transient bleeding from the needle tract can potentially allow the escape of malignant cells into the peritoneal cavity (Leow and Lau, 1997). In a comparative study on the efficacy of cytological versus microhistological diagnosis of hepatocellular carcinoma on fine-needle biopsy specimens, Caturelli *et al.* (1996) demonstrated that smear cytology yielded a much higher percentage of correct diagnosis compared to microhistology (85.6 versus 66.1%). This provides further evidence that seeding of malignant cells is a definite possibility. In the presence of a space-occupying lesion, positive serology for hepatitis B infection and a suspicious angiogram, we would proceed to surgical exploration even if the serum AFP level is normal/non-diagnostic. Based on this approach, all 11 specimens removed from patients with a clinical diagnosis of HCC but with normal/non-diagnostic AFP levels had HCC on histologic examination (Leow and Lau, 1997). We would only perform liver biopsy prior to exploration if the biopsy result would alter our management.

9.3.2 EXTENT OF LOCAL AND DISTANT DISEASE

Patients who are deemed to have an operable hepatocellular lesion on the initial ultrasound scan and with no evidence of lung metastasis on the chest X-ray are subjected to hepatic angiography and computed tomography (CT) prior to resection. We do not perform isotope bone scan, CT of the brain and thorax prior to resection because the diagnostic yield is low.

In the presence of distant metastases, the prognosis is poor despite liver resection. Although Fortner *et al.* (1978) do not advocate hepatic angiography, we, like others (Williamson *et al.*, 1980; Voyles *et al.*, 1983), have found it invaluable in providing a 'road map' of the vasculature of the liver prior to undertaking liver resection. In our experience, approximately 30–40% of patients have angiographic evidence of hepatic vasculature anomalies. A prior knowledge of the vascular anatomy will facilitate dissection at surgery. In addition, if the radiologist has any doubt about the initial lesion, or is suspicious of the presence of other intrahepatic lesions during angiography, he can inject lipiodol at the same session and perform a subsequent day 10 postlipiodol CT of the liver. CT scans provide information on the site and size of the lesion, and its relationship to the portal vessels. Size of the tumor alone is not a contraindication to resection (Adson and Weiland, 1981; Starzl *et al.*, 1982; Okamoto *et al.*, 1984a). Of greater importance to surgeons operating on a cirrhotic liver is the information a CT scan provides on the size of the whole liver and the amount of liver tissue that can be left behind after resection. Diaphragmatic involvement is not a contraindication to resection (Foster and Berman, 1977; Lau *et al.*, 1995). Equally, involvement of adjacent organs, such as the stomach and the colon, is not an absolute contraindication to resection, provided an *en bloc* resection can be achieved.

9.3.3   ASSESSMENT OF THE GENERAL CONDITION OF THE PATIENT

In addition to the radiological investigations stated above, all patients about to undergo liver resection must have a chest X-ray, full blood count, liver and renal function tests, full clotting profile and cross matching. It is routine to perform cardiopulmonary assessment in all patients over the age of 65 years.

9.4   ASSESSING THE RISK TO THE PATIENT

The prevalence of cirrhosis in patients with HCC ranges from 60 to 90% (Kew and Popper, 1984). Although surgery is widely acknowledged as the treatment of choice for HCC, the degree and extent of surgical resectability are limited by the underlying cirrhosis which is intrinsically associated with reduced functional liver reserve and depressed hepatic regenerative capacity.

One of the major risks of liver resection is hemorrhage from the hepatic wound edge, branches of the vessels at the porta hepatis and the hepatic veins or inferior vena cava posteriorly. The risk of hemorrhage in cirrhotic patients is compounded by the presence of portal hypertension, thrombocytopenia and derangement of clotting functions. Measurement of the hepatic-dependent plasma clotting factors gives the surgeon a useful and precise appreciation of the underlying hepatic synthetic functions (Koller, 1973). In our experience with cirrhotic patients, a platelet count < 50 and a prolonged prothrombin time > 4s over control is associated with an adverse outcome following liver resection. An isolated platelet count < 50 or prolonged prothrombin time > 4s over control would not necessarily deter us from proceeding with hepatic resection (Lau *et al.*, 1996). However, we would decline surgical intervention in patients with both abnormalities.

The other major risk of liver resection is the development of postoperative liver insufficiency, failure and death. To improve patient survival and decrease the risk of developing liver failure following liver resection, especially in cirrhotics, it is necessary to have a reliable method or methods for assessing liver function and reserve. However, evaluating the preoperative liver function with a view to predicting functional reserve following liver resection is an imprecise science. Clinical experience has shown that resection of > 80% of functional liver parenchyma in a normal liver is associated with a risk of severe liver insufficiency (Bismuth *et al.*, 1983). A minor resection in a cirrhotic patient with intrinsic impairment of liver function can lead to severe postresection liver insufficiency due to the poor functional liver reserve and the impaired regenerative response of the cirrhotic liver to surgical insults (Nagasue *et al.*, 1987, 1993; Takenaka *et al.*, 1990; Tanabe *et al.*, 1995; Vauthey *et al.*, 1995).

In a retrospective analysis of 108 Child–Pugh class A cirrhotic patients who underwent resection of an underlying hepatocellular carcinoma, Noun *et al.* (1997) found that preoperative serum alanine aminotransferase (ALT) level is a reliable predictor of in-hospital mortality and morbidity. Patients with serum ALT levels less than twice the normal limit (2N) had an in-hospital mortality rate of 3.8% compared with 19.3% ($p = 0.008$) of those with a serum ALT level > 2N. Equally, the incidence of postoperative massive ascites (58 versus 38%, $p = 0.01$), renal failure (16 versus 0%, $p = 0.0003$) and upper gastrointestinal hemorrhage (6.4 versus 0%, $p = 0.02$) were higher in patients with a serum ALT level > 2N. However, it is important to bear in mind that several previous reports had failed to find the preoperative ALT level a reliable independent prognostic factor (Okamoto *et al.*, 1984b; Takenaka *et al.*, 1990; Sitzmann and Greene, 1994; Tanabe *et al.*, 1995).

It has been suggested that the preoperative serum bilirubin level may be the single most important prognostic factor and Hasegawa *et al.*, (1987) have stated that no liver resection should be undertaken in patients with a twofold increase in serum bilirubin. In contrast, several investigators have found that the preoperative bilirubin level did not predict the development of liver failure following liver resection in their patients (Okamoto *et al.*, 1984b; Takenaka *et al.*, 1990).

In an attempt to find a satisfactory method for preoperative estimation of the extent of liver resection which will be tolerated by a patient with impaired liver function, Oka-moto *et al.* (1984b) found a close correlation between the CT volumetric measurements of the liver and tumor and the indocyanine green retention rate at 15 min (ICG R15). These measurements could predict the safe limit of hepatectomy and the development of posthepatectomy liver failure. Although others have also shown it to be useful (Hemming *et al.*, 1992), Takenaka *et al.* (1990) found ICG R15 to be unhelpful in predicting those patients who would develop liver failure following resection of the underlying hepatocellular carcinoma. In an attempt better to predict outcome postoperatively, Yamanaka *et al.* (1984) derived two regression equations using a combination of the age of patient, ICG R15 rate, maximal removal rate of ICG (ICG R_{max}) and parenchymal hepatic resection rate as variables. Another test of intrinsic hepatic function, the [^{14}C] aminopyrine breath test, a measure of hepatic microsomal function, has been shown to be of use in predicting the development of liver failure following various forms of elective surgery in patients with underlying impaired liver function (Gill *et al.*, 1983). The redox tolerance index (RTI), presumed to correlate with hepatic mitochondrial function, is derived from the hepatic ketone body ratio and changes in glucose levels after an oral glucose load. Although the investigators claimed that RTI was predictive of postoperative hepatic failure, 40 patients classified as being high risk of dying after liver resection did not succumb (Mori *et al.*, 1990).

The limitations of all these methods of assessing liver function to predict postoperative liver failure and death resides in our inability to accurately predict the functional liver reserve of the remnant liver which is a product of the balance between the supply of and demand on the liver function. Experimentally, the remnant normal liver regenerates to almost its original size following 70% hepatectomy in 7–14 days (Higgins and Anderson, 1931). Following an uncomplicated hemihepatectomy, the liver function is reduced by approximately 50% while the basal metabolic demand on the liver is increased secondary to the operative trauma. The difference between the remnant liver function and the increased metabolic demands is the functional liver reserve. Postoperatively, with the process of liver regeneration, the functional reserve recovers towards normality while the metabolic demands return to basal level. Although the liver function of a cirrhotic liver is compromised compared with a normal liver, the functional liver reserve following an uneventful hemi-hepatectomy is still adequate. The process of liver regeneration is impaired in cirrhotics, thus the recovery of liver function is prolonged and eventually may not return to its original level (Fig. 9.5). The more severe the underlying cirrhosis, the worse is the functional liver reserve. Removing a portion of a severely cirrhotic liver may leave an insufficient amount of parenchyma in the remnant liver to meet physiological demands. Furthermore, the remaining parenchyma may not function and/or regenerate as expected due to ischemic insults sustained during the Pringle's manuvre, periods of perioperative hypotension or because part of the remaining parenchyma has been devascularized. The impaired and inadequate 'supply' of liver function coupled with excessive metabolic demand due to sepsis, extensive tissue trauma and/or gastrointestinal hemorrhage from stress ulceration and varices thus lead to a state of 'negative' functional liver reserve (Fig. 9.6). Liver failure ensues and death occurs.

Using a point scoring system based on the levels of serum bilirubin, serum albumin, presence or absence of ascites and encephalopathy, and nutritional status, a classification system for hepatic functional reserve, named Child's classification, was created (Child and Turcotte, 1964). This system of classification was modified by Pugh *et al.* (1973). The Pugh–Child's classification indicates whether the cirrhotic liver is compensated (grade A), decompensating (grade B), or decompensated (grade C) and acts as a prognostic index. In our practice, we do not perform any test of the

intrinsic functional liver reserve but instead use the Pugh–Child's classification (Table 9.2) (Pugh *et al.*, 1973) to assess all our potential surgical candidates. We will offer surgical exploration and resection to all Pugh–Child's

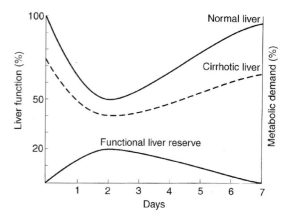

Fig. 9.5   Liver function – 'supply and demand'.

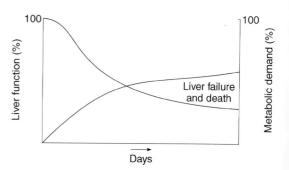

Fig. 9.6   Postresection liver failure.

Table 9.2   Pugh–Child's classification of hepatic functional reserve.

Score	1	2	3
Parameters			
Bilirubin (μmol/l)	<30	30–45	>45
Albumin (g/l)	>35	28–35	<28
Prothrombin time (seconds prolonged)	<4	4–6	>6
Ascites	none	slight	moderate
Encephalopathy	none	1–2	3–4

Grades A, 5–6; B, 7–9; C ≥ 10.

A and B patients; a position not unlike that of Franco *et al.* (1990) who stated that liver resection in patients with a Pugh's score > 8 is hazardous.

9.5   POSTOPERATIVE FOLLOW UP

The half life of AFP is 6 days. Postoperative measurement of AFP provides an indication of whether the underlying tumour has been completely excised. A slower than expected fall or static AFP level implies residual disease and a poor prognosis.

Following discharge, in the first 6 months, we review the patient at 2-weekly intervals with serial AFP measurements. Any patient who develops a rising trend in the AFP levels will be investigated by a chest X-ray and an abdominal ultrasound scan. A suspicious scan is followed by a hepatic angiogram and abdominal CT scan, which also allow assessment of re-resectability. Doubtful lesions are subjected to fine-needle biopsy for histological examination.

9.6   LIVER RESECTION

Detailed description of the techniques of performing liver resection is beyond the scope of this chapter. Our intentions are to highlight aspects of liver resection which we feel are of particular importance and relevance to surgeons with special reference to operating on cirrhotic livers.

9.6.1   INCISIONS

The bilateral subcostal incision with a midline vertical extension to the xiphoid process (also called a 'Mercedes–Benz incision') is the standard incision used by most surgeons. Other incisions used include a midline incision with a right thoracic extension, bilateral subcostal (also called a 'rooftop incision') with or without a right thoracic extension, right subcostal incision extending to the sternum medially and into the right flank laterally

(Sitzmann and Greene, 1994) and a transrectus incision (Ekberg *et al.*, 1986). We, like Launois and Jamieson (1993), believe that the use of the Mercedes–Benz incision will make it most unlikely that a surgeon will ever need to add a thoracic incision to the abdominal incision for liver resection. If there is doubt about resectability, a right subcostal incision is made initially to allow exploration of the abdomen. When the lesion is deemed resectable the incision is converted to a Mercedes–Benz incision.

Apart from the incision, intraoperative access to the liver is greatly enhanced by the retractors. The retractors routinely used include Brook's Water, Turner–Warwick and a paediatric miniretractor system (commonly known as the Omni retractor manufactured by Omnitrak Surgical Company, USA) but we prefer the Gray's retractor (designed by Professor Bruce Gray, Perth, Australia; manufactured by Pilling Wack, Australia). This retractor provides the ideal upwards, outwards and cephalad retraction of the costal margins which gives excellent exposure of the liver. As the retractor is attached to the operating table, the excellent exposure provided can be maintained for the duration of the operation.

9.6.2   MOBILIZATION OF THE LIVER

Franco and Borgonovo (1994) recommend that mobilization should be kept to the minimum to avoid blood and lymph spillage from the transected liver ligaments. Kanematsu *et al.* (1985) emphasized that the round ligament of the liver should only be sacrificed during left hepatectomy as the umbilical vein, if patent, provides portal blood diversion. We routinely divide the ligamentum teres and fully mobilize the relevant lobe of the liver by dividing the falciform, triangular and coronary ligaments. We believe adequate mobilization is paramount to the performance of a safe hepatectomy especially when operating on a cirrhotic liver. Troublesome bleeding from the cut edge of the ligaments has not been a problem in our experience. When performing a left lateral segmentectomy, we divide the falciform ligament closer to the abdominal and diaphragmatic side to leave a flap of ligament. Subsequently this can be sutured over the hepatic stump to provide added hemostasis especially in the presence of a cirrhotic liver with a moderate degree of portal hypertension.

9.6.3   INTRAOPERATIVE ULTRASOUND

Although there are no obvious landmarks on the liver surface to help surgeons to locate each segmental vessel and duct accurately, limited liver resection such as segmentectomy or bisegmentectomy can be performed successfully based on a good knowledge of the anatomy of the liver. The task of locating these structures is made significantly more difficult when the procedure is performed on a cirrhotic liver because the intrahepatic position of the vessels and duct can be grossly distorted by the underlying cirrhosis. Fortunately, the task of locating these structures is greatly enhanced by the advent of intraoperative ultrasound (IOUS) which can clearly demonstrate the portal and hepatic veins. IOUS can precisely identify the tumor relationship to the different segmental portal venous branches, to facilitate the delineation of the boundary of resection and to allow removal of entire tumor-bearing segment which is considered necessary for cure. Makuuchi *et al.* (1985) described their technique of 'systematic subsegmentectomy' whereby the portal unit containing the tumour is 'tattooed' by injecting patent blue into the portal vein supplying the area under ultrasound guidance. The area supplied by the corresponding vein becomes stained and the area marked with diathermy before transection. Another problem is that small hepatocellular carcinomas within a cirrhotic liver are frequently not visible and not palpable

(65% in one study) (Makuuchi *et al.*, 1987) and preoperative imaging by ultrasound (USS) and computed tomography (CT) may fail to pick up other lesions within the liver. In a series of 152 patients with hepatocellular carcinoma, IOUS detected 198 of 203 small hepatocellular carcinoma (99% sensitivity) while the sensitivity of preoperative USS, angiography and CT was 89.3, 84.1 and 89.6%, respectively. In addition IOUS detected 70% of tumour thrombi in the portal system whereas preoperative USS and angiography only revealed 21% of the cases (Makuuchi *et al.*, 1987). Of 77 patients who had preoperative USS, CT and hepatic angiography for hepatocellular carcinoma, IOUS provided additional information in 26 cases (33%) and in 21 cases the IOUS findings altered the intended surgical procedure (Bismuth *et al.*, 1987). Similarly, we have shown that IOUS altered the original surgery planned in 18% of cirrhotic patients (Lau *et al.*, 1993). We believe that the performance of IOUS prior to any liver resection is mandatory. We routinely use IOUS to mark the boundary of our resection margin. In cirrhotics, we aim for a 2 cm margin since the plane of transection will not be a straight line due to the presence of regenerative nodules of various sizes in the line of transection. This leads to a jagged plane of transection, where in some areas the distance of the transection margin to the tumor would be <2 cm, while in other areas the distance would be >2 cm. If initially a 1 cm margin was adopted, the distance of the transection margin to the tumor in some areas would definitely be <1 cm in the pathological specimen. (For significance of depth of resection margin see discussion on prognostic factors.)

9.6.4   ANATOMICAL VERSUS NON-ANATOMICAL RESECTION

As the dissemination of hepatocellular carcinoma occurs by retrograde invasion of distal portal branches (Makuuchi *et al.*, 1985), a curative resection must remove the entire parenchymal area (inclusive of the lesion) supplied by its main portal branch in order that any satellite nodules would be included in the specimen. Moreover, the lesion should be removed with an adequate tumor free margin of parenchyma to reduce or avoid the risk of early cancer recurrence (Franco *et al.*, 1990; Nagao *et al.*, 1990). An anatomical resection will achieve these considerations and by following anatomical planes, injuries to the major vessels and bile ducts can be avoided. Proponents of non-anatomical resection argue that parenchyma resection should be as limited as possible because of the risk of postoperative liver failure and portal hypertension, especially in the presence of cirrhosis. Indeed some authors state that major hepatic resection should not be performed in cirrhotic patients. Achieving an adequate margin while performing a non-anatomical resection may be easy in a normal liver but it can be difficult to achieve in a cirrhotic liver. Transecting the parenchyma outside anatomical planes carries the risk of injuring major blood vessels and bile ducts and more bleeding is encountered as one is transecting across, rather than along, vessels. Consequently, devascularized tissue and undrained liver segments will be left behind. There are occasions when non-anatomical resection is the only or better option, for example in the case of a small tumor at the junction of several segments in a small cirrhotic liver, or a small tumor at the periphery of the liver. In general, an anatomical resection is preferred when technically feasible. We fully endorse the approach of Bismuth (1982) who stated that 'the time when liver surgery was confined to atypical hepatectomies or wedge resections, according to location or volume of a lesion, belongs to the past'.

9.6.5 TRANSECTING THE LIVER AND VASCULAR CONTROL

Since the introduction of the finger-fracture technique by Lin *et al.* (1958) for transecting the liver parenchyma, other tools such as the haemostats (Ekberg *et al.*, 1986), Kelly clamp (Bismuth, 1982), suction knife (Almersjo and Hafstrom, 1974), Cavitron Ultrasonic Surgical Aspirator (CUSA) (Putnam, 1983), laser, microwave coagulator and water-jet dissector (Une *et al.*, 1989) have been used. We routinely employ the CUSA in conjunction with the diathermy forcep for transection. As the CUSA skeletonizes the vascular and biliary pedicles, the diathermy forceps, controlled by the assistant, is applied to the minor structures while larger structures are ligated. While some surgeons favor the use of absorbable clips, we do not use them because they can be dislodged accidentally during the course of liver transection.

The risk of developing intra- and postoperative complications for cirrhotic patients is increased by the amount of intraoperative bleeding (Nagasue *et al.*, 1985; Takenaka *et al.*, 1990). Several techniques have been described to reduce bleeding during liver transection. Temporary hepatic inflow arrest, also known as the 'Pringle maneuver' (Pringle, 1908), is a technique often used to decrease bleeding. The potential detrimental effect of the warm ischemic insult to the liver, especially for the cirrhotic liver, has given rise to two methods of temporary hepatic inflow arrest: intermittent clamping and continuous clamping. No harmful effects on postoperative liver function could be demonstrated when the portal triad in cirrhotic patients was continuously clamped for up to 32 min (Nagasue *et al.*, 1984). We do not routinely adopt the technique of intermittent declamping and reclamping during resection and, in our experience, a period of continuous clamping lasting up to 35 min is generally well tolerated by both cirrhotic and non-cirrhotic livers. A variation of the Pringle maneuver is selective portal venous occlusion under ultrasound guidance coupled with control of the corresponding branch of the hepatic artery at the hilum. This elegant 'selective Pringle maneuver' technique mandates superior expertise in interventional ultrasonography and can only be performed by a minority of liver surgeons (Shimamura *et al.*, 1986; Castaing *et al.*, 1989).

The Pringle maneuver stops portal and arterial inflows but does not prevent 'back-bleeding' from the hepatic veins. As a result, the technique of total vascular exclusion with cross-clamping of the infra- and suprahepatic inferior vena cava (IVC) was developed (Bismuth *et al.*, 1989). As this led to hemodynamic instability, Stephen *et al.* (1990) reported that cross-clamping the aorta and IVC essentially solved this hemodynamic problem. However, this method of total vascular exclusion is not without significant complications (Emre *et al.*, 1992). We practice the method of 'selective' and/or total vascular exclusion of the liver without vena cava and aortic clamping to avoid all the associated complications reported. To gain access to the right and right inferior hepatic veins, or the common trunk of the middle and left hepatic veins or to all hepatic veins, the liver is mobilized accordingly by dividing the relevant ligaments. The extrahepatic portion of the hepatic vein(s), before its/their insertion(s) into the suprahepatic vena cava, can be isolated sufficiently with a right-angle dissector for the application of the vascular clamp(s). Together with the Pringle maneuver, the selective application of vascular clamps to some or all hepatic veins allows partial or total vascular exclusion of the liver without the need of IVC and aortic clamping (Leow *et al.*, 1997).

Potential risk of severe bleeding while transecting the liver has led to the development of different approaches for hepatic vascular inflow and outflow control (Lau, 1997). During left or right hepatectomy, hilar vessels and bile ducts to the resected lobe can be ligated prior to transection of the liver parenchyma (preresection ligation, described by Lortat–Jacob and colleagues initially) or ligated during the course of parenchymal transection (direct parenchymal approach, first described by Ton That Tung). Preresection ligation is said to provide better control

and therefore less bleeding during parenchymal transection. However, it carries the risks of erroneous ligation of hilar vessels (Bismuth, 1982), partial denervation of the liver with the possible risk of increased bleeding (Kullendorff *et al.*, 1984), and inducing warm ischemia in the lobe or segment(s) of the liver to be resected, which in turn may have deleterious effects on the remnant liver (Almersjo *et al.*, 1971). In addition, the hepatic vein can be injured while attempting to control it prior to parenchymal transection.

The direct parenchymal approach allows ligation of the hepatic vein from inside the liver and the hilar vessels to be approached from above the hilum thus obviating the danger of inadvertent ligation of the vessels to the contralateral lobe, especially in the presence of anatomical abnormalities. Furthermore, the amount of liver parenchyma to be resected can be adjusted according to the nature and location of the lesion. Since there is no preliminary vascular control, intraoperative bleeding can be troublesome and temporary clamping of the porta hepatis (Pringle's maneuver) during the procedure is considered necessary by some surgeons. Although the type and rate of complications and the need for intraoperative blood transfusion was similar between the two approaches to isolate hilar structures, Ekberg *et al.* (1986) found that preresection ligation was associated with a significant increase in operative time compared with the direct parenchymal approach. Our practice is to combine the two approaches but to avoid the pitfalls. After gaining full control of the inflow and outflow of the liver as described above, we transect the parenchyma with the CUSA and approach the hepatic vein and hilar structures from within the liver, thus reducing bleeding from the cut surface and avoiding the inadvertent ligation of the structures to the contralateral lobe. Furthermore, not having to ligate the vascular and biliary pedicle at the porta hepatis prior to parenchymal transection will avoid the occasional troublesome bleeding encountered during dissection around the hilar plate in order to gain access to these hilar structures.

9.6.6 EXTENDING THE LIMITS OF RESECTION

A large tumor within a cirrhotic liver would preclude safe resection due to the underlying borderline liver function. By embolizing the tumor with transarterial chemoembolization, the tumor would undergo necrosis leading to reduced tumor bulk. At subsequent operation less non-involved liver parenchyma needs to be resected with the tumor, thus reducing the risk of postresection hepatic failure (Harada *et al.*, 1996). Instead of embolizing the artery, both Japanese and French surgeons embolized the supplying portal vein prior to resection. This allowed compensatory hypertrophy of the non-involved liver, allowing for safer hepatic resection subsequently (Azoulay *et al.*, 1995; Nagino *et al.*, 1996). Sitzman and Abrams (1993) combined preoperative chemotherapy (with doxorubicin and 5-fluorouracil) and radiation therapy (2100 cGy) to downstage initially inoperable HCCs followed by secondary resection. Half of their patients treated in this manner were still alive at 5 years. In a series of 72 patients with initially non-resectable HCC, Tang *et al.* (1995) managed to reduce the size of the tumor by 50% using a combination of hepatic artery ligation, hepatic artery cannulation with infusion of chemotherapeutic agents, radioimmunotherapy and fractionated regional radiotherapy. Five months after the initial treatment, a secondary resection was performed on these patients and the 5-year survival rate was 62.1%. Occasionally, non-resectable large tumors treated with selective internal radiation with yttrium-90 microspheres undergo necrosis, liquefaction and reduction in size. This, coupled with a compensatory hypertrophy of the contralateral lobe, has led to successful resection of the initially non-resectable tumor (Lau *et al.*, 1997).

The absence of the ipsilateral portal vein on USS and/or CT implies possible occlusion by tumor thrombus. We would still proceed to a formal hepatectomy provided that the contralateral portal vein is clear and there is no evidence of locoregional and distant spread. At operation, the involved portal vein is half-opened and the tumor thrombus is gently withdrawn while simultaneously releasing the clamp used for the Pringle maneuver. The gush of portal blood will help to dislodge the tumor thrombus and assist with the extraction – a process not unlike that of uncorking a bottle of champagne! Once removed, the proximal portal vein is clamped and the transection of the vein completed. The portal vein stump is then oversewn. Although these patients are at increased risk of having disseminated disease due to the spread of tumor cells into the portal bloodstream (Yamanaka *et al.*, 1992), in our experience, surgery with thrombus extraction provides better palliation and longer survival than treatment with chemotherapy.

Synchronous involvement of adjacent organs (e.g. diaphragm, stomach) and venous structures (e.g. portal vein, vena cava) (Sitzmann and Abrams, 1993) is not an absolute contraindication to resection. We have performed an *en-bloc* resection of the hepatoma together with the involved diaphragm in 14 patients. The 3- and 5-year survival rates of this group of patients was no different from those patients without diaphragmatic involvement (Lau *et al.*, 1995). Interestingly, histological examination of the diaphragm consistently revealed a substantial layer of fibroconnective tissue separating the diaphragm and the underlying hepatoma with no obvious evidence of direct invasion (Fig. 9.7). Despite this observation, we still resect the tumor with a cuff of the diaphragm as attempts to separate the attached diaphragm from the tumor can lead to bleeding, tumor rupture and tumor seeding into the peritoneal cavity.

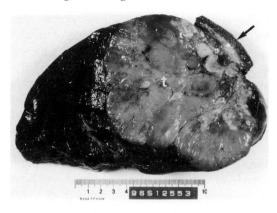 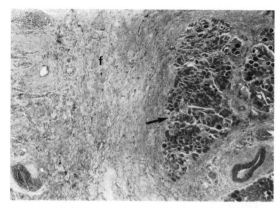

Fig. 9.7 Histological section of a hepatoma separated from the diaphragm by a layer of fibroconnective tissue. There is no evidence of direct tumor invasion of the diaphragm.

9.7 POSTOPERATIVE COMPLICATIONS

The overall morbidity rate in posthepatic resection cirrhotic patients is high. Most investigators have reported a complication rate <30% (Bismuth *et al.*, 1995, Nagasue *et al.*, 1986, 1993) but others have reported a rate as high as 50% (MacIntosh and Minuk, 1992). The overall incidence of postoperative complications in elderly patients (> 70 years old) is higher (Takenaka *et al.*, 1994). Significant complications include upper gastrointestinal

bleeding (peptic ulceration or mucosal erosions), postoperative bleeding, biliary leakage or fistulation, massive ascites, and liver failure (Table 9.3).

As a precaution against the development of acute mucosal erosions or stress ulceration, we routinely start all patients on prophylactic proton pump inhibitor treatment on the day of operation. Those who present with active peptic ulcer disease are treated with an intensive course of H_2 antagonist and undergo liver resection only when repeat gastroscopy shows

Table 9.3 Postoperative complications.

	Nagasue et al. (1986)	Nagasue et al. (1993)	Nagasue et al. (1993)	Takenaka et al. (1994)	Takenaka et al. (1994)	Bismuth et al. (1995)	Takenaka et al. (1996)	Fuster et al. (1996)
Number of cases	118	177[a]	52[b]	229[c]	39[d]	68[b]	280	48[a]
Upper GI bleed (%)	4.2	2.25	1.9	1	5	–	2	–
Postoperative bleeding (%)	3.4	4.5	1.9	3	8	1.5	4	–
Liver failure (%)	8.5	8.5	0	2	10	–	4	–
Biliary leak (%)	3.4	2.8	0	4	5	7.35	5	–
Massive ascites (%)	–	–	–	18	10	–	19	60
Pleural effusion (%)	–	–	–	25	21	–	24	–
Overall complications (%)	28	23.2	11.5	–	–	19	–	–

[a]Cirrhosis; [b]non-cirrhosis; [c]< 70 years old; [d]> 70 years old.

complete healing of the ulcer. Oesophageal variceal bleeding after liver resection is rare (0.4%) (Nagasue *et al.*, 1993) but it can be devastating. Although it has been demonstrated that portal pressure increased significantly after extensive liver resection, there was no correlation between the degree of portal pressure elevation and adverse patient outcome (Kanematsu *et al.*, 1985).

Cirrhotic patients with accompanying coagulopathy and portal hypertension are predisposed to bleeding during the perioperative period. Preoperatively, they should be given vitamin K and postoperatively coagulopathy should be corrected with fresh frozen plasma and platelets infusion. Postoperative bleeding from the hepatic stump is associated with a grave outcome in cirrhotic patients. This can be due to the high portal pressure dislodging a clot or due to a missed arterial bleeder which has been in spasm at the end of the liver resection. After oversewing all obvious bleeding points with 4/0 prolene and ensuring that only minimal oozing is present on the hepatic stump, we overlay the stump with Surgicel and take a mandatory 15-min tea/coffee break (Leow *et al.*, 1997). This not only prevents the surgeons from premature 'peeping' at and tampering with the hepatic wound, but also it allows any vascular spasm to pass, bleeding to recommence and thus permits the surgeon to detect and deal with it after the break.

Postoperative sepsis in the liver bed is not uncommon. The potential dead space permits blood and bile to collect and provides a good medium for bacterial growth. In addition, cirrhotic patients are more susceptible to infection. This is further aggravated by the diabetic state known to complicate cirrhosis.

Minor biliary leakage following hepatic resection can occur and is usually not problematic. The biliary leaks often seal spontaneously and require no intervention. Kohno *et al.* (1992) and Noun *et al.* (1996) demonstrated that the application of fibrin glue to the liver cut surface led to a reduction in bile leakage following liver resection. Biliary fistulation can result from inadequate ligation of the bile ducts at the liver cut surface but often follows sequestration and sloughing of areas of infected, necrotic liver tissue. The incidence of fistulation is much higher following resections involving or close to the liver hilum (Vaccaro *et al.*, 1991). Thompson *et al.* (1983) reported an 11% incidence of biliary fistulation following liver resection among 134 patients. The management of biliary fistulation is the establishment of a controlled fistula and the facilitation of drainage of bile internally by endoscopic means or externally via radiological intervention. Endoscopic sphincterotomy with or without stenting and nasobiliary drainage have been shown to be effective in treating biliary fistulation complicating liver surgery (Liguory *et al.*, 1991; Sherman *et al.*, 1992). Percutaneous transhepatic biliary drainage is another means of diverting the biliary secretion but the risk of hemorrhage complicating the procedure makes the endoscopic approach safer for cirrhotic patients.

Massive ascites complicating liver resection in the cirrhotic population is a significant problem. Apart from the respiratory embarrassment which it can cause, persistent leakage of ascitic fluid from the drain site or the main wound can be a potential source of bacterial contamination with the development of infected ascites and the development of peritonitis. Sodium and water restriction coupled with judicious use of diuretics may reduce the amount of ascites and prevent the development of ascitic fistula.

Sympathetic pleural effusion on the right side is common following hepatic resection. We routinely perform a chest X-ray on postoperative day 7 to check on the presence and size of the effusion. In most cases the effusion is small, asymptomatic and it can be treated expectantly. Thoracocentesis is only necessary when the patient is symptomatic or when the effusion is infected.

Hypoglycemic episodes tend to complicate patients who have had extensive liver resections or with underlying sepsis. As a preventive measure, some authors recommended giving hypocaloric glucose solutions for the first postoperative days (Vajrabukka *et al.*, 1975) while others advocated the infusion of 100 g glucose the night before surgery to replenish the glycogen store (Ekberg *et al.*, 1986). To guard against this potential complication, our normal practice postoperatively is to monitor the blood glucose level every 4 h for the first 48 h and to recommence the patient on a fluid diet on the first or second postoperative day.

In a non-cirrhotic liver, postresection liver insufficiency is rare except after massive liver resection. Although Monaco *et al.* (1964) have claimed success with 90% hepatectomy, in man, with minimal liver dysfunction, this is the exception rather than the rule. Liver insufficiency followed by liver failure is the most dreaded postoperative complication following the resection of a cirrhotic liver. The increased incidence of postoperative hepatic insufficiency in cirrhotics (Nagasue *et al.*, 1993) is a consequence of the pre-existing impaired liver function with poor reserve and the inefficient or absent regenerative process within the remnant liver (Bismuth *et al.*, 1982). Recent experimental studies have shown that the altered hemodynamics within the portal system following hepatectomy can lead to a relative increase in portal flow per unit of liver tissue (Hanna *et al.*, 1988; Kawasaki *et al.*, 1991). Once the portal flow exceeds the capacity of the remnant liver, flow injury to sinusoidal endothelial cells occurs and the Kupffer cells become activated with the liberation of inflammatory cytokines. The increased delivery of gut-derived endotoxin via the portal blood further activates the Kupffer cells with the release of tumor necrosis factor-α (TNF-α) and interleukin 6 (Cornell, 1985; Decker, 1990; Callery *et al.*, 1991). Recently, Panis *et al.* have demonstrated, in rat, the presence of progressive liver necrosis in the remnant liver after 85% hepatectomy and a concomitant massive elevation of serum TNF-α which is injurious to hepatocytes. Resection of the cirrhotic liver will inevitably lead to increased portal flow within an existing portal hypertensive state, activation of Kupffer cells followed by the liberation of the inflammatory cytokine TNF-α, which causes liver necrosis in the cirrhotic remnant liver.

Although derangement of postoperative serum bilirubin levels from the normal pattern has not been found to be a reliable early indicator of liver insufficiency in patients with normal liver (Ekberg *et al.*, 1986), a persistent but gradual rise in bilirubin level coupled with a worsening clotting profile in the presence of background cirrhosis should raise alarm bells. This tends to set in at 7–10 days after resection. A strenuous effort to identify an underlying septic focus must be undertaken and, if found, should be treated vigorously. Portal vein thrombosis following liver resection can occur. In their series of 229 liver resections, Nagasue *et al.* (1993) reported two cases (0.9%) of portal vein thrombosis and a single case of mesenteric artery thrombosis. Spontaneous portal vein thrombosis is a rare but recognized cause of sudden deterioration in liver function after liver resection. In those patients with no identifiable cause for deterioration in their liver function, their clinical state merely reflects insufficient liver parenchyma and insufficient liver reserve to maintain daily physiological demands. The only treatment option available then is supportive measures.

9.8 PROGNOSIS

The operative mortality ranges from 0.9 to 21%. The overall posthepatic resection survival figures range from 74.4 to 92.4% at 1 year, 51.3–78.9% at 3 years, 20–75.9% at 5 years and 19.4–26.4% at 10 years. However the disease-free survival figures are less and range from 68.6 to 80.2% at 1 year, 32.2–45.6% at 3 years, 29–58% at 5 years and 19.5% at 10 years (Table 9.4). Due to the increased frequency of tumor recurrence the disease-free survival figures in cirrhotics are worse than non-cirrhotics.

Table 9.4 Mortality and survival rates after liver resection.

	N (cirrhosis, %)	Operative mortality (%)	30-day mortality (%)	In-hospital mortality (%)	1 year (%) (disease free)	3 years (%)	5 years (%)	10 years (%)
Yamanaka (1990)	295 (79.5)	–	–	–	76	44	31	–
Sasaki (1992)	186[a]	–	–	–	–	–	44 (37)	–
Sasaki (1992)	57[b]	–	–	–	–	–	68 (58)	
Nagasue (1993)	229 (77)	–	7.0	10.5	79.8	51.3	26.4	19.4
Takenaka (1994)	229[c]	–	1.0	–	89.2 (80.2)	75.9 (45.6)	75.9 (30.4)	–
Takenaka (1994)	39[d]	–	5	–	87.4 (77.0)	70.3 (39.1)	51.6 (31.4)	–
Bismuth (1995)	68[b]	2.9	–	–	74.4 (70.5)	51.6 (42.8)	40.2 (33.4)	26.4 (19.5)
Kawasaki (1995)	112 (67.9)	0.9	–	1.8	92.4 (68.6)	78.9 (32.6)	–	–
Fuster (1996)	48 (100)	4.0	–	–	–	64	–	–
Takenaka (1996)	280 (52)	–	2.0	–	88 (78)	70 (41)	50 (29)	–
Nadig (1997)	71 (24)	21	–	–	–	–	20	–

[a]Cirrhosis; [b]non-cirrhosis; [c]< 70 years old; [d]> 70 years old.

Almost every parameter has been tested as a prognostic factor to predict long-term outcome. Factors such as age, tumor size (<5 versus >5 cm), presence of cirrhosis, vascular invasion (including portal and/or hepatic vein invasion, microvascular invasion), presence or absence of tumor capsule, degree of tumor differentiation, number of tumors, minor or major resection, involved or tumor-free resection margin and many others have been studied. On univariate analysis some investigators have been shown these factors to be related to outcome while others have not (Lehnert *et al.*, 1995). This confusing and conflicting state of affairs may be a statistical quirk of performing univariate analysis, which is affected by sample size, multiple testing and interrelated prognostic factors. Multivariate analysis produces more reliable data but this is still conflicting (Table 9.5).

While some surgeons recommend a 1 cm margin, others have suggested a margin >1 cm (Lau *et al.*, 1996). The 7-year survival rate was 100% when the surgical resection margin was 1 cm but it dropped to 25% when the margin was <1 cm. However, this observation is true only when the tumor size was <2 cm. With bigger lesions, a resection margin of ≤1 cm did not influence survival (Masutani *et al.*, 1994). The only factor which a liver surgeon can control is the resection margin. Most authors reporting on resection margin refer to the pathological margin and not the operative resection margin. In cirrhotic livers, we adopt a 2 cm operative resection margin (see above) while in the normal liver, a 1 cm margin is adequate.

Table 9.5 Multivariate analysis demonstrating the association of prognostic factors with survival after liver resection.

Prognostic factor	Positive association	No association
Size of tumor	Lehnert *et al.* (1995)	Yamanaka *et al.* (1990), Sugioka *et al.* (1993)
Cirrhosis	Iwatsuki *et al.* (1991)	Sugioka *et al.* (1993), Nagorney *et al.* (1989)
Infiltrative growth	Iwatsuki *et al.* (1991)	–
Vascular invasion	Yamanaka *et al.* (1990)	Iwatsuki *et al.* (1991), Ringe *et al.* (1991)
TNM stage	Ringe *et al.* (1991)	Iwatsuki *et al.* (1991)
Intrahepatic metastases	Yamanaka *et al.* (1990)	–
Multiple tumors	–	Iwatsuki *et al.* (1991), Ringe *et al.* (1991)
Capsule formation	Kim *et al.* (1992)	Iwatsuki *et al.* (1991), Sugioka *et al.* (1993)
Lymph node metastasis	–	Ringe *et al.* (1991), Nagorney *et al.* (1989)
Margin < 1 cm	Yamanaka *et al.* (1990), Sugioka *et al.* (1993), Lehnert *et al.* (1995)	Iwatsuki *et al.* (1991)

9.9 ADJUVANT THERAPY

Following 'curative' liver resection for HCC, 50–90% of postoperative death is due to recurrent disease (Friedman, 1983; Okuda *et al.*, 1985; Rustgi, 1988). Thus, any treatment which can decrease or delay the incidence of recurrence can dramatically improve the results of liver resection. Using a combination of hepatic lipiodolization (with doxorubicin and mitomycin C) and hepatic arterial 5-fluorouracil, Nonami *et al.* (1991) significantly improved the survival rate of 19 patients considered to be at high risk of developing recurrent disease following resection. Takenaka *et al.* (1995), in a prospective non-randomized study, compared the effect of orally administered chemotherapy and prophylactic lipiodolization (with epirubicin) in patients who have had hepatic resection against patients who had had resection alone. Although the disease-free survival rate of patients who underwent lipiodolization was significantly better than those treated with oral chemotherapy or surgery alone, the overall survival rate between the three groups of patients was not different. Instead of postoperative adjuvant treatment, Harada and colleagues (1996) routinely performed preoperative transarterial chemoembolization (TACE) prior to liver resection in an attempt to reduce the incidence of intrahepatic recurrence. In approximately half of those patients treated with TACE, the tumor size was reduced but just over half of these patients experienced significant TACE-related complications which significantly prolonged the interval between TACE and resection. Moreover, TACE did not alter the survival and disease-free survival rates when compared with those treated with resection alone. Based on the results of their animal studies which demonstrated that an acyclic retinoid, polyprenoic acid, inhibited chemically induced hepatocarcinogenesis in rats and spontaneous hepatomas in mice, Muto *et al.* (1996) randomly assigned patients, who had curative resection or percutaneous ethanol injection for hepatocellular carcinoma, to receive either polyprenoic acid or placebo for 12 months. After a median follow-up of 38 months, only 12 patients (27%) treated with polyprenoic acid compared with 22 placebo-treated patients (49%) developed recurrent or new hepatomas. The potential role of polyprenoic acid and other retinoid derivatives in the chemoprevention of hepatocellular carcinoma will require further and bigger randomized studies.

9.10 PALLIATIVE RESECTION

Inoperable HCC diagnosed at presentation or unexpectedly at laparotomy can be palliated with prolongation and an improved quality of life. In an attempt to improve the quality of life, palliative cytoreductive surgery was offered for symptomatic relief to 26 patients with inoperable hepatocellular carcinoma. Apart from providing excellent symptomatic relief to all patients, the median survival of these patients (10 months) was better than that in 26 control patients who received systemic chemotherapy (2.3 months) instead (Lau *et al.*, 1994). In an attempt to clarify the indications for palliative reduction surgery in patients with advanced disease, Yamamoto *et al.* (1997), using a remnant tumor index (RTI) for selecting suitable patients, demonstrated that palliative cytoreductive surgery can be efficacious since it led to a 1-year survival rate of 67% in patients with a RTI of <5.0.

Patients with unexpected multiple and/or bilobar disease at the time of surgery can be palliated with cryosurgery. Adam *et al.* (1997) using a combination of palliative resection and cryosurgery, demonstrated that at a mean follow-up of 16 months, none of the patients showed any evidence of recurrent disease. The cumulative survival at 24 months was 63% and two-thirds of the patients were disease-free. However the procedure of cryoablation is slow, frequently taking >4 h (Horton *et al.*, 1992). The maximal size of the lesion suitable for cryoablation is 5 cm in diameter (Leow *et al.*, 1996). Although it is now possible to place multiple cryoprobes into a much larger lesion to save time and allow treatment of lesions >5 cm in diameter, the amount of surrounding normal parenchyma destroyed is correspondingly more with an increased risk of precipitating liver insufficiency and failure, especially in patients with underlying cirrhosis.

The efficacy of intralesional ethanol injection for the treatment of hepatocellular carcinoma has been proven (Livraghi *et al.*, 1995) and can be used intraoperatively. It is easy to use, quick, cheap and effective. Microwave tissue coagulation is another form of interstitial treatment applied to induce tumor necrosis (Lau *et al.*, 1994; Hamazoe *et al.*, 1995).

9.11 LIVER TRANSPLANTATION FOR IRRESECTABLE HCC

There is consensus that whenever feasible liver resection is the treatment of choice for liver cancer (Farmer *et al.*, 1994; Kawarada *et al.*, 1994; Langer *et al.*, 1994). Despite better early recognition of those patients with subclinical HCC and the advances in surgical techniques which have led to an increase in the resection rate of otherwise non-resectable HCC (Huguet *et al.*, 1994; Jeng *et al.*, 1994; Pichlmayr *et al.*, 1994), most patients still present with irresectable tumors because of the underlying poor functional reserve (as in patients with cirrhotic liver) or anatomical restrictions such as interlobar or multiple bilobar disease. Indeed liver transplantation can provide a therapeutic answer to these cases but in most centers liver transplantation for HCC only accounts for ≤10% of all liver transplantations performed (Arnold *et al.*, 1988; Jenkins *et al.*, 1989; Pichlmayr *et al.*, 1995).

Two-thirds of the patients with hepatocellular carcinoma treated by liver transplantation have an underlying cirrhotic liver (Pichlmayr *et al.*, 1995; Selby *et al.*, 1995). The evidence on whether non-cirrhotic patients with hepatocellular carcinoma do better than their cirrhotic counterparts after liver transplantation is controversial. While O'Grady *et al.* (1988) observed better outcome in cirrhotic and Haug *et al.* (1992) in non-cirrhotic patients, Pichlmayr *et al.* (1995), in a much larger series, found no difference in survival rates between the two groups of patients.

The reported 1-, 3- and 5-year survival rates of liver transplantation for hepatocellular carcinoma are 40–80, 16–56 and 19.6–36% respectively (Table 9.6) (O'Grady *et al.*, 1988; Haug *et al.*, 1992; Moreno-Gonzales *et al.*, 1992; Pichlmayr *et al.*, 1992, 1995; Bismuth *et al.*, 1993; Chung *et al.*, 1994; Dalgic *et al.*, 1994; Selby *et al.*, 1995). Data from the Cincinatti Transplant Tumor Registry (Penn, 1991) indicated that best results are seen in patients with the fibrolamellar type of HCC and 'incidentoma' found within the explanted liver. The 1-, 3- and 5-year survival rates of transplanted patients with the fibrolamellar type of hepatocellular carcinoma were 72.9, 58.3 and 48.8% respectively (Pichlmayr *et al.*, 1995). Several investigators have shown a strong correlation between post-transplantation survival and International Union against Cancer (UICC) tumor stage of the ordinary HCC. Patients with stage I and II tumors have significantly better survival when compared with those with stages II and IV disease (Pichlmayr *et al.*, 1995; Selby *et al.*, 1995). In one series of 105 patients with HCC treated by liver transplantation, approximately 20% of patients with stage II disease had survived >5 years while there were only two (of 59 patients) 5-year survivors among those patients with stage IVa disease. These two patients had the fibrolamellar type of HCC. Of deaths among stage IVa patients,

64% was related to tumor recurrence compared with 5.3% among stage II patients (Selby *et al.*, 1995). In addition to the histological type and stage of disease, the presence of an involved margin, microscopic and/or macroscopic vascular invasion, and bilobar disease exerts a negative impact on survival (Selby *et al.*, 1995). The size of the tumor and the number of tumor nodules also adversely affect the prognosis. When the tumor is <3 cm in diameter with no more than two nodules, 83% of the patients survived 3 years. The 3-year survival rate falls to 44% if the tumor is >3 cm in diameter with three or more nodules present (Bismuth *et al.*, 1993).

The high incidence of recurrence, up to 65% (Farmer *et al.*, 1994), in the transplanted liver has led to the use of multimodality treatment approaches in an attempt to increase the 5-year survival rate. Cherqui *et al.* (1994) tried a combination of pretransplant chemoembolization with ethiodized oil, doxorubicin and gelatin sponge and one preoperative session of 5-Gy fraction radiotherapy with mithoxanthrone chemotherapy post-transplant for patients with advanced HCC. Using a neoadjuvant, intratransplant and post-transplant chemotherapy regime, Stone *et al.* (1993) achieved a tumor-free 3-year survival of 54% in a

Table 9.6   Liver transplantation for HCC–overall survival.

Reference	Number of patients	1 year	3 year	5 year
O'Grady *et al.* (1988)	50	~40%	–	–
Pichlmayr *et al.* (1992)	87	–	–	19.6%
Haug *et al.* (1992)	24	71%	42%	–
Moreno-Gonzalez *et al.* (1992)	12	80%	16%	–
Bismuth *et al.* (1993)	60	–	49%	–
Chung *et al.* (1994)	29	61%	46%	–
Dalgic *et al.* (1994)	39	56%	32%	26%
Selby *et al.* (1995)	105	66%	39%	36%
Pichlmayr *et al.* (1995)	78	49.9%	26.9%	22.5%
	36[a]	57.1%	31.0%	27.1%

[a]Non-cirrhotic patients.

group of 20 patients with HCC of which 11 had stage IV disease. Seventeen patients with HCC undergoing liver transplantation received 6 months of adjuvant chemotherapy of continuous infusions of 5-fluouracil and intermittent cisplatin and doxorubicin. When compared with a historical group of 27 patients without or with low-dose chemotherapy, the group treated with neoadjuvant chemotherapy fared better with a recurrence rate of 18 versus 37% and a 4-year survival rate of 61 versus 22% (Farmer *et al.*, 1994). In spite of these promising results, the question of when, i.e. pre-, intra-, post-transplant or a combination of all three stages, to commence adjuvant treatment remains unanswered.

9.12 CONCLUSIONS

Surgery on the normal liver is taxing but it becomes much more challenging when performed on a liver with cirrhosis. Although surgery is the only treatment which can cure, the high recurrence rate following liver resection suggests that surgical extirpation is not the complete answer. Other forms of treatment in conjunction with surgery are most likely necessary if we are striving to achieve truly long-term disease-free survival for our patients. Orthotopic liver transplantation (OLT) is an effective treatment for HCC found to be confined to the liver. It not only replaces the diseased liver with a normal one, prevents the development of a metachronous hepatoma within the remnant cirrhotic liver after resection, relieves portal hypertension and its related complications, but also it produces less operative mortality and morbidity than cirrhotic liver resection (Bismuth *et al.*, 1993). In fact OLT appears to be better for treating patients with a single tumor < 5 cm in diameter, or no more than two tumors of diameter < 3 cm or those with inoperable HCC because of the position of the lesion or insufficient liver reserve to withstand surgery (Bismuth *et al.*, 1993; Romani *et al.*, 1994). Novel antiviral drugs such as lamivudine or famciclovir have

been used to specifically inhibit hepatitis B replication and re-infection of the graft, thus improving the graft survival rate in these patients with underlying HBV infection. However, the recent discovery of drug-resistant viral mutants should temper our optimism (Grellier and Dusheiko, 1997). Perhaps we should pause and reflect on our enthusiasm since OLT is associated with a high recurrence rate (up to 65%) and a 5-year survival rate of only 19.6–36%. In addition to the associated morbidity and mortality of being immunosuppressed, OLT on average costs US$150 000 and is associated with an overall mortality rate of 13–32% (Farmer *et al.*, 1994). In the USA, there are >2000 patients with benign end-stage liver disease on the United Network for Organ Sharing (UNOS) list waiting for a suitable liver (Venook, 1994). In Asian countries liver resection is still the preferred method of treatment because of the high prevalence of hepatoma and the lack of cadaveric organs due to a cultural reluctance to consider and accept organ donations. Due to the shortage of suitable organ donors and the high cost of OLT, the impetus should be to find ways of detecting HCC at a stage early enough to permit curative resection without the fear of causing postoperative liver failure. We should also strive to gain insight into the cause and treatment of the impaired regenerative capability of the cirrhotic liver. This should take place in tandem with research in identifying the causes of recurrent HCC in the remnant liver and ways to prevent or delay such recurrence. Surgical intervention is but one of the many jigsaw pieces which makes up the complete clinical management picture of HCC in man.

REFERENCES

Adam, R., Akpiner, E., Johann, M. *et al.* (1997) Place of cryosurgery in the treatment of malignant liver tumors. *Annals of Surgery*, **225**, 39–50.

Adson, M., Weiland, L.H. (1981) Resection of primary solid hepatic tumors. *American Journal of Surgery*, **141**, 18–21.

Almersjo, O., Bengmark, S., Domellof, L. *et al.* (1971) Immediate effects of short-term hepatic and splanchnic ischemia in pigs. *American Journal of Surgery*, **122**, 91–4.

Almersjo, O. and Hafstrom, L. (1974) The 'suction knife'. A new device for dividing liver parenchyma. *Acta Chirurgica Scandinavica*, **140**, 581–3.

Arnold, J.C., O'Grady, J.G., Polson, R.J. *et al.* (1988) Liver transplantation for malignant disease: results in 93 consecutive patients. *Annals of Surgery*, **207**, 373–9.

Azoulay, D., Raccuia, J.S., Castaing, D. *et al.* (1995) Right portal vein embolization in preparation for major hepatic resection. *Journal of the American College of Surgeons*, **181**, 267–9.

Bismuth, H. (1982) Surgical anatomy and anatomical surgery of the liver. *World Journal of Surgery*, **6**, 3–9.

Bismuth, H., Castaing, D. and Garden, O.J. (1987) The use of operative ultrasound in surgery of primary liver tumors. *World Journal of Surgery*, **11**, 610–14.

Bismuth, H., Castaing, D. and Garden, O.J. (1989) Major hepatic resection under total vascular exclusion. *Annals of Surgery*, **210**, 13–19.

Bismuth, H., Chiche, L., Adam, R. *et al.* (1993) Liver resection versus transplantation for hepatocellular carcinoma in cirrhotic patients. *Annals of Surgery*, **218**, 145–51.

Bismuth, H., Chiche, L. and Castaing, D. (1995) Surgical treatment of hepatocellular carcinomas in non-cirrhotic liver: experience with 68 liver resections. *World Journal of Surgery*, **19**, 35–41.

Bismuth, H., Houssin, D. and Castaing, D. (1982) Major and minor segmentectomies 'reglees' in liver surgery. *World Journal of Surgery*, **6**, 10–24.

Bismuth, H., Houssin, D. and Mazmanian, G. (1983) Postoperative liver insufficiency; prevention and management. *World Journal of Surgery*, **7**, 505–10.

Callery, R.P., Mangino, M.J. and Flye, M.W. (1991) A biologic basis for limited Kupffer cell reactivity to portal-derived endotoxin. *Surgery*, **110**, 221–30.

Cantlie, J. (1897–98) On a new arrangement of the right and left lobes of the liver. *Journal of Anatomy and Physiology*, **32**, 4–9.

Castaing, D., Garden, O.J. and Bismuth, H. (1989) Segmental liver resection using ultrasound guided selective portal venous occlusion. *Annals of Surgery*, **210**, 20–3.

Caturelli, E., Bisceglia, M., Fusilli, S. *et al.* (1996) Cytological vs microhistological diagnosis of hepatocellular carcinoma. Comparative accuracies in the same fine-needle biopsy specimen. *Digestive Diseases and Sciences*, **41**, 2326–31.

Cherqui, D., Piedbois, P., Pierga, J.Y. *et al.* (1994) Multimodal adjuvant treatment and liver transplantation for advanced hepatocellular carcinoma. A pilot study. *Cancer*, **73**, 2721–6.

Child, C.G. and Turcotte, J.G. (1964) Surgery and portal hypertension, in *The Liver and Portal Hypertension* (ed. J.E. Dunphy), W.B., Saunders, Philadelphia, pp. 50–2.

Chung, S.W., Toth, J.L., Rezieg, M. *et al.* (1994) Liver transplantation for hepatocellular carcinoma. *American Journal of Surgery*, **167**, 317–21.

Cornell, R.P. (1985) Gut-derived endotoxin elicits hepatotrophic factor secretion for liver regeneration. *American Journal of Physiology*, **249**, R551–62.

Couinaud, C. (1954) Lobes et segments hepatiques: notes sur l'architecture anatomique et chirurgicale du foie. *Presse Medicale*, **62**, 709–12.

Couinaud, C. (1957) Le foie. *Etudes anatomiques et chirurgicales*, Masson, Paris.

Dalgic, A., Mirza, D.F., Gunson, B.K. *et al.* (1994) Role of total hepatectomy and transplantation in hepatocellular carcinoma. *Transplantation Proceedings*, **26**, 3564–5.

Decker, K. (1990) Biologically active products of stimulated liver macrophages (Kupffer cells). *European Journal of Biochemistry*, **192**, 245–61.

Ekberg, H., Tranberg, K.G., Andersson, R. *et al.* (1986) Major liver resection: perioperative course and management. *Surgery*, **100**, 1–8.

Emre, S., Schwartz, M.D., Katz, E. *et al.* (1992) Liver resection under total vascular isolation. Variations on a theme. *American Surgeon*, **217**, 11–19.

Farmer, D.G., Rosove, M.H., Shaked, A. *et al.* (1994) Current treatment modalities for hepatocellular carcinoma. *Annals of Surgery*, **219**, 236–47.

Fortner, J.S., Kim, D.K., Maclean, B.J. *et al.* (1978) Major hepatic resection for neoplasia: personal experience in 108 patients. *Annals of Surgery*, **188**, 363–71.

Foster, J.H. and Berman, M.M. (1977) Solid liver tumours, in *Major Problems in Clinical Surgery*, vol. 1. (ed. P. Ebert), W.B. Saunders, London, p. 342.

Franco, D. and Borgonovo, G. (1994) Liver resection in cirrhosis of the liver, in *Surgery of the Liver and Biliary Tract*, vol. 2. (ed. L.H. Blumgart), Churchill Livingstone, Edinburgh, pp. 1539–55.

Franco, D., Capussotti, L., Smadja, C. *et al.* (1990) Resection of hepatocellular carcinoma: results in 72 European patients with cirrhosis. *Gastroenterology*, **98**, 733–8.

Friedman, M. (1983) Primary hepatocellular cancer: present results and future prospects. *International Journal of Radiation Oncology, Biology, Physics*, **9**, 1841–50.

Fuster, J., Garcia-Valdecasas, J.C., Grande, L. *et al.* (1996) Hepatocellular carcinoma and cirrhosis. Result of surgical treatment in a European series. *Annals of Surgery*, **223**, 297-302.

Gill, R.A., Goodman, M.W., Golfus, G.R. *et al.* (1983) Aminopyrine breath test predicts surgical risk for patients with liver disease. *Annals of Surgery*, **198**, 701–4.

Goldsmith, N.A. and Woodburne, R.T. (1957) The surgical anatomy pertaining to liver resection. *Surgery, Gynecology and Obstetrics*, **105**, 310–18.

Grellier, L. and Dusheiko, G.M. (1997) Hepatitis B virus and liver transplantation: concepts in antiviral prophylaxis. *Journal of Viral Hepatitis*, **4 (Suppl. 1)**, 111–16.

Hamazoe, R., Hirooka, Y., Ohtani, S. *et al.* (1995) Intraoperative microwave tissue coagulation as treatment for patients with nonresectable hepatocellular carcinoma. *Cancer*, **75**, 794–800.

Hanna, S.S., Pagliarello, G. and Ing, A. (1988) Liver blood flow after major hepatic resection. *Canadian Journal of Surgery*, **31**, 363–7.

Harada, T., Matsuo, K., Inoue, T. *et al.* (1996) Is preoperative hepatic arterial chemoembolization safe and effective for hepatocellular carcinoma? *Annals of Surgery*, **224**, 4–9.

Hasegawa, H., Yamazaki, S., Makuuchi, M. *et al.* (1987) Hepatectomies pour hepatocarcinome sur foie cirrhotique: schemas decisionnels et principes de reanimation peri-operatoire. Experience de 204 cas. *Journal de Chirurgie*, **124**, 425–31.

Haug, C.E., Jenkins, R.L., Rohrer, R.J. *et al.* (1992) Liver transplantation for primary hepatic cancer. *Transplantation*, **53**, 376–82.

Healey, J.E., Jr. and Schroy, P.C. (1953) Anatomy of biliary ducts within human liver: analysis of prevailing pattern of branchings and major variations of biliary ducts. *Archives of Surgery*, **66**, 599–616.

Hemming, A.W., Scudamore, C.H., Schackleton, C.R. *et al.* (1992) Indocyanine green clearance as a predictor of successful hepatic resection in cirrhotic patients. *American Journal of Surgery*, **163**, 515–18.

Higgins, G.M. and Anderson, R.M. (1931) Experimental pathology of the liver. I. Restoration of the liver of the white rat following partial surgical removal. *Archives of Pathology*, **12**, 186–202.

Horton, M.D.A., Warlters, A., Dilley, A.V. *et al.* (1992) Survival after hepatic cryotherapy for hepatic metastases. *British Journal of Surgery*, **79**, 452.

Huguet, C., Gavelli, A. and Bona, S. (1994) Hepatic resection with ischemia of the liver exceeding one hour. *Journal of the American College of Surgeons*, **178**, 454–8.

Iwatsuki, S., Starzl, T., Sheahan, D.G. *et al.* (1991) Hepatic resection versus transplantation for hepatocellular carcinoma. *Annals of Surgery*, **214**, 221–8.

Jeng, K.S., Chen, B.F. and Lin, H.J. (1994) En bloc resection for extensive hepatocellular carcinoma: is it advisable? *World Journal of Surgery*, **18**, 834–9.

Jenkins, R.L., Pinson, C.W. and Stone, M.D. (1989) Experience with transplantation in the treatment of liver cancer. *Cancer Chemotherapy and Pharmacology*, **23 (Suppl.)**, 104–9.

Kanematsu, T., Takenaka, K., Furata, T. *et al.* (1985) Acute portal hypertension associated with liver resection: analysis of early post-operative death. *Archives of Surgery*, **120**, 1303–5.

Kawarda, Y., Ito, F., Sakurai, H. *et al.* (1994) Surgical treatment of hepatocellular carcinoma. *Cancer Chemotherapy and Pharmacololgy*, **33 (Suppl.)**, S12–17.

Kawasaki, S., Makuuchi, M., Miyagawa, S. *et al.* (1995) Results of hepatic resection for hepatocellular carcinoma. *World Journal of Surgery*, **19**, 31–4

Kew, M.C. and Popper, H. (1984) Relationship between hepatocellualr carcinoma and cirrhosis. *Seminars in Liver Disease*, **4**, 136–46.

Kim, S.T., Kim, P.H. and Noh, D.Y. (1992) Prognostic factors in surgical patients with hepatocellular carcinoma, in *Primary Liver Cancer in Japan*, (eds Tobe *et al.*), Springer, Tokyo, pp. 421–6.

Kohno, H., Nagasue, N., Chang, Y.C. *et al.* (1992) Comparison of topical hemostatic agents in elective hepatic resection: a clinical prospective randomized trial. *World Journal of Surgery*, **16**, 966–70.

Koller, F. (1973) Theory and experience behind the use of coagulation tests in diagnosis and prognosis of liver disease. *Scandinavian Journal of Gastroenterology*, **19 (Suppl.)**, 51–61.

Kullendorff, C.M., Zoucas, E., Lindfeldt, J. *et al.* (1984) Excessive bleeding at hepatic resection after experimental liver denervation. *World Journal of Surgery*, **8**, 123–8

Langer, B., Greig, P.D. and Taylor, B.R. (1994) Surgical resection and transplantation for hepatocellular carcinoma. *Cancer Treatment Research*, **69**, 231–40.

Lau, W.Y. (1997) The history of liver surgery. *Journal of The Royal College of Surgeons of Edinburgh*, **42**, 303–9.

Lau, W.Y., Leow, C.K. and Li, A.K.C. (1996) Hepatocellular carcinoma–current management and treatment. *GI Cancer*, **2**, 35–42.

Lau, W.Y., Leow, C.K. and Li, A.K.C. (1997) Hepatocellular carcinoma. *British Journal of Hospital Medicine*, **57**, 101–4.

Lau, W.Y., Leung, K.L., Lee, T.W. and Li, A.K.C. (1993) Ultrasonography during liver resection for hepatocellular carcinoma. *British Journal of Surgery*, **80**, 493–4.

Lau, W.Y., Leung, K.L., Leung, T.W.T. *et al.* (1995) Resection of hepatocellular carcinoma with diaphragmatic invasion. *British Journal of Surgery*, **82**, 264–6.

Launois, B. and Jamieson, G.G. (1993) *Modern Operative Techniques in Liver Surgery*, Churchill Livingstone, Edinburgh.

Lehnert, T., Otto, G. and Herfarth, C. (1995) Therapeutic modalities and prognostic factors for primary and secondary tumors. *World Journal of Surgery*, **19**, 252–63.

Leow, C.K. and Lau, W.Y. (1997) Diagnosis of HCC. *Digestive Diseases and Sciences*, **42**, 2033–4.

Leow, C.K., Lau, W.Y. and Li, A.K.C. (1997) Hepatic resection with vascular isolation and routine supraceliac aortic clamping. *American Journal of Surgery*, **173**, 149.

Liguory, C., Vitale, G.C., Lefebre, F. *et al.* (1991) Endoscopic treatment of postoperative biliary fistulae. *Surgery*, **110**, 779–84.

Lin, T.Y., Hsu, K.Y., Hsieh, C.M. *et al.* (1958) Study on lobectomy of the liver; a new technical suggestion on hemihepatectomy and reports of three cases of primary hepatoma treated with total left lobectomy of the liver. *Journal of the Formosan Medical Association*, **57**, 742–59.

Livraghi, T., Lazzaroni, S., Meloni, F. *et al.* (1995) Intralesional ethanol in the treatment of unresectable liver cancer. *World Journal of Surgery*, **19**, 801–6.

MacIntosh, E.L. and Minuk, G.Y. (1992) Hepatic resection in patients with cirrhosis and hepatocellular carcinoma. *Surgery, Gynecology and Obstetrics*, **174**, 245–54.

Makuuchi, M., Hasegawa, H. and Yamazaki, S. (1985) Ultrasonically guided subsegmentectomy. *Surgery, Gynecology and Obstetrics*, **161**, 346–50.

Makuuchi, M., Hasegawa, H., Yamazaki, S. *et al.* (1987) The use of operative ultrasound as an aid to liver resection in patients with hepatocellular carcinoma. *World Journal of Surgery*, **11**, 615–21.

Masutani, S., Sasaki, Y., Imaoka, S. *et al.* (1994) The prognostic significance of surgical margin in liver resection of patietns with hepatocellular carcinoma. *Archives of Surgery*, **129**, 1025–30.

Monaco, A.P., Halgrimson, J. and McDermott, W.V. (1964) Multiple adenoma (hamartoma) of the liver treated by subtotal (90%) resection: morphological and fuctional studies of regeneration. *Annals of Surgery*, **159**, 513–19.

Moreno-Gonzalez, E.M., Gomez, R., Garcia, I. *et al.* (1992) Liver transplantation in malignant hepatic neoplasms. *American Journal of Surgery*, **163**, 395–400.

Mori, K., Ozawa, K., Yamamoto, Y. *et al.* (1990) Response of hepatic mitochondrial redox tolerance test as a new prediction of surgical risk in hepatectomy. *Annals of Surgery*, **211**, 438–46.

Muto, Y., Moriwaki, H., Ninomiya, M. *et al.* (1996) Prevention of second primary tumors by an acyclic retinoid, polyprenoic acid, in patients with hepatocellular carcinoma. *New England Journal of Medicine*, **334**, 1561–7.

Nadig, D.E., Wade, J.P., Fairchild, R.B., Virgo, K.S. and Johnson, F.E. (1997) Major hepatic reszection. Indications and results in a national hospital system from 1988 to 1992. *Archives of Surgery*, **132**, 115–9.

Nagao, T., Inoue, S., Yoshimi, F. *et al.* (1990) Postoperative recurrence of hepatocellular carcinoma. *Annals of Surgery*, **211**, 28–33.

Nagasue, N., Yukaya H., Ogawa, Y. *et al.* (1986) Clinical experience with 118 hepatic resections for hepatocellular carcinoma. *Surgery*, **99**, 664–70.

Nagasue, N., Kohno, H., Chang, Y.C. *et al.* (1993) Liver resection for hepatocellular carcinoma. Results of 229 consecutive patients during 11 years. *Annals of Surgery*, **217**, 375–84.

Nagasue, N., Yukaya, H., Ogawa, Y. *et al.* (1987) Human liver regeneration after major hepatic resection. A study of normal liver and livers with chronic hepatitis and cirrhosis. *Annals of Surgery*, **206**, 30–9.

Nagasue, N., Yukaya, H., Ogawa, Y. *et al.* (1985) Segmental and subsegmental resections of the cirrhotic liver under hepatic inflow and outflow occlusion. *British Journal of Surgery*, **72**, 565–8.

Nagasue, N., Yukaya, H., Suehiro, S. *et al.* (1984) Tolerance of the cirrhotic liver to normothermic ischaemia. A clinical study of 15 patients. *American Journal of Surgery*, **147**, 772–5.

Nagino, M., Nimura, Y., Kamiya, J. *et al.* (1996) Selective percutaneous transhepatic embolization of the portal vein in preparation for extensive liver resection: the ipsilateral approach. *Radiology*, **200**, 559–63.

Nagorney, D.M., van Heerden, J.A., Ilstrup, D.M. *et al.* (1989) Primary hepatic malignancy: surgical management and determinants of survival. *Surgery*, **106**, 740–8.

Nonami, T., Isshiki, K., Katoh, H. *et al.* (1991) The potential role of postoperative hepatic artery chemotherapy in patients with high-risk hepatomas. *Annals of Surgery*, **213**, 222–6.

Noun, R., Elias, D., Balladur, P. *et al.* (1996) Fibrin glue effectiveness and tolerance after elective liver resection: a randomized trial. *Hepatogastroenterology*, **43**, 221–4.

Noun, R., Jagot, P., Farges, O. *et al.* (1997) High preoperative serum alanine transferase levels: effect on the risk of liver resection in child grade A cirrhotic patients. *World Journal of Surgery*, **21**, 390–4.

O'Grady, J.G., Polson, R.J., Rolles, K. *et al.* (1988) Liver transplantation for malignant disease. Results in 93 consecutive patients. *Annals of Surgery*, **207**, 373–9.

Okamoto, E., Kyo, A., Yamanaka, N. *et al.* (1984b) Prediction of the safe limits of hepatectomy by combined volumetric and functional measurements in patients with impaired hepatic function. *Surgery*, **95**, 586–92.

Okamoto, E., Tanaka, N., Vamanaka, N. *et al.* (1984a) Result of surgical treatments of primary hepatocellular carcinoma. Some aspects to improve long–term survival. *World Journal of Surgery*, **8**, 360–6.

Okuda, K., Ohtsuki, T., Obata, H. *et al.* (1985) Natural history of hepatocellular carcinoma and prognosis in relation to treatment: study of 850 patients. *Cancer*, **56**, 918–28.

Panis, Y., McMullan, M.D. and Emond, J.C. (1997) Progressive necrosis after hepatectomy and the pathophysiology of liver failure after massive resection. *Surgery*, **121**, 142–9.

Penn I. (1991) Hepatic transplantation for primary and metastatic cancers of the liver. *Surgery*, **110**, 726–34.

Pichlmayr, R., Weimann, A., Lamesch, P. *et al.* (1994) Liver transplantation for hepatocellular carcinoma and additional reference to bench surgery. *Journal of Hepatic, Biliary and Pancreatic Surgery*, **2**, 133.

Pichlmayr, R., Weimann, A., Oldhafer, K.J. *et al.* (1995) Role of liver transplantation in the treatment of unresectable liver cancer. *World Journal of Surgery*, **19**, 807–13.

Pichlmayr, R., Weimann, A., Steinhoff, G. *et al.* (1992) Liver transplantation for hepatocellular carcinoma: clinical results and future aspects. *Cancer Chemotherapy and Pharmacology*, **31 (Suppl. 1)**, S157–61.

Pringle, J.H. (1908) Notes on the arrest of hepatic hemorrhage due to trauma. *Annals of Surgery*, **48**, 541–9.

Pugh, R.N.H., Murray-Lyon, I.M., Dawson, J.L. *et al.* (1973) Transection of the oesophagus for bleeding oesophageal varices. *British Journal of Surgery*, **60**, 646–9.

Putnam, C.W. (1983) Techniques of ultrasonic dissection in resection of the liver. *Surgery, Gynecology and Obstetrics*, **157**, 475–8.

Ringe, B., Pichlmayr, R., Wittekind, C. *et al.* (1991) Surgical treatment of hepatocellular carcinoma: experience with liver resection and transplantation in 198 patients. *World Journal of Surgery*, **15**, 270–85.

Romani, F., Belli, L.S., Rondinara, G.F. *et al.* (1994) The role of transplantation in small hepatocellular carcinoma complicating cirrhosis of the liver. *Journal of The American College of Surgeons*, **178**, 379–84.

Rustgi, V.K. (1988) Epidemiology of hepatocellular carcinoma, in *Hepatocellular Carcinoma*. NIH conference (ed. A.M. Di Bisceglie), *Annals of Internal Medicine*, **108**, 390–401.

Sasaki, Y., Imaoka, S., Masutami, S. *et al.* (1992) Influence of coexisting cirrhosis on long-term prognosis after surgery in patients with hepatocellular carcinoma. *Surgery*, **112**, 515–21.

Scheele, J. and Stangl, R. (1994) Segment oriented anatomical liver resections. In: Surgery of the liver and biliary tract (ed. H. Blumgart) Churchill Livingstone, Edinburgh, pp. 1557–8.

Selby, R., Kadry, Z., Carr, B. *et al.* (1995) Liver transplantation for hepatocellular carcinoma. *World Journal of Surgery*, **19**, 53–8.

Sherman, S., Shaked, A., Cryer, H.M. *et al.* (1992) Endoscopic management of biliary fistulas complicating liver transplantation and other hepatobiliary operations. *Annals of Surgery*, **218**, 167–75.

Shimamura, Y., Gunven, P., Takenaka, Y. *et al.* (1986) Selective portal branch occlusion by balloon catheter during liver resection. *Surgery*, **100**, 938–41.

Sitzmann, J.V. and Abrams, R. (1993) Improved survival for hepatocellular cancer with combination surgery and multimodality treatment. *Annals of Surgery*, **217**, 149–54.

Sitzmann, J.V. and Greene, P.S. (1994) Perioperative predictors of morbidity following hepatic resection for neoplasm: a multivariate analysis of a single surgeon experience with 105 patients. *Annals of Surgery*, **219**, 13–17.

Starzl, T.E., Iwatsuki, S., Shaw, B.W. *et al.* (1982) Left hepatic trisegmentectomy. *Surgery, Gynecology and Obstetrics*, **155**, 21–7.

Starzl, T.E., Koep, L.J., Weil, R., III. *et al.* (1980) Right trisegmentectomy for hepatic neoplasms. *Surgery, Gynecology and Obstetrics*, **150**, 208–14.

Stephen, M.S., Sheil, A.G.R., Thompson, J.F. *et al.* (1990) Aortic occlusion and vascular isolation allowing avascular hepatic resection. *Archives of Surgery*, **125**, 1482–5.

Stone, M.J., Goran, B.G., Klintmalm, G. *et al.* (1993) Neoadjuvant chemotherapy and liver transplantation for hepatocellular carcinoma: a pilot study in 20 patients. *Gastroenterology*, **104**, 196–202.

Strasberg, S.M. (1997) Terminology of liver anatomy and liver resections: Coming to grips with hepatic babel. *Journal of the American College of Surgeons*, **184**, 413–34.

Sugioka, A., Tsuzuki, T., Kanai, T. *et al.* (1993) Postresection prognosis of patients with hepatocellular carcinoma. *Surgery*, **113**, 612–18.

Takenaka, K., Kanematsu, T., Fukuzawa, K. *et al.* (1990) Can hepatic failure after surgery for hepatocellular carcinoma in cirrhotic patients be prevented? *World Journal of Surgery*, **14**, 123–7.

Takenaka, K., Kawahara, N., Yamamoto, K. *et al.* (1996) Results of 280 liver resections for hepatocellular carcinoma. *Archives of Surgery*, **131**, 71–6.

Takenaka, K., Shimada, M., Higashi, H. *et al.* (1994) Liver resection for hepatocellular carcinoma in the elderly. *Archives of Surgery*, **129**, 846–50.

Takenaka, K., Yoshida, K., Nishizaki, T. *et al.* (1995) Intraoperative risk factors associated with hepatic resection. *British Journal of Surgery*, **82**, 1262–5.

Tanabe, G., Sakamoto, M., Akazawa, K. *et al.* (1995) Intraoperative risk factors associated with hepatic resection. *British Journal of Surgery*, **82**, 1262–5.

Tang, Z.Y., Yu, Y.Q., Zhou, X.D. *et al.* (1995) Treatment of unresectable primary liver cancer: with reference to cytoreduction and sequential resection. *World Journal of Surgery*, **19**, 47–52.

Thompson, H.H., Tompkins, T.K. and Longmire, W.P. (1983) Major hepatic resections–a 25-year experience. *Annals of Surgery*, **197**, 375–87.

Ton That Tung (1979) *Les resections majeures et mineures du foie*, Masson, Paris.

Une, Y., Uchino, J., Horie, T. *et al.* (1989) Liver resection using a water jet. *Cancer Chemotherapy and Pharmacology*, **23 (Suppl.)**, S74–7.

Vaccaro, J.P., Dorfman, G.A. and Lambaise, R.E. (1991) Treatment of biliary leaks and fistulas by simultaneous percutaneous drainage and diversion. *Cardiovascular and Interventional Radiology*, **14**, 109–12.

Vajrabukka, T., Bloom, A.L., Wood, C.B. *et al.* (1975) Postoperative problems and management after hepatic resection for blunt injury to the liver. *British Journal of Surgery*, **62**, 189–200.

Vauthey, J.N., Klimstra, D., Franceschi, D. *et al.* (1995) Factors affecting long-term outcome after hepatic resection for hepatocellular carcinoma. *American Journal of Surgery*, **169**, 28–34.

Venook, A.P. (1994) Treatment of hepatocellular carcinoma: too many options? *Journal of Clinical Oncology*, **12**, 1323–34.

Voyles, C.R., Bowley, N.B., Allison, D.J. *et al.* (1983) Carcinoma of the proximal extrahepatic biliary tree. Radiological assessment and therapeutic alternatives. *Annals of Surgery*, **197**, 188–94.

Williamson, B.W., Blumgart, L.H. and McKellar, N.J. (1980) Management of tumors of the liver. Combined use of arteriography and venography in the assessment of resectability especially in hilar tumours. *American Journal of Surgery*, **139**, 210–15.

Yamamoto, K., Takenaka, K., Kawahara, N. *et al.* (1997) Indications for palliative reduction surgery in advanced hepatocellular carcinoma. The use of a remnant tumor index. *Archives of Surgery*, **132**, 120–3.

Yamanaka, N., Okamoto, E., Fujihara, S. *et al.* (1992) Do the tumor cells of hepatocellular carcinomas dislodge into the portal venous stream during hepatic resection? *Cancer*, **70**, 2263–7.

Yamanaka, N., Okamoto, E., Kuwatak, K. *et al.* (1984) Multiple regression equation for prediction of post-hepatectomy liver failure. *Annals of Surgery*, **200**, 658–63.

Yamanaka, N., Okamoto, E., Toyosaka, A. *et al.* (1990) Prognostic factors after hepatectomy for hepatocellular carcinomas. A univariate and multivariate analysis. *Cancer*

NON-SURGICAL MANAGEMENT 10

T.W.T. Leung

10.1 INTRODUCTION

Surgical resection is the only treatment for hepatocellular carcinoma (HCC) that consistently offers the hope of cure. However, only 9–27% patients are suitable for resection (Okuda, 1980; Shiu *et al.*, 1990; Lee *et al.*, 1982), the reasons mainly being advanced stage disease or poor liver function. Many patients with inoperable HCC have reasonable general condition and liver function at presentation. Such patients are commonly considered for various forms of non-surgical treatment. The goals of treatment are mainly palliative but occasionally such treatment may produce lasting progression-free survival, or rarely, even cure if the disease is rendered operable after treatment. As there are more patients with inoperable disease, non-surgical treatment is more frequently applied to treat HCC than surgery.

Types of non-surgical treatment for HCC are listed in Table 10.1. The long list reflects the fact that there is, so far, no proven single standard non-surgical treatment for inoperable HCC. The choice depends on the general condition of the patient, stage of disease and also treatment protocol of individual oncology centers.

10.2 SYSTEMIC CHEMOTHERAPY

Cytotoxic drugs have been extensively tested in HCC; however, the tumor is relatively

Table 10.1 Types of non-surgical treatment for HCC.

Systemic chemotherapy
1. Cytotoxic and hormonal therapy

Immunotherapy
1. Monoclonal antibody
2. Biological response modifier

Regional intra-arterial treatment
1. Intra-arterial chemotherapy
2. Lipiodolization
3. Chemoembolization

Radiotherapy
1. External radiotherapy
2. Internal radiotherapy

Direct intralesional treatment
1. Percutaneous ethanol injection

Other radiological management
1. Hepatic arterial embolization

resistant to most agents. It was found that MDR1 (multiple drug resistance) gene (Chenivesse *et al.*, 1993) and the gene product P-glycoprotein (Soini *et al.*, 1996) are both over-expressed in HCC which explains its relative resistance to chemotherapeutic agents. Even in selected patients, single agent objective response rate is <35% (Table 10.2) and combination chemotherapy does not appear to be better (Table 10.3). Responses are commonly incomplete and short lasting. Some

Hepatocellular Carcinoma: Diagnosis, investigation and management. Edited by Anthony S.-Y. Leong, Choong-Tsek Liew, Joseph W.Y. Lau and Philip J. Johnson. Published in 1999 by Arnold, London. ISBN 0 340 74096 5.

Table 10.2   Single-agent activity in HCC.

Investigators	Drug	No. of patients	Response (%)
Falkson *et al.* (1981)	amsacrine	35	3
Falkson *et al.* (1984a)	neocarzinostatin	28	7
Damrongsak *et al.* (1973)	vinblastine	25	8
Melia *et al.* (1983)	VP-16	24	13
Falkson *et al.* (1987)	cisplatinum	35	17
Hochster *et al.* (1985)	4'-epidoxorubicin	18	17
Dunk *et al.* (1985)	mitoxantrone	22	27
Choi *et al.* (1984)	doxorubicin	45	24
Johnson *et al.* (1978)	doxorubicin	44	32
Williams *et al.* (1980)	doxorubicin	60	35

phase II studies reported high response rate but it has not been confirmed by subsequent studies. It is also difficult to compare activity among different drugs and to determine whether chemotherapy is better than no treatment because most chemotherapy trials were uncontrolled. They have also used different response criteria, making interpretation and comparison of results difficult. The consensus is that the average response rate for various single or combination chemotherapy is around 15–20%. Whether combination is better than a single agent has yet to be proved. Such a low response rate has a minimal impact on overall survival. Therefore, systemic chemotherapy should not be recommended as standard therapy for HCC outside a clinical trial protocol. The general indications for systemic chemotherapy are: inoperable disease, reasonable liver function (total bilirubin $<50\,\mu mol/l$), Karnofsky Performance Score >70% and age <70 years.

The anthracyclines and anthraquinones, namely, doxorubicin (Johnson *et al.*, 1978; Williams, 1980; Choi *et al.*, 1984), 4'-epidoxorubicin (Hochster *et al.*, 1985) and mitoxantrone (Dunk *et al.*, 1985), are the drugs that have consistently produced response rates of

Table 10.3   Combination chemotherapy in HCC.

Investigators	Drug	No. of patients	Response (%)
Gailani *et al.* (1972)	5-FU, Ara-C	22	5
Falkson *et al.* (1984b)	5-FU, MeCCNU	49	8
Baker *et al.* (1977)	doxorubicin, 5-FU	38	13
Al-Idrissi *et al.* (1985)	doxorubicin, 5-FU, mitomycin C	40	13
Falkson *et al.* (1984b)	5-FU, streptozotocin	55	13
Ravry *et al.* (1984)	doxorubicin, bleomycin	60	16
Patt *et al.* (1993)	5-FU, interferon	28	18
Falkson *et al.* (1984b)	doxorubicin, 5-FU, MeCCNU	38	21
Bezwods and Berman (1982)	doxorubicin, 5-FU, VM26	36	44

around 20%. Complete remission is possible but not lasting (Johnson *et al.*, 1978). The difference among the anthracyclines is probably the cost of the drug and not clinical efficacy. Doxorubicin is the most popular drug either in single agent or combination. The overall response rate from 13 published doxorubicin trials is about 19% and median survival is only 4 months (Nerenstone *et al.*, 1988). A study from Hong Kong which randomized 60 patients to receive either doxorubicin or no treatment reported a small increase in survival from median survival of 10.6 weeks for the doxorubicin arm to 7.5 weeks for no treatment arm (Lai *et al.*, 1988). The dose-limiting toxicities of doxorubicin are mainly cardiac toxicity and bone marrow suppression. Treatment with doxorubicin is relatively contraindicated in patients with concomitant heart disease and the dosage should be reduced if the liver function is poor.

Hormonal therapy can be considered as a form of systemic chemotherapy. As HCC occurs more commonly in males and the tumor cells have been shown to express estrogen and androgen (Nagasue *et al.*, 1985) receptors in HCC tissues, it was hypothesized that some form of hormonal manipulation may be useful. Tamoxifen, an anti-estrogen, was shown to inhibit growth of hepatoma cells *in vitro*, but probably through an estrogen receptor-independent mechanism (Jiang *et al.*, 1995). Tamoxifen used to treat HCC was shown to be inactive in one clinical trial (Paliard *et al.*, 1984). Three randomized studies which compared tamoxifen with no treatment or placebo showed that tamoxifen significantly prolonged survival (Farinati *et al.*, 1992; Martinez Cerezo *et al.*, 1994; Manesis *et al.*, 1995). However, another larger randomized study with 120 patients showed no benefit of tamoxifen over placebo in terms of antitumor effect, survival and probability of disease progression (Castells *et al.*, 1995). Another prospective controlled study randomized 59 patients with inoperable HCC to receive either single-agent doxorubicin or

tamoxifen with doxorubicin, and it showed no difference in response rates or survival duration between the two arms (Melia *et al.*, 1987). These few randomized studies are from non-Oriental populations. Further tamoxifen trials have to be randomized control studies and carried out in high-incidence areas, especially among Oriental populations. The benefit of tamoxifen therapy remains controversial. In general, tamoxifen may have minimal growth restraining activity against HCC as reflected by a small increase in survival.

The results from systemic cytotoxic or hormonal therapy for treatment of inoperable HCC are, in general, depressing. There is so far no large randomized study looking at systemic chemotherapy versus supportive treatment except the one by Lai *et al.* (1988) which showed only a small improvement in survival but with significant toxicity of treatment. Therefore, patients should be carefully chosen before being given systemic chemotherapy or entered into treatment protocols for new drugs, new combinations, dosage, route of administration and scheduling.

10.3 IMMUNOTHERAPY

Immunotherapy using biological response modifiers and monoclonal antibodies is another form of systemic therapy for HCC. Interferons are proteins produced by cells in response to viral infection and foreign antigens. They also have many immunomodulatory and antiproliferative effects and have seen to be effective in the treatment of chronic leukemia and indolent lymphomas. Recombinant α-interferon had been tested for activity in HCC. Lai *et al.* (1989) reported that high-dose interferon (25–25 mU/m^2 three times weekly) induced more tumor regression (10% partial response), less toxicity and fatal complication than doxorubicin. Another study showed that high-dose interferon is better than no treatment in terms of survival and tumor regression. The median survival duration reported was only 14.5 weeks for the treatment arm (Lai *et al.*, 1993). Toxicity was considerable in this study as about one third of the patients required dose-reduction because of persistent fatigue after interferon therapy. However, a similar study by The Gastrointestinal Tumor Study Group (1990) showed that recombinant α-interferon has no significant antitumor activity in HCC. Recombinant α-interferon was also tested in two trials and both reported no activity in HCC (Yoshida *et al.*, 1990; Forbes *et al.*, 1985). It seems that α-interferon may have some activity in HCC but a high dose is required to produce an optimal response rate. Systemic toxicity is an important consideration when using interferon at such high dosages. Another attempt employed was with lower doses of interferon and combined with other cytotoxic agents. Patt *et al.* (1993) used combination 5-FU and α-interferon (5 mU/m² on days 1, 2 and 3) to treat 28 patients with inoperable HCC and a documented partial response of 18%. The treatment was well-tolerated and achieved a similar response rate when compared with high-dose interferon.

The use of monoclonal antibodies (anti-AFP, anti-ferritin) in the treatment of HCC is usually coupled with radioisotopes and will be discussed in the section on radiotherapy.

10.4 REGIONAL INTRA-ARTERIAL TREATMENT

10.4.1 INTRA-ARTERIAL CHEMOTHERAPY

Systemic chemotherapy for HCC is generally unsatisfactory. Before new drugs are used for clinical testing, attempts are made to give existing drugs through a different route and to improve efficacy. The liver has a dual blood supply both from the portal venous and systemic arterial systems. It is also known that large liver tumors such as HCC derive their blood supply mainly from the hepatic artery (Breedis and Young, 1954; Ackerman, 1972). Therefore, infusion of cytotoxic drugs into the feeding hepatic artery has the theoretical advantage of increased total drug exposure to the tumor which may in turn improve tumor cell kill. The aim of intra-arterial chemotherapy is to obtain higher concentrations of cytotoxic drugs within the tumor relative to the systemic circulation. This depends on the blood supply of the tumor and also extraction of the drug by the liver. Regional intra-arterial chemotherapy for HCC can either be through hepatic angiography or an implantable arterial port inserted intraoperatively. Drugs such as 5-FU, 5-FUDR, cisplatin, doxorubicin and 4'-epidoxorubicin are commonly used in intra-arterial treatment because they have high liver extraction rates and short plasma half-life (Civalleri, 1992). The fluoropyrimidines (5-FU and 5-FUDR) are perhaps the best agents for intra-arterial chemotherapy because they have a high rate of systemic clearance and also have prolonged drug exposure to hepatic tumors. From various phase II clinical trials, intra-arterial doxorubicin seems to be most active with a better response rate and survival than intravenous treatment (Table 10.4)

It is worth noting that only a few studies have reported pharmacokinetic data. One study showed only a small relative pharmacokinetic advantage in man of intra-arterial cisplatin compared with intravenous administration (Campbell *et al.*, 1983). Another study found no difference in the pharmacokinetics and tumor response rates between intra-arterial and intravenous doxorubicin (Johnson *et al.*, 1991a).

Intra-arterial chemotherapy using combination chemotherapy was tested by three different groups using mainly a doxorubicin-containing regimen. The results from these three trials are listed in Table 10.5.

The response and survival rates appeared to be better than single agents in the studies by Carr *et al.* (1991) and Patt *et al.* (1994). However, significant toxicity such as cholangitis and bone marrow suppression was reported. The treatment also required an operation to insert an injection device for prolonged infusion of drugs.

Table 10.4   Intra-arterial chemotherapy with single agents.

Investigators	Drug	No. of patients	Response (%)	Survival (months)
Olweny *et al.* (1980)	doxorubicin	10	60	–
Urist and Balch (1984)	doxorubicin	13	47	20
Chearanai *et al.* (1974)	mechloethamine	60	33	–
Kinami *et al.* (1978)	mitomycin C	14	50	7
Cheng *et al.* (1982)	cisplatin	16	19	–
Ansfield *et al.* (1971)	5-FU	11	27	–
Wellwood *et al.* (1979)	FUDR	28	54	7

Although it appears that intra-arterial chemotherapy, as a single agent or in combination, produced a better response rate, interpretation of the results from different studies is hampered by a difference in the response criteria and a lack of a randomized study. It is also worth noting that toxicity associated with more optimal intra-arterial chemotherapy is considerable and results are no different from intravenous treatment.

10.4.2 LIPIODOLIZATION AND CHEMOEMBOLIZATION

To increase selectively the tumor drug exposure to HCC, it is logical to look for a drug carrier which can target and be retained by it. Lipiodol or ethiodol is an oily X-ray contrast medium which was found to be retained selectively by HCC for many weeks after intra-arterial administration (Yumoto *et al.*, 1985; Okayasu *et al.*, 1988). A preliminary study in Japan using styrene maleic acid neocarzinostatin (SMANCS) solubilized in lipiodol administered intra-arterially to HCC patients yielded some encouraging results (Tashiro and Muedu, 1985). Hydrophilic drugs such as doxorubicin (Kanematsu *et al.*, 1989) and cisplatin (Kasugai *et al.*, 1989) may also be mixed with lipiodol in an emulsion and given intra-arterially. Results from selected studies are listed in Table 10.6.

Despite promising results from single-arm studies on intra-arterial chemotherapy with lipiodol, there are few randomized trials to test whether the addition of lipiodol makes a difference. Madden *et al.* (1993) randomized 136 HCC patients to receive intra-arterial epirubicin lipiodol emulsion versus symptomatic treatment. They found no survival benefit but inst ead an increased morbidity for the treatment arm. Another randomized study found prolonged survival favoring intra-arterial cisplatin, doxorubicin and lipiodol (Carr *et*

Table 10.5   Regional intra-arterial chemotherapy with combinations.

Investigators	Drug	No. of patients	Response (%)	Survival (months)
Shildt *et al.* (1984)	FUDR, doxorubicin, streptozotocin	30	10	–
Carr *et al.* (1991)	doxorubicin, cisplatin	25	50	12
Patt *et al.* (1994)	FUDR, leucovorin, doxorubicin, cisplatin	29	41	15

Table 10.6   Intra-arterial chemotherapy with lipiodol.

Investigators	Drugs	No. of patients	Response (%)
Konno *et al.* (1983)	SMANCS + ethiodol	44	90
Kanematsu *et al.* (1989)	doxorubicin + ethiodol	70	47
Shibata *et al.* (1989)	cisplatin + ethiodol	71	47
Carr *et al.* (1994)	cisplatin + doxorubicin with lipiodol versus without lipiodol	56	57 (with lipiodol) 44 (without lipiodol)
Ryder *et al.* (1996)	doxorubicin + lipiodol	67	22

al., 1994). In a more recent study, a better response was found for smaller tumors using intra-arterial doxorubicin and lipiodol (Ryder *et al.*, 1996). Another prospective randomized study from Japan showed a better response rate and survival for the intra-arterial lipiodol and 4'-epidoxorubicin arm than for 4'-epidoxorubicin alone (Yoshikawa *et al.*, 1994). However, our own study, which compared intravenous 4'-epidoxorubicin and intra-arterial lipiodol to 4'-epidoxorubicin, did not find any difference in response rate and survival (Leung *et al.*, 1992). A study from the UK compared intra-arterial doxorubicin and lipiodol with intravenous doxorubicin at the same dosage, found no difference in response and survival (Kalayci *et al.*, 1990). The pharmacokinetic part of this study reported separately found no difference in plasma drug levels in terms of area under the curve, among the three groups of patients receiving intra-arterial doxorubicin alone, intra-arterial doxorubicin with lipiodol, or intravenous doxorubicin (Johnson *et al.*, 1991b). However, our own study comparing intra-arterial 4'-epidoxorubicin with or without lipiodol showed that the mean serum concentration time profile of 4'-epidoxorubicin with lipiodol was lower than without lipiodol (Lee *et al.*, 1992). We also found that the bioavailability of 4'-epidoxorubicin in the systemic circulation after intra-arterial lipiodol-epidoxorubicin was lower than that after intravenous injection. This suggested some

form of targeting of the lipiodol-epidoxorubicin emulsion.

To increase drug exposure to the tumor after intra-arterial chemotherapy, attempts have been made to slow down arterial blood flow by temporary or permanent occlusion of the hepatic artery. Infusion of gelfoam pellets, ivalon particles or degradable starch particles into the hepatic artery can achieve this immediately after intra-arterial chemotherapy. Such treatment is called chemoembolization. The theoretical advantage is greater cytotoxic drug concentration in the tumor as the arterial blood flow is slowed down or even stopped. The approach was supported by a pharmacokinetic study of distribution of doxorubicin after a chemoembolization procedure which showed that the addition of ethiodol and gelfoam lowered the peak concentration of the drug in peripheral blood more than intravenous treatment (Raoul *et al.*, 1992b). Results from selected studies are listed in Table 10.7. Reported response rates vary from 17 to 56% which seem better than systemic chemotherapy and intra-arterial chemotherapy.

Despite the favorable response rates reported, two randomized studies (Pelletier *et al.*, 1990; Trinchet *et al.*, 1995) did not find any improvement in survival when compared with no treatment. The French multicentre randomized study in 1997 found no difference in survival rates between chemoembolization (cisplatin + lipiodol + gelfoam) plus tamoxifen

Table 10.7 Chemoembolization for HCC.

Investigators	Drugs	No. of patients	Response (%)
Pelletier *et al.* (1990)*	doxorubicin + gelfoam	42	17
Venook *et al.* (1990)	doxorubicin/cisplatin/mitomycin C + gelfoam	50	24
Rougier *et al.* (1993)	doxorubicin + gelfoam +/– lipiodol	232	41
Stuart *et al.* (1993)	doxorubicin + ethiodol + gelatin powder	52	43
Trinchet *et al.* (1995)*	cisplatin + ethiodol + gelfoam	43	16
Carr *et al.* (1995)	cisplatin + doxorubicin + degradable starch particles	26	58
Ngan *et al.* (1996)	cisplatin + lipiodol + gelfoam	132	56

*Randomized studies.

and tamoxifen alone (Rougier *et al.*, 1997). It is also worth noting that one study (Ngan *et al.*, 1996) only used a relatively small dose of cisplatin of 10 mg which is five to six times lower than other studies but produced similar response rates with the same technique.

The benefit of chemoembolization in terms of tumor response and survival is still controversial and more randomized studies should be done to compare with other modalities and different drug dosages. Chemoembolization is not free of morbidity. Side-effects such as fever, abdominal pain and transient elevation of transaminases are often seen. Therefore, chemoembolization should be considered only for patients with good general condition, favorable liver function, patent portal venous system and those free of extrahepatic disease. Chemoembolization has in general little activity in large tumors >9 cm.

10.5 RADIOTHERAPY

10.5.1 EXTERNAL BEAM IRRADIATION

Radiotherapy is seldom given for liver tumors because normal hepatocytes are sensitive to radiation. Indeed, as early as 1940 it was recognized that normal liver cells are as radiosensitive as are the malignant ones (Pack and Livingstone, 1940). In a review of 11 patients who received whole liver irradiation

and boost treatment of 53–70 Gy equivalent, it was recommended that no more than 30% of the liver should be irradiated in excess of 30–35 Gy (2-Gy fractions) to avoid radiation hepatitis (Austin-Seymour *et al.*, 1986). Schacter *et al.* (1986) reviewed 32 cases from the literature and noted a mortality of nearly 50% from radiation hepatitis. Therefore, external beam radiotherapy cannot be delivered to the tumor without jeopardizing the non-tumorous liver.

Recently, in an attempt to improve the therapeutic ratio, several new approaches have been developed. The aim is to increase radiation dose to the tumor while sparing the normal liver. These include the use of external irradiation with conformal radiotherapy, radiosensitizers, and internal irradiation with radioisotopes.

Conformal radiotherapy can increase the radiation dose to target tumor volume, at the same time allowing adjacent normal tissue to be excluded from the treatment volume. The application of conformal radiotherapy with intra-arterial 5-FUDR as radiosensitizer was found to be effective in treatment of hepatobiliary cancers (Robertson *et al.*, 1993). The radiation dose to the tumor was between 48 and 72.6 Gy. Objective responses were seen in all patients with localized tumors. Median survival was 11 months. Only two patients had non-fatal radiation hepatitis. This suggests that tumor regression with durable response is possible with an adequate dose of radiation and reduced radiation dose to non-tumorous liver tissue can reduce the incidence of radiation hepatitis.

In the search for a better method to deliver an even higher radiation dose selectively to a tumor, internal irradiation using radioisotopic sources seems an attractive approach. Internal irradiation treatment for hepatic tumors can be done by administration of unsealed radioactive sources. There are two methods of internal irradiation: systemic radiolabeled monoclonal antibodies or regional intra-arterial targeting therapy with a tumor-seeking carrier labeled with radioisotopes.

10.5.2   INTERNAL IRRADIATION WITH RADIOIMMUNOGLOBULINS

With the development of monoclonal antibodies such as anti-ferritin and anti-AFP, which are tumor-selective, HCC can be targeted after systemic administration of the appropriate antibodies. By labeling the antibodies with iodine-131 or yttrium-90, a therapeutic dose of radiation can be delivered to the tumor specifically. A partial remission rate of 41% and a complete remission rate of 7% were achieved after iodine-131-antiferritin treatment (Order *et al.*, 1985). Median survival was up to 5 months for patients with raised AFP levels and 10 months for AFP-negative patients. The treatment was preceded by whole liver external beam irradiation, and radio-sensitizers (doxorubicin and 5-FU) were added in the latter phase of the trial. Hence, the radio-immunoglobulins served as a 'boost' to the tumor, but it is difficult to be certain about the specific cytotoxic role of the radio-labelled antibodies. Taking into account the tumor-effective half-life and administered dose of radio-immunoglobulins, the radiation dose to the tumor was calculated to be in the order of 10 to 12 Gy. Since the treatment is given systemically, bone marrow toxicity is to be expected. The side effects tend to be

cumulative after repeated treatments. Host reaction to the antibody and the development of anti-antibodies were also recognised side effects. The treatment was compared with systemic chemotherapy in a randomized trial, which showed comparable response rates and survival duration. Those failing chemotherapy could still respond to iodine-131- anti-ferritin treatment (Order *et al.*, 1991).

10.5.3   SELECTIVE INTERNAL RADIATION

Regional treatment with chemotherapeutic drugs which are mixed or tagged with a targeting substance (e.g. lipiodol or microspheres) through the hepatic artery has been advocated as a form of treatment for localized HCC because the tumor is mainly supplied by the hepatic artery. A similar approach can be exploited by administering a therapeutic dose of radioisotopes into the hepatic artery thereby irradiating the tumor internally while sparing the non-tumorous liver. This is called selective internal irradiation (SIR) and has the advantage of reducing systemic toxicity. Radiolabeled lipiodol and inert microspheres (in glass, plastic or resin form) are commonly used in SIR. The two radioisotopes that are currently used are yttrium-90 and iodine-131. Yttrium-90 is usually tagged to resin-based or glass microspheres and iodine-131 is usually labeled to lipiodol.

10.5.3.1   SIR with iodine-131-lipiodol

Lipiodol, as mentioned above, is preferentially taken up and retained by HCC. Through an ion to ion exchange reaction, the iodine moiety of lipiodol can be labeled with iodine-131 (Park *et al.*, 1986). By giving the radioactive ^{131}I-lipiodol intra-arterially, a therapeutic dose of irradiation can be delivered to the tumor. Lipiodol-iodine-131 emits γ-radiation with an energy of 364 KeV. The physical half life is 8.04 days. The radioactive lipiodol-iodine-131 is usually given slowly through an angiographic catheter that is placed in the tumor-feeding hepatic artery. Since the substance is radio-opaque, the flow of lipiodol is easily traced during injection. By scanning with a gamma camera, the distribution and kinetics of the radioactive lipiodol can be worked out. Since lipiodol may be degraded within the liver, a trace amount of radioactive iodine is detected in the patient's urine. The thyroid needs to be blocked by non-radioactive iodine before commencement of treatment to prevent uptake of the radioisotope. To allow the radiation to decay to a safe level before discharge, patients need to stay in hospital for approximately 10–14 days, depending on the effective half life of the radioactive lipiodol.

The distribution of lipiodol-iodine-131 within the liver can be detected with a gamma camera. From a dosimetry study, it was shown that HCC would receive on average eight times the irradiation dose of normal liver (Madsen *et al.*, 1988). Hence for a 4cm tumor to receive >100 Gy, about 40 mCi radioactive lipiodol is required and yet the dose to the normal liver is still kept below the maximum tolerable level. Although the radiation dose depends on many factors and may be different from patient to patient, a therapeutic dose of radiation can be delivered to the liver tumor without added external irradiation. Furthermore, radioactivity detected in the peripheral tissue is relatively small so that systemic toxicity is minimal. The treatment was used as a single modality to treat 24 HCC patients in a Korean study. Tumor regression occurred in 89% of patients with small tumors (<4 cm in diameter) and in 65% of patients having a tumor size between 4 and 6cm. All the responsive cases showed a reduction of serum AFP level. The prescribed dose of lipiodol-iodine-131 ranged from 555 to 2220MBq (15–60mCi) (Yoo *et al.*, 1991). Another French multicenter trial using radioactive lipiodol to treat 63 HCC patients produced an objective response in 40% patients with minimal toxicities yet keeping radiation dose to normal liver <20Gy (Raoul *et al.*, 1992a). The treatment was also found to be

useful even in the presence of portal venous thrombosis (Raoul *et al.*, 1994). We have treated 26 patients with inoperable HCC with intra-arterial lipiodol-iodine-131 and found an overall response rate of 52% (Leung *et al.*, 1992). Fig. 10.1 shows a gamma scan picture after lipiodol-iodine-131 injection. There is hot uptake by the HCC. CT scans of one of the responders before and after treatment are shown in Fig. 10.2. The treatment was well tolerated and median survival was 6 months.

The limitation of lipiodol-iodine-131 is difficulty in the treatment of large (>5 cm) tumors. To give a huge dose of radioactive lipiodol for large tumors may not be technically feasible because of radiation hazard to medical personnel and too large a volume of lipiodol. Therefore, lipiodol-iodine-131 is only suitable for tumors <5 cm in diameter.

10.5.3.2 SIR with yttrium-90 microspheres

Yttrium-90 is also used in the treatment of HCC. A comparison of iodine-131 and yttrium-90 is listed in Table 10.8.

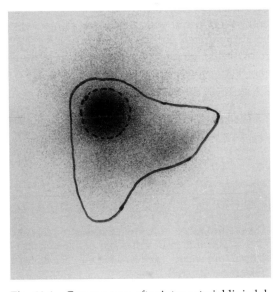

Fig. 10.1 Gamma scan after intra-arterial lipiodol-iodine-131.

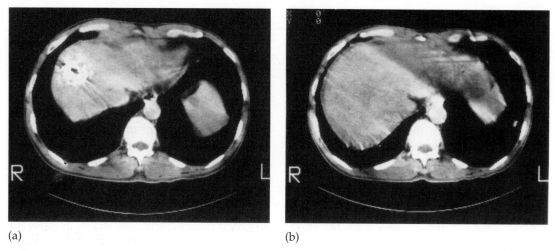

(a)   (b)

Fig. 10.2   (a) CT scan of liver before lipiodol-iodine-131. (b) CT scan of liver after lipiodol-iodine-131.

The physical half life of yttrium-90 is 64.2 h, which is shorter than iodine-131, so that the duration of hospital stay after yttrium-90 therapy can be reduced. It is also a pure β-emitter which makes radiation protection easier. The mean energy and mean penetration of yttrium-90 is also greater for yttrium-90 so that it can be used to treat larger tumors. Yttrium-90 is commonly used for labeling monoclonal antibodies for systemic targeting therapy. The isotope can also be incorporated either into resin-based (Gray *et al.*, 1989) or glass microspheres (Houle *et al.*, 1989; Anderson *et al.*, 1992) and given intra-arterially to treat HCC. Angiotensin II, which is a vasoconstrictor, has been shown to constrict normal blood vessels to improve flow of the labelled microspheres to the tumor (Burton *et al.*, 1985; Goldberg *et al.*, 1991). With the use of angiotensin II, which is followed by infusion of the radiolabeled microspheres into the feeding hepatic artery of the tumor, the microspheres will preferentially go to the tumor because of increased blood flow. The microspheres are made to a size (32 μm) approximating that of the precapillary diameter and they are not degradable. Fig. 10.3 shows the photomicrograph of

Table 10.8   Comparison between lipiodol-iodine-131 and yttrium-90 microspheres.

	Lipiodol-iodine-131	Yttrium-90 microspheres
β-radiation		
Physical half-life	8.04 days	64.2 h
Maximum range in tissue (cytotoxic range) (mm)	2	11
Mean penetration in tissue (soft tissue density = 1.03) (mm)	0.4	2.5
Maximum energy (KeV)	600	2270
Mean energy (KeV)	187	936.7
γ-radiation (KeV)	364	–

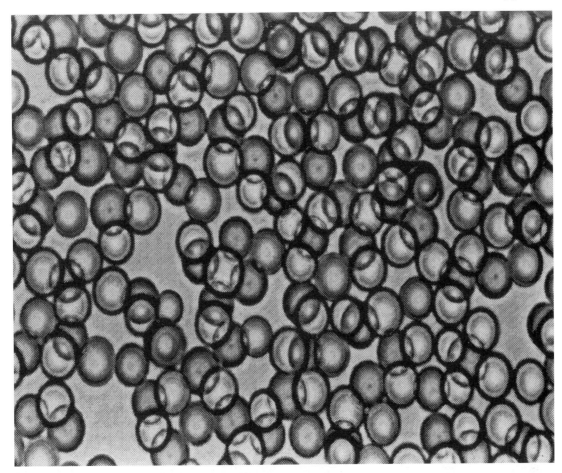

Fig. 10.3   Photomicrograph of yttrium-90 microspheres in suspension (×300).

yttrium-90 microspheres in suspension. They will be lodged within the tumor forever and will deliver the planned radiation dose. With such an approach, it was found that tolerance of the liver to the effects of radiation by yttrium-90 microspheres is higher than that expected from external radiation and a therapeutic dose of radiation is able to be delivered without causing radiation hepatitis (Gray *et al.*, 1990).

Yttrium-90 microspheres can be delivered either through an angiographic catheter during hepatic angiography or an implantable arterial port. To predict the radiation dose to the tumor and non-tumorous liver accurately,

we have developed a simulation test using technetium-99m macroaggregated albumin (Tc-MAA). Tc-MAA is biodegradable and it has a similar size as the microspheres. By injecting a small dose of Tc-MAA into the hepatic artery, a gamma camera can be employed to collect count rates over the tumor, non-tumorous liver, lungs and other organs. The tumor-to-non-tumor ratio and percentage shunting of Tc-MAA to the lungs can then be computed. The ratio was verified by intraoperative dosimetric measurements and liquid scintillation counting of multiple liver biopsies (Lau *et al.*, 1994a). Using a partition model derived by Ho *et al.* (1996), it

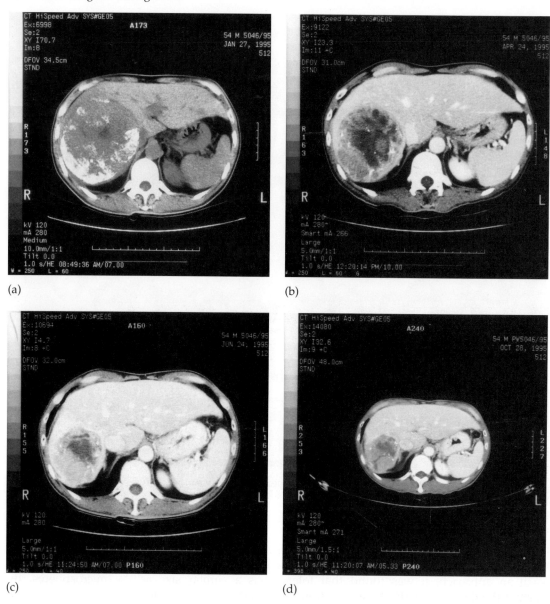

(a)   (b)

(c)   (d)

Fig. 10.4   (a) CT scan of liver before yttrium-90 microspheres. (b) CT scan of liver 3 months after yttrium-90 microspheres. (c) CT scan of liver 5 months after yttrium-90 microspheres. (d) CT scan of liver 9 months after yttrium-90 microspheres.

is possible to predict accurately the radiation dose to the tumor and normal liver. Another consideration is extrahepatic shunting of the microspheres to other organs, especially the lungs, through arteriovenous shunting. The Tc-MAA scan is also able to predict the degree of lung shunting after SIR. When lung shunting is >10%, SIR is usually not considered except when the dose required is very small. Giving SIR to patients with high lung shunting will result in radiation pneumonitis (Leung *et al.*, 1995).

Patients can be considered for yttrium-90-microspheres treatment if they have inoperable HCC but without extrahepatic disease and if the liver function is satisfactory. The lung shunting should, in general, be <10%, and the tumor-to-non-tumor ratio be >2.

In an early phase II study on 15 patients who received intraoperative yttrium-90 microspheres treatment, the partial response rate was 67% (Lau *et al.*, 1994a). Among eight patients with raised AFP, seven had a decrease >50%. Tumor regression on CT scan was usually seen after 2 months. Median survival of the whole group was about 7 months from diagnosis (Lau *et al.*, 1994b). It was also found from this study that optimal tumor regression and reduction of serum AFP levels were seen when the average radiation dose to the tumor was >120 Gy and survival is related to the dose of radiation to the tumor. Although cirrhosis was present in all patients, there was no incidence of radiation hepatitis even when the non-tumorous liver received up to 70 Gy. In a subsequent phase II study from the same group, 71 patients were treated with intra-arterial yttrium-90 microspheres treatment through hepatic angiography (Lau *et al.*, 1997). The dose ranged from 0.8 to 5 GBq as a single treatment. The overall objective response in terms of reduction of AFP was 89%. Tumor volume regression >50% occurred in 27% of all the patients. The median survival of all patients was 9.4 months (Fig. 10.4). Another study from Canada treated 10 patients with yttrium-90 glass microspheres also reported stable disease in all patients after the treatment and tolerable toxicities (Shepherd *et al.*, 1992).

The most common complaint after yttrium-90 microspheres treatment was right upper quadrant discomfort that was easily controlled with simple analgesics. This was due to the embolization effect of the microspheres. However, bone marrow toxicities were not seen.

10.6   DIRECT INTRA-LESIONAL TREATMENT

Small HCCs can be treated with percutaneous intralesional treatment under ultrasound guidance. Ethanol is commonly used for intralesional treatment immediately to fix or coagulate the tissue in a dose-dependent manner. It also causes occlusion of blood vessels and results in coagulative necrosis of tumor nodules, and to a small extent the adjacent hepatic parenchyma. Systemic side effects are usually minimal. It is done under ultrasound guidance, percutaneously, and it requires an experienced ultrasonographer. An early study treated 95 patients and reported 41.8% complete response after percutaneous ethanol injection (PEI) for tumors <3 cm. The 5-year survival rate was 28% (Ebara *et al.*, 1990). The side-effects were mainly pain, fever and a transient rise in liver enzymes. Livraghi *et al.* (1992) published the largest series of 2485 PEI treatment in 207 patients with cirrhosis and HCC. The 1-, 2- and 3-year survival rates were 90, 80 and 63% respectively, which was comparable with a matched group of patients who underwent resection.

Size of tumor is one of the limitations of PEI as penetration of ethanol within liver tissue is limited. It is indicated only in tumors <3 cm in diameter (Vilana *et al.*, 1992). The technique is difficult in cases with multiple tumors and is only suitable for patients with limited disease. The patients are usually not considered for surgical resection because of poor liver function due to cirrhosis. It is also indicated for isolated recurrence after surgery when further resection cannot be performed. Success of treatment is related to the initial size of tumor. The procedure has also been found to be useful during laparotomy to control bleeding HCC (Chung *et al.*, 1990; Sunderland *et al.*, 1992). There are at least one non-randomized (Yamasaki *et al.*, 1991) and one randomized trial (Castells *et al.*, 1993) comparing PEI with surgical resection for small HCCs (<3 cm) which show a similar treatment result. This suggests that surgery can probably be delayed and PEI can be the first treatment of choice for small HCCs. It also confirms the observation that small HCCs behave very much like a local disease with a low systemic metastasis rate. Therefore, an effective locoregional treatment, which is well tolerated, may reduce the morbidity or even mortality which accompanies surgical resection.

10.7   HEPATIC ARTERIAL EMBOLIZATION

Hepatic arterial embolization is another form of palliative treatment for inoperable HCC. Hepatic arterial occlusion can be permanent and this is done by surgical ligation at laparotomy or by embolizing the feeding hepatic artery of the HCC with undegradable particles or coils through during hepatic angiography. The principle of arterial occlusion is to induce ischemia and necrosis of the HCC. Since the liver has a dual blood supply from the hepatic artery and portal venous system, occluding the hepatic artery, which is the major supply of blood to the tumor, does not render the entire liver ischemic. However, it is relatively contraindicated if the portal system is blocked due to tumor invasion or thrombus.

The lack of long-term clinical efficacy of this approach is probably due to the rapid development of collateral vessels. The study by Plengvanit *et al.* (1972) showed that neovascularization can occur within 1 week of hepatic artery ligation. Collaterals originate from any of the nearby arteries. There was one prospective randomized study done in Hong Kong which compared surgical hepatic de-arterialization and a control group receiving no treatment. Despite treatment-related mortality, especially in the embolization group, no survival advantage could be demonstrated when compared with the controls, with median survivals both <3 months (Lai *et al.*, 1986).

Hepatic arterial embolization through hepatic angiography is a safer procedure and has less morbidity than surgical de-arterialization. Several types of foreign materials are used to occlude tumor vessels in HCC. Steel coils, Ivalon (250–590 μm) particles and gelatin sponge particles (Gelfoam, 3 mm cubes) have been used to occlude larger vessels more centrally located. Ivalon and steel coils can produce permanent occlusion of the hepatic artery while the other materials (Gelfoam, degradable starch microspheres) only produce temporary occlusion. A temporary occlusion can allow subsequent intra-arterial treatment after the vessel opens up again. This is widely practised in conjunction with cytotoxic chemotherapy in chemoembolization,

The side-effects of hepatic arterial embolization are usually pain, fever and nausea. There may be a transient increase in liver enzymes (Coldwell and Mortimer, 1991) which is due to enzymes released by the necrotic tumor cells. Despite good symptomatic control for most well-selected cases for embolization, the treatment has failed to improve survival as a whole. It remains as one of the choices of palliative treatment for pain or tumor rupture (Corr *et al.*, 1993).

REFERENCES

Ackerman, N.B. (1972) Experimental studies on the circulatory dynamics of intrahepatic blood flow supply. *Cancer*, **29**, 435–9.

Al-Idrissi, H., Ibrahim, E., Satir, A. *et al.* (1985) Primary hepatocellular carcinoma in the Eastern Province of Saudi Arabia: treatment with combination chemotherapy using 5-fluorouracil, adriamycin and mitomycin-C. *Hepatogastroenterology*, **32**, 8–10.

Anderson, J.H., Goldberg, J.A., Bessent, R.G. *et al.* (1992) Glass yttrium-90 microspheres for patients with colorectal liver metastases. *Radiotherapy and Oncology*, **25**, 137–9.

Ansfield, F., Ramirez, G., Skibba, J. *et al.* (1971) Intrahepatic arterial infusion with 5-fluorouracil. *Cancer*, **28**, 1147–51.

Austin-Seymour, M.M., Chen, G.T., Castro, J.R. *et al.* (1986) Dose volume histogram analysis of liver radiation tolerance. *International Journal of Radiation Oncology, Biology Physics*, **12**, 31–5.

Baker, L., Saiki, J., Jones, S., Hewlett, J. *et al.* (1977) Adriamycin and 5-fluorouracil in the treatment of advanced hepatoma: a Southwest Oncology Group study. *Cancer Treatment Reports*, **61**, 1595–7.

Bezwods, W. and Berman, D. (1982) Treatment of advanced malignant hepatoma with adriamycin or AMSA in combination with VM26 + 5-FU. *Proceedings of the American Society of Clinical Oncology*, **1**, 91.

Breedis, C. and Young, G. (1954) The blood supply of neoplasms in the liver. *American Journal of Pathology*, **30**, 969–85.

Burton, M.A., Gray, B.N., Self, G.W. *et al.* (1985) Manipulation of experimental rat and rabbit liver tumour blood flow with angiotensin-II. *Cancer Research*, **45**, 5390–3.

Campbell, T., Howell, S., Pfeifle, C. *et al.* (1983) Clinical pharmacokinetics of intra-arterial cisplatin in humans. *Journal of Clinical Oncology*, **1**, 755–62.

Carr, B.I., Orons, P., Zajko, A. *et al.* (1994) Prolonged survival with chemotherapy alone for hepatocellular carcinoma (HCC) with intra-arterial chemotherapy. *Proceedings of the Annual Meeting of the American Society of Clinical Oncology*, **13**, A606.

Carr, B.I., Orons, P., Zajko, A. *et al.* (1995) Phase II study of intra-hepatic arterial (I/A) *cis*-platinum, doxorubicin and Spherex for advanced stage hepatocellular carcinoma (HCC) (Meeting abstract). *Proceedings of the Annual Meeting of the American Society of Clinical Oncology*, **14**, A451.

Carr, B.I., Starzl, T.E., Iwatsuki, S. *et al.* (1991) Aggressive treatment for advanced hepatocellular carcinoma (HCC). High response rates and prolonged survival. *Hepatology*, **14**, 243.

Castells, A., Bruix, J., Bru, C. *et al.* (1993) Treatment of small hepatocellular carcinoma in cirrhotic patients: a cohort study comparing surgical resection and percutaneous ethanol injection. *Hepatology*, **18**, 1121–6.

Castells, A., Bruix, J., Bru, C. *et al.* (1995) Treatment of hepatocellular carcinoma with tamoxifen: a double-blind placebo-controlled trial in 120 patients. *Gastroenterology*, **109**, 917–22.

Chearanai, O., Plengvanit, U., Tuchinda, S. *et al.* (1974) Treatment of advanced primary liver carcinoma using intermittent intra-arterial nitrogen mustard. *Southeast Asian Journal of Tropical Medicine and Public Health*, **5**, 96–104.

Cheng, E., Watson, R., Fortner, J. *et al.* (1982) Regional intra-arterial infusion of cisplatin in primary liver cancer: a phase II trial. *Proceedings of the American Society of Clinical Oncology*, **2**, 179 (abstr.).

Chenivesse, X., Franco, D. and Brechot, C. (1993) MDR1 (multidrug resistance) gene expression in human primary liver cancer and cirrhosis. *Journal of Hepatology*, **18**, 168–72.

Choi, T., Lee, N. and Wong, J. (1984) Chemotherapy for advanced hepatocellular carcinoma. Adriamycin versus quadruple chemotherapy. *Cancer*, **53**, 401–5.

Chung, S.C.S., Lee, T.W., Kwok, S.P.Y. and Li, A.K.C. (1990) Injection of alcohol to control bleeding from ruptured hepatomas. *British Medical Journal*, **301**, 421.

Civalleri, D. (1992) Methods to enhance the efficacy of regional chemotherapeutic treatment of liver malignancies, in *An Update on Regional Treatment of Liver Cancer*, Wells Medical Press, pp. 17–34.

Coldwell, D.M. and Mortimer, J.E. (1991) Hepatic artery embolization in the treatment of hepatic malignancies. *Regional Cancer Treatment*, **3**, 298–301.

Corr, P., Chan, M., Lau, W.Y. and Metreweli, C. (1993) The role of hepatic arterial embolization in the management of ruptured hepatocellular carcinoma. *Clinical Radiology*, **48**, 163–5.

Damrongsak, C., Viranuvatti, V., Chearanai, O. and Tuchinda, S. (1973) Vinblastine in the treatment of carcinoma of the liver. *Journal of the Medical Association of Thailand*, **56**, 370–2.

Dunk, A., Scott, S.C., Johnson, P.J. *et al.* (1985) Mitozantrone as single agent therapy in hepatocellular carcinoma. A phase II study. *Journal of Hepatology*, **1**, 395–404.

Ebara, M., Ohto, M., Sugiura, N. *et al.* (1990) Percutaneous ethanol injection for the treatment of small hepatocellular carcinoma. Study of 95 patients. *Journal of Gastroenterology and Hepatology*, **5**, 616–26.

Falkson, G., Coetzer, B. and Klaassen, D. (1981) A phase II study of m-AMSA in patients with primary liver cancer. *Cancer Chemotherapy and Pharmacology*, **6**, 127–9.

Falkson, G., MacIntyre, J., Moertel, C. *et al.* (1984a) Primary liver cancer. An Eastern Cooperative Oncology Group trial. *Cancer*, **54**, 970–7.

Falkson, G., MacIntyre, J., Schutt, A. *et al.* (1984b) Neocarzinostatin versus m-AMSA or doxorubicin in hepatocellular carcinoma. *Journal of Clinical Oncology*, **2**, 581–4.

Falkson, G., Ryan, L.M., Johnson, L.A. *et al.* (1987) A randomized phase II study of mitoxantrone and cisplatin in patients with hepatocellular carcinoma: an ECOG study. *Cancer*, **60**, 2141–5.

Farinati, F., De Maria, N., Fornasiero, A. *et al.* (1992) Prospective controlled trial with anti-estrogen drug tamoxifen in patients with unresectable hepatocellular carcinoma. *Digestive Disease Sciences*, **37**, 659–62.

Forbes, A., Johnson, P.J. and Williams, R. (1985) Recombinant human gamma-interferon in primary hepatocellular carcinoma. *Journal of the Royal Society Medicine*, **78**, 826–9.

Gailani, S., Holland, J., Falkson, G. *et al.* (1972) Comparison of treatment of metastatic gastrointestinal cancer with 5-fluorouracil (5-FU) to a combination of 5-FU with cytosine arabinoside. *Cancer*, **29**, 1308–13.

Goldberg, J.A., Thomson, J.A.K., Bradnam, M.S. *et al.* (1991) Angiotensin II as a potential method of targeting cytotoxic-loaded microspheres in patients with colorectal liver metastases. *British Journal of Cancer*, **64**, 114–19.

Gray, B.N., Burton, M.A., Kelleher, D.K. *et al.* (1989) Selective internal radiation (S.I.R.) therapy for treatment of liver metastases: measurement of response rate. *Journal of Surgical Oncology*, **42**, 192–6.

Gray, B.N., Burton, M.A., Kelleher, D. *et al.* (1990) Tolerance of the liver to the effects of Yttrium-90 radiation. *International Journal of Radiation Oncology, Biology, Physics*, **18**, 619–23.

Ho, S., Lau, W.Y., Leung, W.T. *et al.* (1996) Partition model for estimating radiation doses from Yttrium-90 microspheres in treating hepatomas. *European Journal of Nuclear Medicine*, **23**, 947–52.

Hochster, H., Green, M., Speyer, J. *et al.* (1985) 4′-Epidoxorubicin (Epirubicin): activity in hepatocellular carcinoma. *Journal of Clinical Oncology*, **11**, 1535–40.

Houle, S., Yip, T.K., Shepherd, F.A. *et al.* (1989) Hepatocellular carcinoma: pilot trial of treatment with Y-90 microspheres. *Radiology*, **172**, 857–60.

Jiang, S.Y., Shyu, R.Y., Yeh, M.Y. and Jordan, V.C. (1995) Tamoxifen inhibits hepatoma cell growth through an estrogen receptor independent mechanism. *Journal of Hepatology*, **23**, 712–9.

Johnson, P.J., Kalayci, C., Dobbs, N. *et al.* (1991a) Pharmacokinetics and toxicity of intra-arterial adriamycin for hepatocellular carcinoma: effect of coadministration of lipiodol. *Journal of Hepatology*, **13**, 120–7.

Johnson, P.J., Kalayci, C., Dobbs, N. *et al.* (1991b) Pharmacokinetics and toxicity of intra-arterial adriamycin for hepatocellular carcinoma: effect of coadministration of lipiodol. *Journal of Hepatology*, **13**, 120–7.

Johnson, P.J., Thomas, H., Williams, R. *et al.* (1978) Induction of remission in hepatocellular carcinoma with doxorubicin. *Lancet*, **i**, 1006–9.

Kalayci, C., Johnson, P.J., Raby, N. *et al.* (1990) Intra-arterial adriamycin and lipiodol for inoperable hepatocellular carcinoma: a comparison with intravenous adriamycin. *Journal of Hepatology*, **11**, 345–53.

Kanematsu, T., Furuta, T., Takenaka, K. *et al.* (1989) A 5-year experience of lipiodolisation: selective regional chemotherapy for 200 patients with hepatocellular carcinoma. *Hepatology*, **10**, 89–102.

Kasugai, H., Kojima, J., Tatsuta, M. *et al.* (1989) Treatment of hepatocellular carcinoma by transcatheter arterial embolization combined with intra-arterial infusion of a mixture of cisplatin and ethiodized oil. *Gastroenterology*, **97**, 965–71.

Kinami, Y., Shinmura, K. and Miyazaki, I. (1978) The super-selective and the selective one-shot methods for treating inoperable cancer of the liver. *Cancer*, **41**, 1720–1.

Konno, T., Maeda, H., Iwai, K. *et al.* (1983) Effect of arterial administration of high-molecular-weight anticancer agent SMANCS with lipid lymphographic agent on hepatoma: a preliminary report. *European Journal of Cancer and Clinical Oncology*, **19**, 1053–65.

Lai, C.L., Lau, J.Y., Wu, P.C. *et al.* (1993) Recombinant interferon-alpha in inoperable hepatocellular carcinoma: a randomized controlled trial. *Hepatology*, **17**, 389–94.

Lai, C.L., Wu, P.C., Chan, G.C. *et al.* (1988) Doxorubicin versus no antitumor therapy in inoperable hepatocellular carcinoma. A prospective randomized trial. *Cancer*, **62**, 479–83.

Lai, C.L., Wu, P.C., Lok, A.S. *et al.* (1989) Recombinant alpha 2 interferon is superior to doxorubicin for inoperable hepatocellular carcinoma: a prospective randomised trial. *British Journal of Cancer*, **60**, 928–33.

Lai, E., Choi, T., Tong, S. *et al.* (1986) Treatment of unresectable hepatocellular carcinoma: results of a randomized controlled trial. *World Journal of Surgery*, **10**, 501–9.

Lau, W.Y., Ho, S., Leung, W.T. *et al.* (1998) Selective internal radiation therapy for non-resectable hepatocellular carcinoma with intra-arterial infusion of yttrium-90 microspheres. *International Journal of Radiation Oncology, Biology, Physics*, **40**, 583–92.

Lau, W.Y., Leung, W.T., Ho, S. *et al.* (1994a) Diagnostic pharmaco-scintigraphy with hepatic intra-arterial technetium-99 m macroaggregated albumin in the determination of tumour to non-tumour uptake ratio in hepatocellular carcinoma. *British Journal of Radiology*, **67**, 136–9.

Lau, W.Y., Leung, W.T., Ho, S. *et al.* (1994b) Treatment of inoperable hepatocellular carcinoma with intrahepatic arterial yttrium-90 microspheres: a phase I and II study. *British Journal of Cancer*, **70**, 994–9.

Lee, K., Chan, K., Leung, W.T. *et al.* (1992) Disposition of epirubicin in an oily contrast medium after intravenous and intrahepato-arterial administration in liver cancer: a preliminary report. *European Journal of Drug Metabolism and Pharmacokinetics*, **17**, 221–6.

Lee, N.W., Wong, J. and Ong, G.B. (1982) The surgical management of primary carcinoma of the liver. *World Journal of Surgery*, **6**, 66–75.

Leung, W.T., Lau, W.Y., Ho, S. *et al.* (1995) Radiation pneumonitis after selective internal radiation treatment with intra-arterial [90]yttrium-microspheres for inoperable hepatic tumors. *International Journal of Radiation Oncology, Biology, Physics*, **33**, 919–24.

Leung, W.T., Shiu, W.C., Leung, N. *et al.* (1992) Treatment of inoperable hepatocellular carcinoma by intra-arterial lipiodol and 4'-epidoxorubicin. *Cancer Chemotherapy and Pharmacology*, **29**, 401–4.

Livarghi, T., Bolondi, L., Lazzaroni, S. *et al.* (1992) Percutaneous ethanol injection in the treatment of hepatocellular carcinoma in cirrhosis. *Cancer*, **69**, 925–6.

Madden, M.V., Krige, J.E., Bailey, S. *et al.* (1993) Randomised trial of targeted chemotherapy with lipiodol and 5-epidoxorubicin compared with symptomatic treatment for hepatoma. *Gut*, **34**, 1598–600.

Madsen, M.T., Park, C.H. and Thakur, M.L. (1988) Dosimetry of iodine-131 ethiodol in the treatment of hepatoma. *Journal of Nuclear Medicine*, **29**, 1038–44.

Manesis, E.K., Giannoulis, G., Zoumboulis, P. *et al.* (1995) Treatment of hepatocellular carcinoma with combined suppression and inhibition of sex hormones: a randomized, controlled trial. *Hepatology*, **21**, 1535–42.

Martinez Cerezo, F.J., Tomas, A. *et al.* (1994) Controlled trial of tamoxifen in patients with advanced hepatocellular carcinoma. *Journal of Hepatology*, **20**, 702–6.

Melia, W., Johnson, P. and Williams, R. (1983) Induction of remission in hepatocellular carcinoma. A comparison of VP16 with adriamycin. *Cancer*, **51**, 206–21.

Melia, W.M., Johnson, P.J. and Williams, R. (1987) Controlled clinical trial of doxorubicin and tamoxifen versus doxorubicin alone in hepatocellular carcinoma. *Cancer Treatment Reports*, **71**, 1213–16.

Nagasue, N., Ito, A., Yukaya, H. and Ogawa, Y. (1985) Androgen receptors in hepatocellular carcinoma and surrounding parenchyma. *Gastroenterology*, **89**, 643–7.

Nagasue, N., Ito, A., Yukaya, H. and Ogawa, Y. (1986) Estrogen receptors in hepatocellular carcinoma. *Cancer*, **57**, 87–91.

Nerenstone, S.R., Ihde, D.C. and Friedman, M.A. (1988) Clinical trials in primary hepatocellular carcinoma: current status and future directions. *Cancer Treatment Reviews*, **15**, 1–31.

Ngan, H., Lai, C.L., Fan, S.T. *et al.* (1996) Transcatheter arterial chemoembolization in inoperable hepatocellular carcinoma: four-year follow-up. *Journal of Vascular Interventive Radiology*, **7**, 419–25.

Okayasu, I., Hatakeyama, S., Yoshida, T. *et al.* (1988) Selective and persistent deposition and gradual drainage of iodized oil, Lipiodol in the hepatocellular carcinoma after injection into the feeding hepatic artery. *American Journal of Clinical Pathology*, **90**, 536–44.

Okuda, K. (1980) Primary liver cancers in Japan. *Cancer*, **45**, 2663–72.

Olweny, C., Katongole-Mbidde, E., Bahendeka, S. *et al.* (1980) Further experience in treating patients with hepatocellular carcinoma in Uganda. *Cancer*, **46**, 2717–22.

Order, S., Pajak, T., Leibel, S. *et al.* (1991) A randomized prospective trial comparing full dose chemotherapy to ^{131}I-antiferritin: an RTOG study. *International Journal of Radiation Oncology, Biology, Physics*, **20**, 953–63.

Order, S.E., Stillwagon, G.B. and Klein, J.L. (1985) Iodine-131 antiferritin, a new treatment modality in hepatoma: a Radiation Therapy Oncology Group Study. *Journal of Clinical Oncology*, **3**, 1573–82.

Pack, G.T. and Livingston, E.M. (eds) (1940) *Treatment of Cancer and Allied Diseases*, Paul B. Hoeber, New York, **9**, p. 1092.

Paliard, P., Clement, G., Saez, S. *et al.* (1984) Traitment du carcinome hepato-cellulaire par le tamoxifene. *Gastroenterology, Clinical Biology*, **8–9**, 680–1.

Park, C.H., Suh, J.H., Yoo, H.S. *et al.* (1986) Evaluation of Intrahepatic I-131 ethiodol on a patient with hepatocellular carcinoma. Therapeutic feasibility study. *Clinical Nuclear Medicine*, **11**, 514–17.

Patt, Y.Z., Charnsangavej, C., Yoffe, B. *et al.* (1994) Hepatic arterial infusion of floxuridine, leucovorin, doxorubicin, and cisplatin for hepatocellular carcinoma: effects of hepatitis B and C viral infection on drug toxicity and patient survival. *Journal of Clinical Oncology*, **12**, 1204–11.

Patt, Y.Z., Yoffe, B., Charnsangavej, C. *et al.* (1993) Low serum alpha-fetoprotein level in patients with hepatocellular carcinoma as a predictor of response to 5-FU and interferon-alpha-2b. *Cancer*, **72**, 2574–82.

Pelletier, G., Roche, A. and Ink, O. (1990) A randomized trial of hepatic arterial chemoembolization in patients with unresectable hepatocellular carcinoma. *Journal of Hepatology*, **11**, 181–4.

Plengvanit, U., Chearanai, O., Sindhvananda, K. *et al.* (1972) Collateral arterial blood supply of the liver after hepatic artery ligation. Angiographic study of 20 patients. *Annals of Surgery*, **175**, 105–10.

Raoul, J.I., Bretagne, J.F., Caucanas, J.P. *et al.* (1992a) Internal radiation therapy for hepatocellular carcinoma, results of a French multicentre phase II trial of transarterial injection of iodine 131-labeled Lipiodol. *Cancer*, **69**, 346–52.

Raoul, J.L., Guyader, D., Bretagne, J.F. *et al.* (1994) Randomized controlled trial for hepatocellular carcinoma with portal vein thrombosis: intra-arterial iodine-131-iodized oil versus medical support. *Journal of Nuclear Medicine*, **35**, 1782–7.

Raoul, J.L., Heresbach, D., Bretagne, J.F. *et al.* (1992b) Chemoembolization of hepatocellular carcinomas. A study of the biodistribution and pharmacokinetics of doxorubicin. *Cancer*, **70**, 585–90.

Ravry, M., Omura, G. and Bartolucci, A. (1984) Phase II evaluation of doxorubicin plus bleomycin in hepatocellular carcinoma: a Southeastern Cancer Study Group Trial. *Cancer Treatment Reports*, **68**, 1517–18.

Robertson, J.M., Lawrence, T.S., Dworzanin, L.M. *et al.* (1993) Treatment of primary hepatobiliary cancers with conformal radiation therapy and regional chemotherapy. *Journal of Clinical Oncology*, **11**, 1286–93.

Rougier, P., Pelletier, G., Ducreux, M. *et al.* (1997) Unresectable hepatocellular carcinoma: lack of efficacy of lipiodol chemoembolization. Final results of a multicenter randomized trial. *Proceedings of the Annual Meeting of the American Society of Clinical Oncology*, **16**, A989.

Rougier, P., Roche, A., Pelletier, G. *et al.* (1993) Efficacy of chemoembolization for hepatocellular carcinomas: experience from the Gustave Roussy Institute and the Bicetre Hospital. *Journal of Surgical Oncology*, **3 (Suppl.)**, 94–6.

Ryder, S.D., Rizzi, P.M., Metivier, E. *et al.* (1996) Chemoembolisation with lipiodol and doxorubicin: applicability in British patients with hepatocellular carcinoma. *Gut*, **38**, 125–8.

Schacter, L., Crum, E., Spitzer, T. *et al.* (1986) Fatal radiation hepatitis: a case report and review of the literature. *Gynecological Oncology*, **24**, 373–80.

Shepherd, F.A., Rotstein, L.E., Houle, S. *et al.* (1992) A phase I dose escalation trial of Yttrium-90 microspheres in the treatment of primary hepatocellular carcinoma. *Cancer*, **70**, 2250–4.

Shibata, J., Fujiyama, S., Sata, T. *et al.* (1989) Hepatic arterial injection chemotherapy with cisplatin suspended in an oily lymphographic agent for hepatocellular carcinoma. *Cancer*, **64**, 1586–94.

Shildt, R., Baker, L. and Stuckey, W. (1984) Hepatic artery infusion (HAI) with 5FUDR, adriamycin (A) and streptozotocin (St) in unresectable hepatoma. A Southwest Oncology Group Study. *Proceedings of the American Society of Clinical Oncology*, **3**, 150 (abstr.).

Shiu, W., Dewar, G., Leung, N. *et al.* (1990) Hepatocellular carcinoma in Hong Kong: a clinical study on 340 cases. *Oncology*, **47**, 241–5.

Soini, Y., Virkajarvi, N., Raunio, H. and Paakko, P. (1996) Expression of P-glycoprotein in hepatocellular carcinoma: a potential marker of prognosis. *Journal of Clinical Pathology*, **49**, 470–3.

Stuart, K., Stokes, K., Jenkins, R. *et al.* (1993) Treatment of hepatocellular carcinoma using doxorubicin/ethiodized oil/gelatin powder chemoembolization. *Cancer*, **72**, 3202–9.

Sunderland, G.T., Chisholm, E.M., Lau, W.Y. *et al.* (1992) Alcohol injection: a treatment for ruptured hepatocellular carcinoma. *Surgical Oncology*, **1**, 61–3.

Tashiro, S. and Maeda, H. (1985) Clinical evaluation of arterial administration of SMANCS in oily contrast medium for liver cancer. *Japanese Journal of Medicine*, **24**, 79–80.

The Gastrointestinal Tumor Study Group (1990) A prospective trial of recombinant human interferon-alpha 2b in previously untreated patients with hepatocellular carcinoma. *Cancer*, **66**, 135–9.

Trinchet *et al.* from Groupe d'Etude et de Traitement du Carcinome Hepatocellulaire (1995) A comparison of lipiodol chemoembolization and conservative treatment for unresectable hepatocellular carcinoma. *New England Journal of Medicine*, **332**, 1256–61.

Urist, M. and Balch, C. (1984) Intra-arterial chemotherapy for hepatoma using adriamycin administered via an implantable infusion pump. *Proceedings of the American Society of Clinical Oncology*, **3**, 148 (abstr.).

Venook, A.P., Stagg, R.J., Lewis, B.J. *et al.* (1990) Chemoembolization for hepatocellular carcinoma. *Journal of Clinical Oncology*, **8**, 1108–14.

Vilana, R., Bruix, J., Bru, C. *et al.* (1992) Tumor size determines the efficacy of percutaneous ethanol injection for the treatment of small hepatocellular carcinoma. *Hepatology*, **16**, 354–7.

Wellwood, J., Cady, B. and Oberfield, R. (1979) Treatment of primary liver cancer: response to regional chemotherapy. *Clinical Oncology*, **5**, 25–31.

Williams, R. and Melia, W. (1980) Liver tumors and their management. *Clinical Radiology*, **31**, 1–11.

Yamasaki, S., Hasegawa, H., Makuuchi, M. *et al.* (1991) Choice of treatments for small hepatocellular carcinoma: Hepatectomy, embolization or ethanol injection. *Journal of Gastroenterology and Hepatology*, **6**, 408–13.

Yoo, H.S., Lee, J.T., Kim, K.W. *et al.* (1991) Nodular hepatocellular carcinoma. Treatment with subsegmental intra-arterial injection of iodine 131-labeled iodized oil. *Cancer*, **68**, 1878–84.

Yoshida, T., Okazaki, Yoshino, M. *et al.* (1990) Phase II trial of high dose recombinant gamma-interferon in advanced hepatocellular carcinoma. *European Journal of Cancer*, **26**, 545–6.

Yoshikawa, M., Saisho, H., Ebara, M. *et al.* (1994) A randomized trial of intrahepatic arterial infusion of 4'-epidoxorubicin with lipiodol versus 4'-epidoxorubicin alone in the treatment of hepatocellular carcinoma. *Cancer Chemotherapy and Pharmacology*, **33**, S149–52.

Yumoto, Y., Jinno, K., Tokuyama, K. *et al.* (1985) Hepatocellular carcinoma detected by iodized oil. *Radiology*, **154**, 19–24.

MANAGEMENT OF SPECIFIC TUMOR COMPLICATIONS

C.K. Leow and J.W.Y. Lau

Apart from the presentations common to all malignant tumors, hepatocellular carcinoma (HCC) can give rise to presentations that can confuse and mislead the unwary.

11.1 SPONTANEOUS RUPTURE

Spontaneous rupture of the liver with acute hemoperitoneum can be the result of bleeding from peliosis hepatis and liver cell adenomas in oral contraceptive users (Bagheri and Boyer, 1974), hemangiomas (Sewell and Weiss, 1961), polyarteritis nodosa (Li *et al.*, 1979), metastases (Mokka *et al.*, 1976; Urdneta and Nielsen, 1986) and eclampsia (Baumwol and Park, 1976). However, spontaneous rupture of the liver is rarely due to these causes in Africa and the East. Spontaneous rupture of the HCC presenting as an acute abdomen, though rare, is the most common cause of spontaneous hemoperitoneum in sub-Saharan Africa and the Far East. The incidence ranges from 5 to 15% of patients with hepatoma (Leading Article, 1976; Nagasue and Inokuchi, 1979; Chearanai *et al.*, 1983; Chen *et al.*, 1988). In contrast, spontaneous rupture of HCC is rare in the West with an incidence of only 2.7% in England (Kew *et al.*, 1971). The incidence at our institution is 9.7% (Dewar *et al.*, 1991). Ruptured HCC is more common in males and is associated with underlying cirrhosis (Ong

and Taw, 1972; Chearanai *et al.*, 1983; Dewar *et al.*, 1991). The exact mechanism for spontaneous rupture of HCC remains unproven. While cirrhosis (with its attendant portal hypertension and coagulopathy) and maleness (a reflection of robust physical activity or hormonal influences) are probable co-contributory factors, venous hypertension secondary to thrombi obstructing the draining hepatic veins of the tumor, together with a rich and fragile arterial supply may be important mechanistic factors in the spontaneous rupture of HCC (Nagasue and Inokuchi, 1979; Chearanai *et al.*, 1983).

The majority of patients with spontaneous rupture of HCC present with acute abdominal pain, peritonitis with or without evidence of hypovolemic shock. There may be a history of ill health, esophageal varices treated endoscopically or a diagnosis of hepatic malignancy. Physical examination may reveal signs of hypovolemic shock, jaundice and abdominal distension. Abdominal paracentesis will confirm the presence of hemoperitoneum and urgent resuscitation is required in unstable patients. Those patients not in shock can have the diagnosis confirmed urgently by abdominal ultrasonography or computed tomography. However, a minority of patients present with malaise, marked pallor and increasing abdominal girth.

Hepatocellular Carcinoma: Diagnosis, investigation and management. Edited by Anthony S.-Y. Leong, Choong-Tsek Liew, Joseph W.Y. Lau and Philip J. Johnson. Published in 1999 by Arnold, London. ISBN 0 340 74096 5.

Abdominal paracentesis will confirm the presence of hemorrhagic ascites from tumor oozing into the peritoneal cavity over a period of days. These patients are hemodynamically compensated but have marked pallor from the hemodilution.

Traditionally, the treatment of spontaneous rupture of HCC in Hong Kong has been aggressive surgical intervention in the form of laparotomy and hepatic resection following resuscitation (Ong *et al.*, 1965; Ong and Taw, 1972). These resections were mostly palliative and one-third was accompanied by operative death (Ong and Taw, 1972). While some investigators have reported similar operative mortality (Chen *et al.*, 1988), others, including

us, have reported a much higher operative mortality rate of 55–75% (Dewar *et al.*, 1991; Muhammed and Mabogunje, 1991).

Bleeding from ruptured HCC is neither invariably exsanguinating nor progressive in nature. At our institution, these patients are managed according to the algorithm shown in Fig. 11.1. After the initial resuscitation, these patients can be divided into two groups, namely, hemodynamically labile and hemodynamically stable.

Patients with stable blood pressure undergo urgent ultrasonography to confirm the diagnosis and they proceed to selective hepatic angiogram. If the source of bleeding is demonstrated, the lesion(s) is embolized.

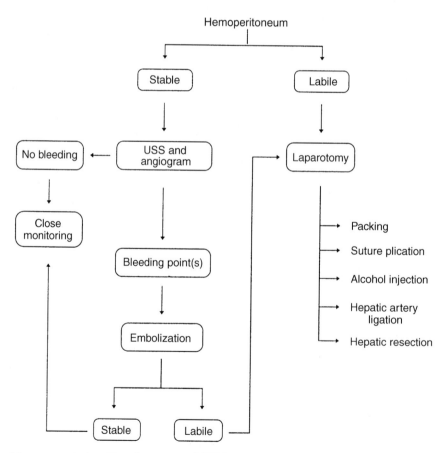

Fig. 11.1 Management algorithm for ruptured HCC.

Treatment of ruptured HCC by angiographic embolization is advocated by others (Sato *et al.*, 1985; Hirai *et al.*, 1986; Hsieh *et al.*, 1987) provided the patient is adequately resuscitated and the procedure performed with an experienced hepatic surgeon in attendance.

Unstable patients, despite resuscitation, undergo immediate laparotomy for hemostasis. Previously we resorted to the application of local pressure, suture plication of the bleeding lesion, packing, hepatic artery ligation or formal hepatic resection as a last resort for hemostasis. In the presence of cirrhosis, impaired liver function and acute hemorrhage, the majority of these patients tolerate hepatic artery ligation or hepatic resection poorly. In our series of emergency surgical intervention for control of spontaneous rupture of HCC, the operative mortality for emergency hepatic resection was 55%. Twelve patients were managed by hepatic artery ligation but eight died postoperatively from liver failure. Although three of the 12 patients managed to survive for 6 months, they too died from subsequent liver failure (Dewar *et al.*, 1991). Presently, our preferred treatment modality is direct injection of absolute alcohol into and around the bleeding site until blanching of the tumor occurs and the bleeding stops. In our series of patients treated with intralesional alcohol injection for ruptured HCC, hepatic artery ligation as an additional procedure for hemostasis was only necessary in 44% of cases. None required emergency hepatic resection (Sunderland *et al.*, 1992) and there was only one in-hospital death.

Following the acute episode, patients with potentially resectable lesions undergo further evaluation with computed tomography and hepatic angiography with a view to hepatic resection. In most large series of patients with ruptured HCC, it is not unusual to find the occasional long-term survivor following hepatic resection. Thus, a history of previous rupture does not equate invariably to the presence of peritoneal dissemination of tumor.

11.2 OBSTRUCTIVE JAUNDICE

Jaundice as a presenting symptom of hepatocellular carcinoma occurs in 5–44% of cases (Edmonson and Steiner, 1954; Kappel and Miller, 1972; Ihde *et al.*, 1974; Kew and Geddes, 1982). The majority of these icteric patients have underlying parenchymal insufficiency and a percutaneous ultrasound scan will reveal a non-dilated biliary ductal system. For these patients, the presence of jaundice merely reflects the end-stage nature of the disease. HCC can rarely present as obstructive jaundice due to obstruction of the biliary tract by intraluminal tumor cast, tumor fragments or blood clots, extraluminal compression of the bile ducts by the tumor or enlarged lymph nodes with metastases in the porta hepatis. The reported incidence varies from 0.7 to 11.7% (Ihde *et al.*, 1974; Lin, 1976; Okuda, 1976; Kojiro *et al.*, 1982; Lee *et al.*, 1984; Lau *et al.*, 1990). Lin (1976) coined the term 'icteric type' HCC for these rare cases and stressed their peculiarity which can give rise to diagnostic difficulty.

After demonstrating the presence of a dilated system by ultrasonography, an endoscopic retrograde cholangiography or a percutaneous transhepatic cholangiogram is performed. Based on the cholangiographic appearance, we classify the cases into obstructive icteric HCC type 1, 2 or 3.

11.2.1 CLASSIFICATION OF OBSTRUCTIVE ICTERIC TYPE HCC

11.2.1.1 Type 1

This type of obstruction is due to intraluminal bile duct obstruction (Fig. 11.2). The tumor, having invaded into a peripheral bile duct, grows into and along the hepatic duct until the confluence of the right and left hepatic ducts, causing partial or complete biliary obstruction. Further extension of the biliary tumor cast into the common hepatic and bile duct will cause complete obstruction of the biliary system. The appearance of the intra-luminal cast on ERCP resembles that of a cork in the neck of a bottle, termed the 'cork sign'. Occasionally, the tumor cast is within one of the main hepatic ducts and in itself would not lead to obstructive jaundice. However, tumor fragments shed within the main hepatic duct can drop into the common bile duct, causing biliary obstruction. The filling defects are similar to those seen in choledocholithiasis but the edges of the filling defects secondary to tumor fragments are irregular and less well-defined than those of stones. Patients with obstructive icteric HCC type 1 should undergo further assessment by selective hepatic angiography and computed tomography since a proportion of these patients have potentially resectable tumors.

11.2.1.2 Type 2

This type of obstruction is due to hemobilia. The tumor within the biliary ducts can bleed and part or whole of the common bile duct and common hepatic duct becomes filled with blood clots. These blood clots give rise to a cholangiographic appearance of fluffy intra-luminal filling defects that obscure the under-lying tumor. The obstructed system should be temporized with a nasobiliary drain. Once the hemobilia has settled, the patient is subjected to another cholangiographic examination to clarify the underlying cause of the obstruction.

11.2.1.3 Type 3

This type of obstruction is due to extraluminal bile duct obstruction (Fig. 11.3). Tumor inva-sion and/or encasement of the hepatic ducts will give rise to localized stricture and prox-imal intrahepatic ductal dilatation. The pres-ence of enlarged, involved malignant porta hepatis lymph nodes can compress the com-mon hepatic/bile duct, leading to obstructive jaundice. Patients with obstructive icteric HCC type 3 have inoperable disease and are best palliated with endoscopic or percuta-neous stents, unless they are terminally ill.

In our series of 49 patients with obstructive icteric type HCC, nine patients were explored surgically and had curative resection (Lau *et al.*, 1997). The survival of these patients was significantly better than those who were trea-ted by stenting alone. The 5-year survival was approximately 45%.

Obstructive icteric type HCC is rare but prompt intervention in the appropriate patient in the form of palliative drainage of

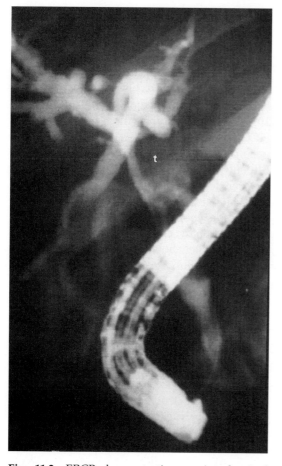

Fig. 11.2 ERCP demonstrating an intraluminal tumor thrombus (t) in the common hepatic duct. The appearance of the intraluminal cast resembles that of a cork in the neck of a bottle, termed the 'cork sign'.

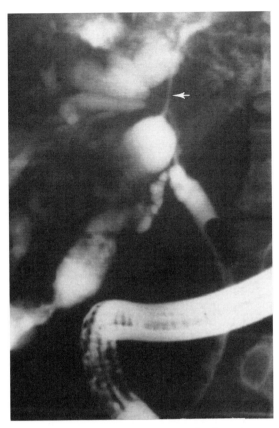

Fig. 11.3 ERCP demonstrating multiple strictures affecting the intrahepatic bile ducts. Encasement of the bile duct leads to localized stricture (arrow) and dilatation of proximal intrahepatic ducts.

the obstructed system or surgical resection can lead to prolonged survival and potential cure (Afroudakis *et al.*, 1978; van Sonnenberg and Ferucci, 1979; Kojiro *et al.*, 1982; Lee *et al.*, 1984; Roslyn *et al.*, 1984; Wu *et al.*, 1994; Lau *et al.*, 1997).

11.3 VARICEAL HEMORRHAGE

In a post-mortem study of 287 cirrhotic patients with HCC, 61 patients died from massive variceal hemorrhage (Ho *et al.*, 1981). At our institution, 13% of HCC patients presented with upper gastrointestinal hemorrhage. Although 71% of these patients had

endoscopic evidence of varices, only 47% of the bleeding was variceal in origin (Yeo *et al.*, 1995). The median survival of these patients was 21 days from the initial bleed. This is comparable with the figure of 3.5 weeks (mean) previously reported (Ng *et al.*, 1989).

The poor survival of these patients is related to uncontrollable hemorrhage or rebleed soon after endoscopic sclerotherapy. A high percentage of these patients (50–86%) have tumor thrombi within the portal venous system, demonstrated at post-mortem or by ultrasonography (Ho *et al.*, 1981; Ng *et al.*, 1989; Yeo *et al.*, 1995). The risk of variceal bleed is highest when the main portal trunk contains tumor thrombi. In contrast tumor thrombus in the splenic vein is associated with a very low risk of variceal hemorrhage (Arakawa *et al.*, 1979; Akiba *et al.*, 1983). The presence of tumor thrombi within the portal venous system leads to venous obstruction and increased pressure. This aggravates the underlying portal hypertension from the associated cirrhosis and predisposes the patient to variceal rupture. In addition, the existence of a hepatic artery-portal venous shunt within the hepatoma allows the direct transmission of the arterial pressure to the splanchnic venous system (Nagasue *et al.*, 1977). This increased pressure will not only cause and aggravate variceal rupture but will also perpetuate the variceal hemorrhage. In addition to uncontrollable hemorrhage, the hemodynamic disturbance of an acute bleed, coupled with the presence of a large hepatoma in a cirrhotic liver, can decompensate the already suboptimal liver function leading to liver failure and death.

11.4 PARANEOPLASTIC SYNDROMES

It can be said that HCC is a great 'imitator' as patients with this tumor can develop a variety of clinical syndromes as part of the paraneoplactic manifestations of HCC. These phenomena may be present long before any local effects of the tumor are apparent and can thus mislead and delay diagnosis. The most important and 'common' paraneoplastic syndromes are hypoglycemia, erythrocytosis, hypercalcemia and hypercholesterolemia. Other rare syndromes include porphyria cutanea tarda, virilization and feminization syndromes, carcinoid syndrome, hypertrophic osteoarthropathy, hyperthyroidism and osteoporosis.

11.4.1   HYPOGLYCEMIA

The prevalence of hypoglycemia associated with HCC is variable and has been reported to vary from 4.6% in North American patients, to 6.7% in Southern African blacks and 27% in Hong Kong Chinese (McFazdean and Yeung, 1969; Ihde *et al.*, 1974; Kew and Paterson, 1985).

McFazdean and Yeung (1969) described two different forms of hypoglycemia in such patients. Type A hypoglycemia occurs in the last few weeks of the disease, amid rapidly progressing cachexia and tumor growth. The hypoglycemia is mild-to-moderate in degree, slowly progressive, mainly asymptomatic and may be overlooked easily if it is not assessed systematically. The development of hypoglycemia in these patients is attributed to increased insulin sensitivity secondary to some putative factors secreted by the tumor which might act as a sponge for glucose. The hypoglycemic state may be due in part to undernutrition and can be remedied with ease. Type B hypoglycemia occurs early in the course of the disease and is characterized by severe symptomatic hypoglycemia which leads to neuropsychiatric syndromes, coma, convulsions and occasionally death. Type B hypoglycemia is common among Hong Kong Chinese with HCC (13%) but is thought to be rare in Western countries (McFazdean and Yeung, 1969). It is too obvious to overlook and the hypoglycemia is difficult to control with glucose infusion, glucagon, corticosteroids and diazoxide.

The mechanism for type B hypoglycemia is thought to be related to tumor production of peptides with insulin-like activity and insulin-like growth factor II (IGF-II) has been implicated (Megyesi *et al.*, 1974; Gordon *et al.*, 1981). However, the plasma level of IGF-II is frequently not elevated (Megyesi *et al.*, 1974; Gordon *et al.*, 1981; Merimee, 1986). The serum of these patients contains predominantly 'big' IGF-II rather than 7.5 kDa IGF-II and the problem is a consistent abnormality in IGF-II transport. Normally, about 75% of serum IGFs are carried in a ternary complex which includes the IGFs, IGF binding protein 3 (IGFBP-3) and an acid-labile α-subunit. The remainder of the IGF is carried as complexes <50 kDa (Daughaday and Kapadia, 1989). The failure of the IGF-II and IGFBP-3 complex to bind with the acid-labile α-subunit results in smaller IGFBP complexes which facilitates transport across the capillary membrane and increases access to target tissues (Binoux and Hossenlopp, 1988). The net result is to increase the bioavailability of the 'big' IGF-II. Growth hormone therapy is useful in treating the severe hypoglycaemia in these patients while more definitive treatment such as hepatic resection or chemotherapy is being planned (Hunter *et al.*, 1994).

11.4.2   ERYTHROCYTOSIS

A low hemoglobin level is common in chronic liver disease and HCC patients (Jacobson *et al.*, 1978; Hwang *et al.*, 1994). Of southern African blacks with HCC, 58% are anemic at presentation (Jacobson *et al.*, 1978). However, a proportion of these HCC patients present with high normal or elevated levels of hemoglobin. McFadzean *et al.* (1958) defined erythrocytosis as a hemoglobin level >16 gm/dl (2 SD above the mean hemoglobin level of 12 normal controls) while Kan *et al.* (1961) defined it as a hematocrit >48%. The association between erythrocytosis and hepatocellular carcinoma was first reported from Hong Kong in 1958. Some degree of polycythemia, as measured by red cell counts and hemoglobin concentrations, was found in 10% of patients with HCC (McFadzean *et al.*, 1958). The reported incidence varies from 2.5 to 12% (McFadzean *et al.*, 1958; Kan *et al.*, 1961; Brownstein and Ballard, 1964; Jacobson *et al.*, 1978; Hwang *et al.*, 1994) and it is the second most common paraneoplastic syndrome (after hypoglycemia) associated with HCC.

Ectopic production of erythropoietin (Epo) by the tumor has been suggested as a cause of the erythrocytosis. Epo is produced by the fetal liver *in utero* (Fried, 1972). After birth, the kidney is the main source of Epo in man but the liver can produce Epo in the presence of uremia, in particular in anephric individuals, in response to hypoxia or hemolysis, or when the hepatocytes are regenerating (Anagnostov *et al.*, 1977; Simon *et al.*, 1980). Not all patients with erythrocytosis and HCC have raised Epo levels. Kew and Fisher (1986) found that only 15 of 65 patients with erythrocytosis had raised serum Epo concentrations. There appears to be an association between ectopic production of Epo and large tumor volume within a single lobe or both lobes of the liver. In their series of 20 patients, Hwang *et al.* (1994) showed that the mean tumor volume was 50% that of the entire liver. In addition to the raised level of Epo, these patients also have high serum levels of α-fetoprotein (AFP). Recently, Sakisaka *et al.* (1993), using immunohistochemical techniques, demonstrated that AFP was localized in the malignant hepatocyte which was also erythropoietin-positive. Not unlike the abnormal production of AFP, Epo production by HCC probably represents the de-differentiation of malignant hepatocytes with the abnormal secretion of Epo and AFP.

11.4.3 HYPERCALCEMIA

The incidence of hypercalcemia associated with HCC ranges from 5.3 to 40% (Knill-Jones *et al.*, 1970; Hwang *et al.*, 1989; van Leeuwen *et al.*, 1991). This increased to 69% in patients with sclerosing HCC (Omata *et al.*, 1981).

Based on the pathogenesis, Martin and Mundy (1987) classified hypercalcemia in malignancy into three subtypes: (1) tumors with bony metastases, (2) hematological malignancies and (3) tumors without bony metastases. The development of hypercalcemia in malignancy in the absence of metastases is thought to be secondary to the liberation of humoral factor(s), a main factor being parathyroid hormone-related peptide (PTHrP) (Martin and Mundy, 1987; Broadus *et al.*, 1988). The majority of HCC patients with hypercalcemia do not have bony metastases (Shek *et al.*, 1990) and PTHrP may mediate the development of hypercalcemia through an increased rate of bone resorption (Knill-Jones *et al.*, 1970; Panesar *et al.*, 1991). It is noteworthy that in patients with chronic viral hepatitis without HCC, hypercalcemia can occur without the presence of PTHrP factor and other bone resorptive factors such as osteoclast-activating factor, tumor necrosis factor, interleukin 1, prostaglandin and transforming growth factor may be responsible (Cadranel *et al.*, 1989).

11.4.4 HYPERCHOLESTEROLEMIA

Approximately 11–38% of patients with HCC have accompanying hypercholesterolemia (Alpert *et al.*, 1969; Goldberg *et al.*, 1975, Hwang *et al.*, 1992). In a series of 91 patients with HCC with hypercholesterolemia, there was no difference in survival between those with and those without hypercholesterolemia. The associated incidence of hypoglycemia was significantly higher in those with hypercholesterolemia. In 19 hypercholesterolemic HCC patients, the serum cholesterol level fell to normal following surgical resection or transhepatic arterial chemoembolization of the tumor. With tumor recurrence the cholesterol level rose to abnormal levels again. The change in the serum cholesterol parallels that of serum AFP, raising the possibility of employing cholesterol levels as another marker to monitor treatment response and/or identify tumor recurrence (Hwang *et al.*, 1992).

11.4.5   RARE SYNDROMES

Cutaneous signs in patients with HCC include vitiligo (Curth, 1969), thrombophlebitis migrans (Nusbacher, 1964; Bismuth *et al.*, 1995), pitiriasis rotunda (circumscripta) in blacks and Japanese (Ito and Tanaka, 1961; DiBisceglie *et al.*, 1986).

Primack *et al.* (1971) described a patient with HCC who presented with diarrhoea and fainting, increased urinary 5-hydroxy indole acetic acid and total 5-hydroxy indoles, features compatible with the diagnosis of carcinoid syndrome. Porphyria cutanea tarda, hypertrophic pulmonary osteoarthropathy, and clinically evident hyperthyroidism with elevated serum concentrations of thyroid-stimulating hormone, T4, T3 and free T3 have all been reported in patients with HCC (Keczkes and Barker, 1976; Kew and Dusheiko, 1981; Pierach *et al.*, 1984). Sexual changes occasionally occur in patients with HCC. These include isosexual precocious puberty, feminization and virilization. Isosexual precocious puberty tends to complicate hepatoblastoma, rarely it does afflict patients with HCC. It occurs only in males, with high testosterone levels, attributed to ectopic tumor production of gonadotrophin (Schwarz *et al.*, 1982). Kew and Dusheiko (1981) reported four cases of feminization and HCC in the absence of cirrhosis and in one well documented case feminization was attributed to trophoblastic activity of the tumor leading to high levels of serum estrone, estradiol, estriol and placental lactogen (Kew *et al.*, 1977). Bismuth *et al.* (1995), in their series of 68 non-cirrhotic patients with HCC who underwent resection, had two patients presenting with a syndrome of thrombophlebitis and virilization.

11.5   CONCLUSION

HCC can present in varying guises and forms. In low-incidence areas, this can lead to a delay in its diagnosis. As the mean survival time of untreated patients with HCC, from diagnosis to death, is 2–3 months (Nakamura *et al.*, 1993), the delay in arriving at a definitive diagnosis can make the difference between a potentially resectable lesion and an irresectable tumor. Awareness of the unusual presentations of HCC is even more relevant and is crucial for the management of patients in high incidence areas, in order to increase the chances of early treatment and improvement of survival.

REFERENCES

Afroudakis, A., Bhuta, S.M., Ranganath, K.A. *et al.* (1978) Obstructive jaundice caused by hepatocellular carcinoma. Report of three cases. *Digestive Diseases*, **23**, 609–17.

Akiba, M., Fujita, Y., Takahashi, H. *et al.* (1983) Clinical significance of tumor thrombosis of portal vein in hepatocellular carcinoma. *Jikeikai Medical Journal*, **30**, 197–206.

Alpert, M.E., Hutt, M.S.R. and Davidson, C.S. (1969) Primary hepatoma in Uganda. A prospective clinical and epidemiologic study of forty-six patients. *American Journal Medicine*, **46**, 794–802.

Anagnostov, A., Schade, S., Barone, J. *et al.* (1977) Effect of partial hepatectomy on extra-renal erythropoietin production in rats. *Blood*, **50**, 457–62.

Arakawa, M., Koga, M. and Kage, M. (1979) Pathomorphological study on primary liver cancers–relationship between tumor thrombus of portal vein and esophageal varices. *Kanzo Acta Hepatologica Japanica*, **20**, 941–7.

Bagheri, S.A. and Boyer, J.L. (1974) Peliosis hepatis associated with androgenic-anabolic steroid therapy. A severe form of hepatic injury. *Annals of Internal Medicine*, **81**, 610–18.

Baumwol, M. and Park, W. (1976) An acute abdomen: spontaneous rupture of liver during pregnancy. *British Journal of Surgery*, **63**, 718–20.

Binoux, M. and Hossenlopp, P. (1988) Insulin-like growth factor (IGF) and IGF-binding proteins: comparison of human serum and lymph. *Journal of Clinical Endocrinology and Metabolism*, **67**, 505–14.

Bismuth, H., Chiche, L. and Castaing, D. (1995) Surgical treatment of hepatocellular carcinomas in noncirrhotic liver: experience with 68 liver resections. *World Journal of Surgery*, **19**, 35–41.

Broadus, A.E., Mangin, M. and Ikeda, K. (1988) Humoral hypercalcaemia of cancer: identification of a novel parathyroid hormone-like peptide. *New England Journal of Medicine*, **319**, 556–63.

Brownstein, M.H. and Ballard, H.S. (1964) Hepatoma associated with erythrocytosis. *American Journal of Medicine*, **40**, 204–10.

Cadranel, J.F., Cadranel, J., Buffet, C. *et al.* (1989) Hypercalcaemia associated with chronic viral hepatitis. *Postgraduate Medical Journal*, **65**, 678–80.

Chearanai, O., Plengvanit, U., Asavanichi, C. *et al.* (1983) Spontaneous rupture of primary hepatoma; Report of 63 cases with particular reference to the pathogenesis and rationale treatment by hepatic artery ligation. *Cancer*, **51**, 1532–6.

Chen, M.F., Hwang, T.L., Jeng, L.B. *et al.* (1988) Surgical treatment for spontaneous rupture of hepatocellular carcinoma. *Surgery, Gynecology and Obstetrics*, **167**, 99–102.

Curth, W. (1969) Vitiligo hepatoma. *Archives of Dermatology*, **99**, 374–5.

Daughaday, W.H. and Kapadia, M. (1989) Significance of abnormal serum binding of insulin-like growth factor II in the development of hypoglycaemia in patients with non-islet cell tumours. *Proceedings of the National Academy of Sciences, USA*, **86**, 6778–82.

Dewar, G.A., Griffin, S.M., Ku, K.W. *et al.* (1991) Management of bleeding liver tumours in Hong Kong. *British Journal of Surgery*, **78**, 463–6.

DiBisceglie, A.M., Hodkinson, H.J., Berkowitz, I. *et al.* (1986) Pityriasis rotunda. A cutaneous marker of hepatocellular carcinoma in southern African blacks. *Archives of Dermatology*, **122**, 802–4.

Edmonson, H.A. and Steiner, P.E. (1954) Primary carcinoma of the liver. A study of 100 cases among 48,900 necropsies. *Cancer*, **7**, 462–503.

Fried, W. (1972) The liver as a source of extra-renal erythropoietin production. *Blood*, **40**, 671–7.

Goldberg, R.B., Bersohn, I. and Kew, M.C. (1975) Hypercholesterolemia in primary cancer of the liver. *South African Medical Journal*, **49**, 1464–6.

Gordon, P., Hendricks, C.M., Kahn, C.R. *et al.* (1981) Hypoglycemia associated with non-islet cell tumors and insulin-like growth factors: a study of tumor types. *New England Journal of Medicine*, **305**, 1452–5.

Hirai, K., Kawazoe, Y., Yamashita, K. *et al.* (1986) Transcatheter arterial embolization for spontaneous rupture of hepatocellular carcinoma. *American Journal of Gastroenterology*, **81**, 275–9.

Ho, J., Wu, P.C. and Kung, T.M. (1981) An autopsy study of hepatocellular carcinoma in Hong Kong. *Pathology*, **13**, 409–15.

Hsieh, J.S., Huang, C.J., Huang, Y.S. *et al.* (1987) Intraperitoneal hemorrhage due to spontaneous rupture of hepatocellular carcinoma: treatment by hepatic artery embolization. *American Journal of Roentgenology*, **149**, 715–17.

Hunter, S.J., Daughaday, W.H., Callender, M.E. *et al.* (1994) A case of hepatoma associated with hypoglycaemia and overproduction of IGF-II (E-21): beneficial effects of treatment with growth hormone and intrahepatic adriamycin. *Clinical Endocrinology*, **41**, 397–401.

Hwang, S.J., Chan, C.Y., Wu, J.C. *et al.* (1989) Clinical study of hypercalcaemia in Chinese patient with hepatocellular carcinoma. *Chinese Journal of Gastroenterology*, **6**, 182–6.

Hwang, S.J., Lee, S.D., Chang, C.F. *et al.* (1992) Hypercholesterolaemia in patients with hepatocellular carcinoma. *Journal of Gastroenterology and Hepatology*, **7**, 491–6.

Hwang, S.J., Lee, S.D., Wu, J.C. *et al.* (1994) Clinical evaluation of erythrocytosis in patients with hepatocellular carcinoma. *Chinese Medical Journal (Taipei)*, **53**, 262–9.

Ihde, D.C., Sherlock, P., Winamer, S.J. *et al.* (1974) Clinical manifestations of hepatoma. A review of 6 years' experience at a cancer hospital. *American Journal of Medicine*, **56**, 83–91.

Ito, M. and Tanaka, T. (1961) Pseudo-ichtyosis acquisita en taches circulaires proposed as a better name for pityriasis circinata Toyama. *Japanese Journal of Dermatology*, **71**, 586–8.

Jacobson, R.J., Lowenthal, M.N. and Kew, M.C. (1978) Erythrocytosis in hepatocellular carcinoma. *South African Medical Journal*, **53**, 658–60.

Kan, Y.W., McFadzean, A.J.S., Todd, D. *et al.* (1961) Further observations on polycythaemia in hepatocellular carcinoma. *Blood*, **18**, 592–8.

Kappel, D.A. and Miller, D.R. (1972) Primary hepatic carcinoma. A review of thirty-seven patients. *American Journal of Surgery*, **124**, 798–802.

Keczkes, K. and Barker, D.J. (1976) Malignant hepatoma associated with acquired hepatic cutaneous porphyria. *Archives of Dermatology*, **112**, 78–82.

Kew, M.C., Dos Santos, H.A. and Sherlock, S. (1971) Diagnosis of primary liver cancer of the liver. *British Medical Journal*, **4**, 408–11.

Kew, M.C. and Dusheiko, G.M. (1981) *Frontiers in Liver Disease*, Thieme-Stratton, New York, p. 305.

Kew, M.C. and Fisher, J.W. (1986) Serum erythropoietin concentrations in patients with hepatocellular carcinoma. *Cancer*, **58**, 2485–8.

Kew, M.C. and Geddes, E.W. (1982) Hepatocellular carcinoma in rural Southern African Blacks. *Medicine*, **61**, 98–108.

Kew, M.C., Kirschner, M.A., Abrahams, G.E. *et al.* (1977) Mechanisms of feminization in primary liver cancer. *New England Journal of Medicine*, **296**, 1084–8.

Kew, M.C. and Paterson, A.C. (1985) Unusual clinical presentations of hepatocellular carcinoma. *Tropical Gastroenterology*, **6**, 10–22.

Knill-Jones, R.P., Buckle, R.M., Parsons, V. *et al.* (1970) Hypercalcaemia and increased parathyroid-hormone activity in a primary hepatoma. *New England Journal of Medicine*, **282**, 704–8.

Kojiro, M., Kawabaata, K., Kawano, Y. *et al.* (1982) Hepatocellular carcinoma presenting as intrabile duct tumor growth. A clinicopathologic study of 24 cases. *Cancer*, **49**, 2144–7.

Lau, W.Y., Leung, J.W.C. and Li, A.K.C. (1990) Management of hepatocellular carcinoma presenting as obstructive jaundice. *American Journal of Surgery*, **160**, 280–2.

Lau, W.Y., Leung, K.L., Leung, T.W.T. *et al.* (1997) A logical approach to hepatocellular carcinoma presenting with jaundice. *Annals of Surgery*, **225**, 281–5.

Leading Article (1976) Spontaneous rupture of the liver. *British Medical Journal*, **2**, 1278–9.

Lee, N.W., Wong, K.P., Siu, K.F. *et al.* (1984) Cholangiography in hepatocellular carcinoma with obstructive jaundice. *Clinical Radiology*, **35**, 119–23.

Li, A.K.C., Rhodes, J.M. and Valentine, A.R. (1979) Spontaneous liver rupture in polyarteritis nodosa. *British Journal of Surgery*, **66**, 251–2.

Lin, T.Y. (1976) Tumors of the liver. Part I. Primary malignant tumors, in *Gastroenterology*, vol. 3, 3rd ed (ed. H.L. Bockus), W.B. Saunders, Philadelphia, pp. 522–34.

Martin, T.J. and Mundy, G.R. (1987) Hypercalcaemia of malignancy, in *Clinical Endocrinology of Calcium Metabolism* (eds T.J. Martin and L.C. Raisz) Marcel Dekker, New York, pp. 171–99.

McFadzean, A.J.S., Todd, D. and Tsang, K.C. (1958) Polycythaemia in primary carcinoma of the liver. *Blood*, **8**, 427–35.

McFazdean, A.J.S. and Yeung, R.T.T. (1969) Further observations on hypoglycemia in hepatocellular carcinoma. *American Journal of Medicine*, **47**, 220–35.

Megyesi, K., Kahn, C.R., Roth, J. *et al.* (1974) Hypoglycaemia in association with extrapancreatic tumours: demonstration of elevated plasma NSILA-S by a new radio-receptor assay. *Journal of Clinical Endocrinology and Metabolism*, **38**, 931–4.

Merimee, T.J. (1986) Insulin-like growth factors in patients with non-islet cell tumours and hypoglycaemia. *Metabolism*, **35**, 33–6.

Mokka, R., Seppl, A., Huttunen, R. *et al.* (1976) Spontaneous rupture of liver tumours. *British Journal of Surgery*, **63**, 715–17.

Muhammed, I. and Mabogunje, O. (1991) Spontaneous rupture of primary hepatocellular carcinoma in Zaria, Nigeria. *Journal of the Royal College of Surgeons of Edinburgh*, **36**, 117–20.

Nagasue, N. and Inokuchi, K. (1979) Spontaneous and traumatic rupture of hepatoma. *British Journal of Surgery*, **66**, 248–50.

Nagasue, N., Inokuchi, K., Kabayashi, M. *et al.* (1977) Hepatoportal arteriovenous fistula in primary carcinoma of the liver. *Surgery, Gynecology and Obstetrics*, **145**, 504–8.

Nakamura, Y., Terade, T., Ueda, K. *et al.* (1993) Adenomatous hyperplasia of the liver as a precancerous lesion. *Liver*, **13**, 1–9.

Ng, W.D., Chan, Y.T., Ho, K.K. *et al.* (1989) Injection sclerotherapy for bleeding esophageal varices in cirrhotic patients with hepatocellular carcinoma. *Gastrointestinal Endoscopy*, **35**, 69–70.

Nusbacher, J. (1964) Migratory venous thrombosis and cancer. *New York Journal of Medicine*, **64**, 2166–73.

Okuda, K. (1976) Clinical aspects of hepatocellular carcinoma–analysis of 134 cases, in *Hepatocellular Carcinoma* (eds K.K. Okuda and F.L. Peters) Wiley, New York, pp. 387–436.

Omata, M., Peters, R.L. and Tatter, D. (1981) Sclerosing hepatic carcinoma: relationship to hypercalcaemia. *Liver*, **1**, 33–49.

Ong, G.B., Chu, E.P.H., Yu, F.Y.K. *et al.* (1965) Spontaneous rupture of hepatocellular carcinoma. *British Journal of Surgery*, **52**, 123–9.

Ong, G.B. and Taw, J.L. (1972) Spontaneous rupture of hepatocellular carcinoma. *British Medical Journal*, **4**, 146–9.

Panesar, N.S., Au, K.M., Leung, N.W.Y. *et al.* (1991) Nephrogenous cyclic AMP in primary hepatocellular carcinoma patients with or without hypercalcaemia. *Clinical Endocrinology*, **35**, 527–32.

Pierach, C.A., Bossenmaier, I.C., Cardinal, R.A. *et al.* (1984) Pseudoporphyria in a patient with hepatocellular carcinoma. *American Journal of Medicine*, **76**, 545–8.

Primack, A., Wilson, J., O'Conner, G.T. *et al.* (1971) Hepatocellular carcinoma with the carcinoid syndrome. *Cancer*, **27**, 1182–9.

Roslyn, J.J., Kuchenbecker, S., Longmire, W.P. *et al.* (1984) Floating tumor debris. A cause of intermittent biliary obstruction. *Archives of Surgery*, **119**, 1312–25.

Sakisaka, S., Watanabe, M., Tateishi, H. *et al.* (1993) Erythropoietin production in hepatocellular carcinoma cells associated with polycythemia: immunohistochemical evidence. *Hepatology*, **18**, 1357–62.

Sato, Y., Fujiwara, K., Furui, S. *et al.* (1985) Benefit of transarterial embolization for ruptured hepatocellular carcinoma complicating liver cirrhosis. *Gastroenterology*, **89**, 157–9.

Schwarz, K.O., Schwartz, I.J. and Machervky, A. (1982) Virchow–Trosier's lymph node as a presenting sign of hepatocellular carcinoma. *Mount Sinai Journal of Medicine*, **49**, 59–62.

Sewell, J.H. and Weiss, K. (1961) Spontaneous rupture of haemangioma of the liver. *Archives of Surgery*, **83**, 729–34.

Shek, C.C., Natkunam, A., Tsang, V. *et al.* (1990) Incidence, causes and mechanism of hypercalcaemia in a hospital population in Hong Kong. *Quarterly Journal of Medicine*, **77**, 1277–85.

Simon, P., Meyrier, A., Tanquerel, T. *et al.* (1980) Improvement in anaemia in haemodialysed patients after viral or toxic hepatic cytolysis. *British Medical Journal*, **280**, 892–8.

Sunderland, G.T., Chisholm, E.M., Lau, W.Y. *et al.* (1992) Alcohol injection: a treatment for ruptured hepatocellular carcinoma. *Surgical Oncology*, **1**, 61–3.

Urdneta, L.F. and Nielsen, J.V. (1986) Massive haemoperitoneum secondary to spontaneous rupture of hepatic metastases: report of two cases and review of the literature. *Journal of Surgical Oncology*, **31**, 104–7.

Van Leeuwen, D.J., Bos, R.J. and Vidacovic-Vucic, M.M. (1991) Hepatocellular carcinoma in the Amsterdam area. A retrospective analysis in 61 patients. *Scandinavian Journal of Gastroenterology Suppl.*, **188**, 108–17.

Van Sonnenberg, E. and Ferucci, J.T. (1979) Bile duct obstruction in hepatocellular carcinoma (hepatoma) – clinical and cholangiographic characteristics. Report of 6 cases and review of the literature. *Radiology*, **130**, 7–13.

Wu, C.S., Wu, S.S., Chen, P.C. *et al.* (1994) Cholangiography of icteric type hepatoma. *American Journal of Gastroenterology*, **89**, 774–7.

Yeo, W., Sung, J.Y., Ward, S.C. *et al.* (1995) A prospective study of upper gastrointestinal hemorrhage in patients with hepatocellular carcinoma. *Digestive Diseases and Sciences*, **40**, 2516–21.

PALLIATIVE CARE 12

A.T.C. Chan and P.J. Johnson

12.1 INTRODUCTION

By definition, palliation means relieving of symptoms without curing or affecting the natural history of the underlying disease. Palliative care is an important aspect of the management of hepatocellular carcinoma (HCC) since only 10% of patients are suitable for resection with curative intent and the goal of all other forms of treatment is palliation. Palliative treatment may be disease-oriented and/or symptom-oriented. Disease-oriented measures, including systemic chemotherapy and locoregional therapies such as chemoembolization and internal irradiation, have been described in earlier chapters. To achieve the goal of effective symptom control, it is crucial to have an accurate diagnosis of the cause of the symptoms and a clear understanding of the palliative measures available. Symptom-oriented measures specifically directed at pain, ascites and gastrointestinal bleeding are of particular importance in patients with HCC and will be described later.

Conventional measures of the success of palliative treatment in terms of tumor response rate and prolongation of survival may not be entirely appropriate in the palliative management of patients with HCC. With the median survival of inoperable HCC patients being only 8–10 weeks, it is the quality of life of this short remaining life-span that is particularly crucial as a measure of success. Hence pain control measures can only be considered effective if this can be accurately reflected in patient-based pain scales and quality of life measurements.

12.2 CLINICAL EVALUATION

12.2.1 PAIN SCALES

Adequate palliative management of pain is critical since it is the most common symptom in patients with HCC. In a retrospective series, pain was present in 76% of HCC patients at presentation (Shiu *et al.*, 1990). A questionnaire survey of 1177 oncologists reported that the biggest barrier to adequate cancer pain management is the inadequate assessment of pain and pain relief (von Roenn *et al.*, 1993). Hence validated instruments for pain measurement which can be used in a multidimensional nature have to be employed in the clinical setting.

Two of the most widely used methods are the Wisconsin Brief Pain Inventory (Daut *et al.*, 1983), and the McGill Pain Questionnaire (Graham *et al.*, 1980). These instruments have been translated into several languages and

Hepatocellular Carcinoma: Diagnosis, investigation and management. Edited by Anthony S.-Y. Leong, Choong-Tsek Liew, Joseph W.Y. Lau and Philip J. Johnson. Published in 1999 by Arnold, London. ISBN 0 340 74096 5.

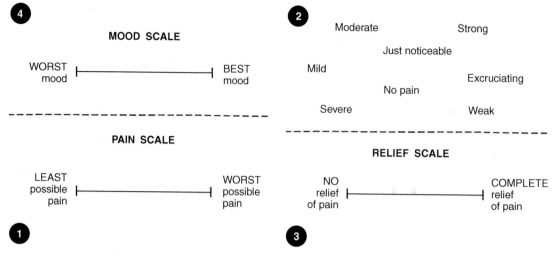

Fig. 12.1 Front side of MPAC. VAS measures of pain intensity and mood. The card is folded along the broken line such that each measure is presented to the patient separately, in the numbered order.

Fig. 12.2 Back side of MPAC. Modified Tursky Pain Descriptors Scale and VAS measure of pain relief.

validated (Cleeland *et al.*, 1988). Another method that has gained wide acceptance is the use of visual analogue scales (VAS). The Memorial Pain Assessment Card (MPAC) (Fishman *et al.*, 1987) is a valid and multidimensional method which includes VAS scales on pain intensity, pain relief and mood, and a set of pain severity descriptors which patients use to describe their subjective experience of pain severity (Figs 12.1 and 12.2).

12.2.2 QUALITY OF LIFE MEASURES

In patients with inoperable HCC, the median survival is short and palliative measures must aim maximally to improve the quality of life during this short duration. The benefit of any palliative treatment, which may be associated with high morbidity and/or extended hospital stays, must be assessed using patient-based quality of life measures. Hence the use of more intensive treatment with the attend-

ant toxicities to achieve higher tumor response rates in the palliative treatment of HCC needs to be justified.

Quality of life measures are, to date, conspicuous by their absence in the treatment of HCC. The Karnofsky Performance Scale, a physician-based assessment of the overall functional state of patients, has been widely used in clinical trials and has reasonably good correlation with the overall medical state of illness (Yates *et al.*, 1980; Mor *et al.*, 1984). However, the scale does not relate well to measures of psychological well-being, sociability, or even somatic discomfort.

For any quality of life measure to be considered for use in the clinical setting, it must be constructed on multiple samples and analysed for content, concurrent, and construct validity. One of the most widely recognized quality of life measures is the Functional Life Index-Cancer (FLIC) scale which comprises of 22 items (Schipper *et al.*, 1984) (Fig. 12.3). In the process of the FLIC's validation, literature review and patient inter-

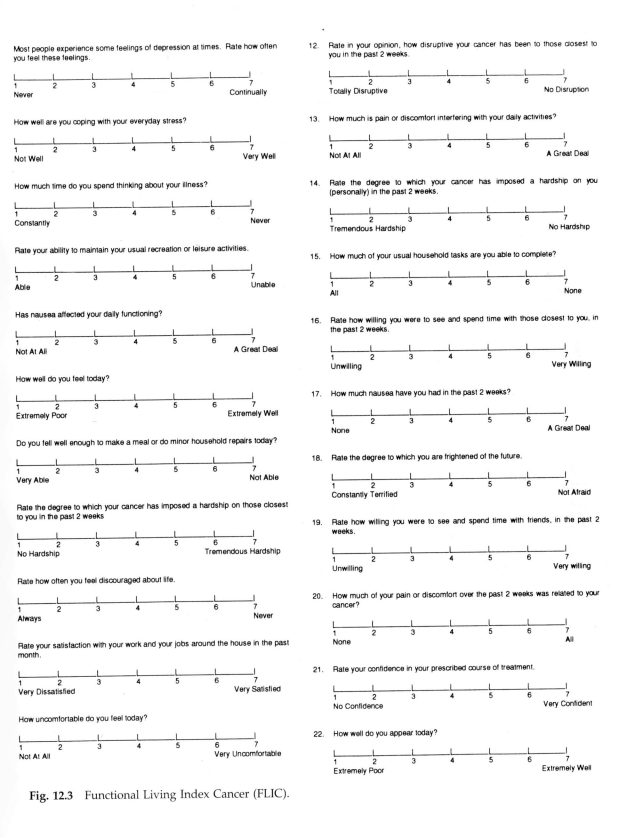

Most people experience some feelings of depression at times. Rate how often you feel these feelings.

1 Never — 2 — 3 — 4 — 5 — 6 — 7 Continually

How well are you coping with your everyday stress?

1 Not Well — 2 — 3 — 4 — 5 — 6 — 7 Very Well

How much time do you spend thinking about your illness?

1 Constantly — 2 — 3 — 4 — 5 — 6 — 7 Never

Rate your ability to maintain your usual recreation or leisure activities.

1 Able — 2 — 3 — 4 — 5 — 6 — 7 Unable

Has nausea affected your daily functioning?

1 Not At All — 2 — 3 — 4 — 5 — 6 — 7 A Great Deal

How well do you feel today?

1 Extremely Poor — 2 — 3 — 4 — 5 — 6 — 7 Extremely Well

Do you fell well enough to make a meal or do minor household repairs today?

1 Very Able — 2 — 3 — 4 — 5 — 6 — 7 Not Able

Rate the degree to which your cancer has imposed a hardship on those closest to you in the past 2 weeks

1 No Hardship — 2 — 3 — 4 — 5 — 6 — 7 Tremendous Hardship

Rate how often you feel discouraged about life.

1 Always — 2 — 3 — 4 — 5 — 6 — 7 Never

Rate your satisfaction with your work and your jobs around the house in the past month.

1 Very Dissatisfied — 2 — 3 — 4 — 5 — 6 — 7 Very Satisfied

How uncomfortable do you feel today?

1 Not At All — 2 — 3 — 4 — 5 — 6 — 7 Very Uncomfortable

12. Rate in your opinion, how disruptive your cancer has been to those closest to you in the past 2 weeks.

1 Totally Disruptive — 2 — 3 — 4 — 5 — 6 — 7 No Disruption

13. How much is pain or discomfort interfering with your daily activities?

1 Not At All — 2 — 3 — 4 — 5 — 6 — 7 A Great Deal

14. Rate the degree to which your cancer has imposed a hardship on you (personally) in the past 2 weeks.

1 Tremendous Hardship — 2 — 3 — 4 — 5 — 6 — 7 No Hardship

15. How much of your usual household tasks are you able to complete?

1 All — 2 — 3 — 4 — 5 — 6 — 7 None

16. Rate how willing you were to see and spend time with those closest to you, in the past 2 weeks.

1 Unwilling — 2 — 3 — 4 — 5 — 6 — 7 Very Willing

17. How much nausea have you had in the past 2 weeks?

1 None — 2 — 3 — 4 — 5 — 6 — 7 A Great Deal

18. Rate the degree to which you are frightened of the future.

1 Constantly Terrified — 2 — 3 — 4 — 5 — 6 — 7 Not Afraid

19. Rate how willing you were to see and spend time with friends, in the past 2 weeks.

1 Unwilling — 2 — 3 — 4 — 5 — 6 — 7 Very willing

20. How much of your pain or discomfort over the past 2 weeks was related to your cancer?

1 None — 2 — 3 — 4 — 5 — 6 — 7 All

21. Rate your confidence in your prescribed course of treatment.

1 No Confidence — 2 — 3 — 4 — 5 — 6 — 7 Very Confident

22. How well do you appear today?

1 Extremely Poor — 2 — 3 — 4 — 5 — 6 — 7 Extremely Well

Fig. 12.3 Functional Living Index Cancer (FLIC).

views were undertaken to define areas of day-to-day function that were deemed of consequence. From this process, four principal areas of functional importance were ultimately defined:

1. vocation/activity;
2. affect/psychological state;
3. social interaction; and
4. somatic sensation.

A questionnaire-design panel was established to review the identified areas and to formulate meaningful questions. Initially 250 questions were developed and some of these underwent four generations of test development. Each item was composed to be answerable in a seven-point Likert format. In the first-generation questionnaire, 250 questions were reduced to 92 by eliminating duplicated, unclear and limited applicability items by the panel of experts. This was further reduced to 42 questions after factor analysing answered questions from 175 patients. In the second-generation questionnaire, 312 patients answered the 42 questions; again using factor analysis, demographic variables were not found to contribute to the dimensions of the original questionnaire and thus were subsequently omitted. In the third generation, the questionnaire, consisting of 20 items, was tested against established and previously accepted measures of quality of life. This questionnaire was again administered to 175 patients in Manitoba, Canada along with other established scales for (1) physical well being (i.e. General Health Questionnaire C scale for social dysfunction, McGill/Melzack Present Pain Index and Karnofsky scale) and (2) psychosocial functioning (i.e. General Health Questionnaire C scale for anxiety and insomnia and D scale for severe depression, Beck Depression scale, Spielberger State and Trait Anxiety Scales).

As desired, the physical function and ability derived factors on the FLIC correlated well with physical attributes or their consequences, but they did not correlate strongly with the psychosocial measures. Further, and again as desired, FLICs derived emotional function factor scores correlated strongly with the measures of depression and anxiety, and poorly with the physical ability measures.

Further factor analysis and correlational studies and modifications of the questionnaire were made based on the scale's use in another region (Alberta). A fourth and final generation test comprised of 22 items and provided clear evidence that the FLIC measured a composite of distinct factors contributing to overall functional living. This FLIC version is answered easily by patients during each test. Since factor analysis solutions were stable through separate trials involving two populations, a strong measure of construct validity was evident.

The FLIC questionnaire has been utilized in other prospective studies demonstrating it to be an easy and repeatable patient self-administration test, and is currently utilized in prospective studies at the authors' institution.

12.3   SPECIFIC MEASURES

12.3.1   PAIN

HCC causes pain by stretching the liver capsule as it enlarges and also it may cause pressure symptoms on adjacent organs. The principles of the approach to pain control in the palliative management in HCC should not be different from pain control in general as recommended by the World Health Organization's three-step ladder (WHO, 1986). The three principal groups of analgesic drugs include non-narcotic analgesics, narcotic analgesics, and adjuvant analgesics. Non-narcotic analgesics include paracetamol, aspirin and non-steroidal anti-inflammatory drugs (NSAIDS). Maximal drug doses at regular intervals should be used before switching. The commonest drugs used in our institution are paracetamol 1 g every 6 h and naproxen 500 mg every 12 h. The gastrointestinal side effects of NSAIDs often limit their long-term use. These drugs form the first step of the analgesic ladder. Narcotic analgesics can be used in combination with non-narcotics and many drug combinations are available. The most widely used combination in our institution is Doloxene Co, one capsule every 6 h. This combination contains dextropropoxyphene napsylate 100 mg, aspirin 375 mg and caffeine 30 mg in each capsule.

The most common narcotic analgesic used as a single agent is morphine. There is no ceiling effect. Effective use of narcotic analgesic requires a balance between adequate pain relief and undesirable side effects particularly in terms of constipation, nausea and sedation. The starting dose of morphine is 5 mg every 4 h with longer acting preparations also widely available. The rapid growth of HCC may necessitate a rapid escalation of doses. In the cirrhotic HCC patients with deranged liver function, narcotic analgesics may precipitate hepatic encephalopathy. However, in the preterminal stages of this disease, palliation of the patients' pain would be the paramount goal of the overall management.

In all three steps of the analgesic ladder, adjuvant analgesic drugs may be added according to the need of the patient. Anticonvulsants including phenytoin 100 mg nocte and carbamazepine 100 mg every 12 h, and antidepressants such as amitriptyline 10 mg nocte are particularly useful in neuropathic pains. In HCC steroids may be particularly useful as an adjuvant analgesic in reducing any associated inflammatory or edematous elements that may be contributing to the pain. In patients whose pain is resistant to analgesics and where the pain is localized to a few dermatomes, regional nerve blocks may be extremely useful as a palliative measure. If the pain is referred to the lower thoracic or upper abdominal wall, a celiac plexus block can be performed. Types of neurolytic agents used include alcohol, which may cause a severe burning pain when injected, and phenol with glycerine, which has a local anesthesia effect when injected.

12.3.2 ASCITES

Malignant ascites is a frequent cause of morbidity and prolonged hospitalization of HCC patients. The pressure effect and abdominal distension caused by the ascites may lead to a compromise of respiratory function and gaseous gastrointestinal dysfunction. Several measures are available for the palliation of ascites.

12.3.2.1 Diuretics

The starting dose of spironolactone is 100 mg/day with escalation of the dosage until an effective result is achieved. High doses of spironolactone of up to 600 mg/day are often required to achieve effective palliation (Campra and Reynolds, 1978). However this may be associated with renal dysfunction and electrolyte disturbances. Other side effects include nausea and gynecomastia.

12.3.2.2 Abdominal paracentesis

Removal of ascites by paracentesis achieves good palliation which is unfortunately often short-lasting. Hence repeated paracentesis is usually required. Sudden removal of a large volume of ascites may result in a fall in right atrial pressure and consequently the systemic vascular resistance (Panos *et al.*, 1990). Another potential morbidity is the risk of peritoneal infection, which may be fatal in this group of debilitated HCC patients.

12.3.2.3 Peritoneovenous shunting

This procedure, first introduced by Le Veen *et al.* in 1974, may be considered in patients with ascites resistant to diuretics and abdominal paracentesis with rapid reaccumulation. The procedure is hazardous particularly in patients with deranged clotting times and platelet functions. The theoretical morbidity associated with implantation of malignant cells is uncommon.

12.3.2.4 Intraperitoneal chemotherapy

There have been reports of the use of bleomycin to reduce reaccumulation of malignant ascites with varying degrees of success (Ostrowski, 1986). The major limitation of this technique is the need for total paracentesis before instillation of bleomycin, which depletes the patient's protein reserves and may not be tolerated by patients with advanced HCC.

12.3.3 GASTROINTESTINAL BLEEDING

Gastrointestinal bleeding is a frequent terminal event in patients with HCC, accounting for one-quarter of deaths in an autopsy series of 287 cases (Ho *et al.*, 1981). Over 80% of HCC patients have underlying cirrhosis, hence variceal bleeding is one of the major causes of gastrointestinal hemorrhage. It has been recognized that there is a strong association between invasion of the portal vein and subsequent variceal hemorrhage. Other causes of upper gastrointestinal hemorrhage in HCC patients include hematobilia, direct tumor invasion and rarely as a complication of Selective Internal Irradiation therapy. Furthermore, in a prospective study of 52 HCC patients with gastrointestinal hemorrhage, 15 patients had peptic ulceration as the cause (Yeo *et al.*, 1995). Hence, apart from supportive measures to stabilize patients hemodynamically, endoscopic diagnosis with appropriate intervention for the control of hemorrhage is recommended for all patients with a good premorbid status. Nevertheless, gastrointestinal hemorrhage in HCC patients represents a grave prognostic sign with a subsequent median survival of only 21 days being reported in a prospective study (Yeo *et al.*, 1995).

12.4 HOSPICE CARE

For most patients with HCC the time will come when locoregional or systemic forms of therapy are no longer feasible and the patients are facing death within a short period. At this stage it is vital that patients do not feel abandoned by care-givers and therefore a hospice with comprehensive physical, psychological, social and spiritual support becomes the ideal setting for the care of these patients.

The goals of hospice care of the dying patient are four fold (Twycross, 1986):

1. Relief of pain and other symptoms.
2. Psychological and spiritual care for patients to prepare them to come to terms with death.
3. A supportive system to maintain personal integrity and self-esteem.
4. A system to support the family members to cope during the patient's final days and also their bereavement.

Increasingly Hospice Home Care Services are provided so that terminally ill patients can spend as much time at home as possible. Healthcare givers are specifically trained to cater for the specific needs of the dying patient. It must be emphasized that terminal patients often require more, rather than less, care. This is frequently the case if patients are left on busy acute medical or surgical wards in general hospitals.

REFERENCES

Campra, J.L. and Reynolds, T.B. (1978) Effectiveness of high dose spironolactone therapy in patients with chronic liver disease and relatively refractory ascites. *American Journal of Digestive Diseases*, **23**, 1025–30.
Cleeland, C.S., Ladinsky, J.L., Serlin, R.C. and Thuy, N.C. (1988) Multidimensional measurement of cancer pain: comparisions of US and Vietnamese patients. *Journal of Pain and Symptom Management*, **3**, 23–7.
Daut, R.L., Cleeland, C.S. and Flanery, R.C. (1983) The development of the Wisconsin Brief Pain Questionnaire to assess pain in cancer and other diseases. *Pain*, **17**, 197–210.
Fishman, B., Pasternak, S., Wallerstein, S.L. *et al.* (1987) The Memorial Pain Assessment Card: a valid instrument for the assessment of cancer pain. *Cancer*, **60**, 1151–7.

Graham, C., Bond, S.S., Gertrovitch, M.M. and Cook, M.R. (1980) Use of the McGill Pain Questionnaire in the management of cancer pain –replicability and consistency. *Pain*, **8**, 377–87.

Ho, J., Wu, P.C. and Kung, T.M. (1981) An autopsy study of hepatocellular carcinoma in Hong Kong. *Pathology*, **13**, 409–16.

Le Veen, H.H., Christoudias, G., Moon, I.P. *et al.* (1974) Peritoneovenous shunting for ascites. *Annals of Surgery*, **180**, 580–90.

Mor, V., Laliberte, L.M., Morris, J.N. and Weimann, M. (1984) The Karnofsky Performance Status Scale: an examination of its reliability and validity in a research setting. *Cancer*, **53**, 2002–7.

Ostrowski, M.J. (1986) An assessment of the long-term results of controlling the reaccumulation of malignant effusions using intracavity bleomycin. *Cancer*, **57**, 721–7.

Panos, M., Moore, K.P. and Vlavianos, P. (1990) Single total paracentesis for tense ascites: sequential haemodynamic changes and right atrial size. *Hepatology*, **11**, 662–7.

Schipper, H., Clinch, J., McMarray, A. and Levitt, M. (1984) Measuring the quality of life of cancer patients: the Functional Living Index–cancer development and validation. *Journal of Clinical Oncology*, **2**, 472–83.

Shiu, W., Dewar, G., Leung, N. *et al.* (1990) Hepatocellular carcinoma in Hong Kong. *Oncology*, **47**, 241–5.

Twycross, R.G. (1986) Hospice care, in *Terminal Care at Home* (ed. R. Spilling), Oxford University Press, Oxford, pp. 96–112.

Von Roenn, J.H., Cleeland, C.S., Gonin, R. *et al.* (1993) Physician attitudes and practice in cancer pain management. A survey from the Eastern Cooperative Oncology Group. *Annals of Internal Medicine*, **119**, 121–6.

WHO (1986) *Cancer Pain Relief*, World Health Organization, Geneva.

Yates, J.W., Chalmer, B. and McKegney, F.P. (1980) Evaluation of patients with advanced cancer using the Karnofsky Performance Status. *Cancer*, **45**, 2220–4.

Yeo, W., Sung, J.Y., Ward, S.C. *et al.* (1995) A prospective study of upper gastrointestinal haemorrhage in patients with hepatocellular carcinoma. *Digestive Disease and Sciences*, **40**, 2516–20.

Africa

A.C. Paterson and K. Cooper

Hepatocellular carcinoma (HCC) is one of the most common and lethal neoplasms seen in Africa. The true incidence is under reported because of the rural origins of many patients as well as the widespread use of non-histological methods, serum α-fetoprotein and sonar in the routine diagnosis of this tumor (Sitas *et al.*, 1992). The incidence increases with age with a significant peak in the third to fifth decades, with the male-to-female ratio ranging from 4:1 to 8:1 (Kew, 1983).

Major risk factors for HCC in Africa have traditionally included chronic hepatitis B virus (HBV) infection, often with associated cirrhosis, and aflatoxin exposure. More recently, other viruses, particularly hepatitis C virus (HCV), membranous obstruction of the inferior vena cava (MOIVC), alcohol and African iron overload (AIO) have been considered possible etiologic agents. In the past, most research into African HCC concentrated on rural and migrant mineworker communities. However, with the emergence of an urban black society, differences have emerged, particularly with respect to age and associated non-tumorous liver pathology.

A viral etiology for HCC was postulated some years before the discovery of the HBV (Higginson, 1963). Shortly after the discovery of the hepatitis B surface antigen (HBsAg), an association was confirmed in many African countries including Uganda (Vogel *et al.*, 1972; Anthony, 1973), Senegal (Prince *et al.*, 1975), Zambia (Tabor *et al.*, 1977) and South Africa (Kew *et al.*, 1974). In recent studies the importance of this association was again stressed in studies from Egypt (Darwish *et al.*, 1993), The Gambia (Ryder *et al.*, 1992), Niger (Cenac *et al.*, 1995) and Rwanda (Mets, 1993).

Initially, there appeared to be a strong association between chronic HBV infection, the development of macronodular cirrhosis and subsequent HCC. However, over the past 40 years the prevalence of cirrhosis associated with HCC has declined significantly in southern Africa (Paterson *et al.*, 1985). This trend has also been observed elsewhere in South Africa. Furthermore, the type of cirrhosis has changed in this region with portal fibrosis and micronodular cirrhosis becoming increasingly common, particularly in urban black populations (Paterson *et al.*, 1985). The contentious subject of large cell liver dysplasia (LCD) and its relationship to cirrhosis and HBV infection was first documented in Uganda (Anthony *et*

Hepatocellular Carcinoma: Diagnosis, investigation and management. Edited by Anthony S.-Y. Leong, Choong-Tsek Liew, Joseph W.Y. Lau and Philip J. Johnson. Published in 1999 by Arnold, London. ISBN 0 340 74096 5.

al., 1973). In South Africa, there is a relationship between LCD and chronic HBV infection, rural domicile, young age and evidence of ongoing viral replication (serum HBeAg and/or tissue HBcAg positivity) (Paterson *et al.*, 1989). LCD of small cell type has not been documented in Africa.

Only 5% of adult southern African blacks are HBeAg-positive as compared with other hyperendemic regions (Kramvis *et al.*, 1997). In Africa, the common mode of transmission of HBV is horizontal with 15–20% of rural children studied in southern Africa being chronically infected by HBV within the first 5 years of life. HCC in these children has been well-documented (Kew *et al.*, 1982).

Chronic exposure to aflatoxins was strongly researched in many regions of Africa since Lancaster *et al.* (1971) first reported their carcinogenic properties in rat. A positive relationship between level of exposure to the toxin and incidence of HCC was observed in Kenya (Peers and Linsell, 1973), Swaziland (Keen and Martin, 1971; Peers *et al.*, 1976), Uganda (Alpert *et al.*, 1971), and South Africa (van Rensburg *et al.*, 1974). Interest in this association declined with the discovery of HbsAg. More recently, there has been a resurgence in interest with the discovery of mutations of the p53 gene, particularly as the point mutation at the third base position of codon 249 seen in African and Chinese HCC (Bressac *et al.*, 1991; Hsu *et al.*, 1991), corresponds with mutations caused by aflatoxin B_1 in experimental mutagenesis.

This specific mutation appears to be most prevalent in Mozambique, as opposed to the Transkei and Natal regions of South Africa (Ozturk *et al.*, 1991; Yap *et al.*, 1993). Using p53 immunohistochemistry, 35% of HCC expressed p53 protein in >10% of tumor cells in urban and rural patients across a wide area of South Africa (Paterson *et al.*, unpublished data). This positivity was not associated with tumor differentiation, age, sex, rural/urban domicile or background liver disease. It is presently not known how many of these patients have the specific codon 249 mutation.

HCV is well known as a cofactor in the development of HCC in Japan. Serum studies have shown antibodies to HCV in up to 2% of South Africans (Soni *et al.*, 1996) and a recent survey by Kew *et al.* (1997) of 231 black southern African patients with HCC has shown HBV alone to confer a relative risk of 23.3 and 6.6 for HCV. However, a synergistic effect was evident when both viruses were present in the same patient (relative risk 82.5). There is no reliable information on HCV elsewhere in Africa at the present time, with the exception of a recent report from Egypt (Darwish *et al.*, 1993) and Niger (Cenac *et al.*, 1995). Chronic infection with hepatitis D virus (HDV) infection does not appear to have any relationship to the development of HCC in southern Africa (Kew *et al.*, 1984).

Membranous obstruction of the inferior vena cava (MOIVC) is a worldwide phenomenon. Its association with HCC was first documented in Africa by Simson (1982) with a reported 101 cases of MOIVC over a 9-year period, 47.5% being associated with HCC. Simson postulated genetic and environmental factors in the development of MOIVC. More recently, Kew and co-workers (1989) have demonstrated MOIVC in African subjects from South Africa, Mozambique, Botswana, Zimbabwe and Malawi, noting that only a small number of patients with MOIVC have associated HCC. Their data support the concept that MOIVC *per se* is not responsible for HCC, but rather its presence renders the individual susceptible to one or more environmental carcinogens.

Alcohol has long been considered a cofactor in the development of HCC, particularly in the presence of cirrhosis. Rural black populations with HCC have traditionally been younger with chronic HBV infection and, often, a typical post-hepatitic macronodular cirrhosis. There is no evidence to implicate alcohol as a cofactor in these patients. However, a study carried out in the urban black city of Soweto in South Africa found alcohol to be a risk factor in men >40 years of age who drank >80 g ethanol daily. This risk remained after adjustment for chronic HBV infection, smoking and sex (Mohamed *et al.*, 1992). Smoking does not appear to represent an unqualified risk factor for HCC in South Africa although there may be a trend in older patients who are not HBV carriers (Kew *et al.*, 1985).

African iron overload (AIO) has traditionally been studied as an alcohol-related phenomenon (Powell *et al.*, 1995). However, review of these cases shows a predominant pattern of portal fibrosis with progressive portal–portal linking without evidence of the liver damage characteristic of alcohol abuse (Isaacson 1978; Paterson, unpublished data). With the development of an urban community, a changing pattern in the age and morphology of associated non-tumorous liver tissue has been described. An increasing number of urbanized black patients with HCC, older than rural cohorts and showing heavy iron overload in the liver with progressive portal fibrosis and cirrhosis, has been observed (Paterson *et al.*, 1985). At the time, the possibility that iron could be carcinogenic was disregarded. Early studies in genetic hemochromatosis (GH) reported that the resultant cirrhosis, rather than iron, was the precipitating factor (MacSween and Scott, 1973). Recently, however, reports of HCC in non-cirrhotic GH, including patients who were considered adequately venesected (Deugnier *et al.*, 1993a), and the presence of putative preneoplastic iron-free foci (Deugnier *et al.*, 1993b), has forced a re-evaluation of this concept. In Africa, a possible genetic (non-HLA) basis for AIO has been postulated (Gordeuk *et al.*, 1992). AIO is responsible for up to 50% of biopsy-related pathology in rural black patients from South Africa (van Rensburg, 1989). Recently, data from Strachan's study on AIO, conducted between 1925 and 1928, have been reviewed and it has been suggested that AIO may be a risk factor in the development of HCC (Gordeuk *et al.*, 1996). HCC associated with heavily iron overloaded livers has been documented in the rural district of Shongwe in South Africa, showing a risk of developing HCC of 10.6 relative to patients with normal iron status, although it is uncertain whether iron loading is an independent cause of the tumor or acts as an indirect carcinogen by inducing chronic necroinflammatory hepatic disease (Mandishona *et al.*, 1998).

With respect to diagnosis and treatment, non-invasive chemotherapeutic and other treatment modalities have met with limited success (Kew, 1983). The only feasible treatment at present is early diagnosis and surgical resection. However, follow-up of South African mineworkers with chronic HBV infection using serial α-fetoprotein and ultrasound, has not been successful, mainly due to the unjustified fear that these individuals would be tested for carriage of HIV (Paterson and Dusheiko, unpublished data). Working in a sophisticated hospital environment, Maraj and co-workers (1988) documented 224 patients with HCC, but only two patients were proved to have resectable tumors.

Survival of South African patients with HCC is shorter than North American subjects (Falkson *et al.*, 1988), probably a reflection of delays in diagnosis in the African group. There is some evidence that African HCC may have different biological properties to that of other hyperendemic regions (Okuda, 1986), e.g. differences in nuclear ploidy (Yoshida *et al.*, 1994). However, this requires confirmation. Ultimately, the only solution for HCC prevention in Africa would appear to be the vaccination of all neonates, a process only beginning in this continent (Ryder, 1992).

REFERENCES

Alpert, M.E., Hutt, M.S., Wogan, G.N. and Davidson, C.S. (1971) Association between aflatoxin content and hepatoma frequency in Uganda. *Cancer*, **28**, 253–60.

Anthony, P.P. (1973) Primary carcinoma of the liver: a study of 282 cases in Ugandan Africans. *Journal of Pathology*, **110**, 37–48.

Anthony, P.P., Vogel, C.L. and Barker, L.F. (1973) Liver cell dysplasia: a premalignant condition. *Journal of Clinical Pathology*, **26**, 217–33.

Bressac, B., Kew, M.C., Wands, J. and Ozturk, M. (1991) Selective G to T mutations of p53 gene in hepatocellular carcinoma from southern Africa. *Nature*, **350**, 429–31.

Cenac, A., Pedroso, M.L., Djibo, A. *et al.* (1995) Hepatitis B, C, and D virus infections in patients with chronic hepatitis, cirrhosis and hepatocellular carcinoma: a comparative study in Niger. *American Journal of Tropical Medicine and Hygiene*, **52**, 293–6.

Darwish, M.A., Issa, S.A., Aziz, A.M. *et al.* (1993) Hepatitis C and B viruses, and their association with hepatocellular carcinoma in Egypt. *Journal of the Egyptian Public Health Asssociation*, **68**, 1–9.

Deugnier, Y.M., Guyader, D., Crantock, L. *et al.* (1993a) Primary liver cancer in genetic hemochromatosis: a clinical, pathological, and pathogenetic study of 54 cases. *Gastroenterology*, **104**, 228–34.

Deugnier, Y.M., Charalambous, P., le Quilleuc, D. *et al.* (1993b) Preneoplastic significance of hepatic iron-free foci in genetic hemochromatosis: a study of 185 patients. *Hepatology*, **1993**, 1363–9.

Falkson, G., Cnaan, A., Schutt, A.J. *et al.* (1988) Prognostic factors for survival in hepatocellular carcinoma. *Cancer Research*, **48**, 7314–18.

Gordeuk, V.R., McLaren, C.E., MacPhail, A.P. *et al.* (1996) Associations of iron overload in Africa with hepatocellular carcinoma and tuberculosis: Strachan's 1929 thesis revisited. *Blood*, **87**, 3470–6.

Gordeuk, V.R., Mukiibe, J., Hasstedt, S.J. *et al.* (1992) Iron overload in Africa: interaction between a gene and dietary iron content. *New England Journal of Medicine*, **326**, 95–100.

Higginson, J. (1963) The geographic pathology of primary liver cancer. *Cancer Research*, **23**, 1624–33.

Hsu, I.C., Metcalf, R.A., Sun, T. *et al.* (1991) Mutational hotspot in the p53 gene in human hepatocellular carcinomas. *Nature*, **350**, 427–8.

Isaacson, C. (1978) The changing pattern of liver disease in South African blacks. *South African Medical Journal*, **53**, 365–8.

Keen, F.G. and Martin, P. (1971) Is aflatoxin carcinogenic in man? The evidence from Swaziland. *Tropical and Geographical Medicine*, **23**, 44–52.

Kew, M.C. (1983) Hepatocellular carcinoma. *Postgraduate Medical Journal*, **59 (Suppl. 4)**, 78–87.

Kew, M.C., DiBisceglie, A.M. and Paterson, A.C. (1985) Smoking as a risk factor in hepatocellular carcinoma: a case-control study in southern African blacks. *Cancer*, **56**, 2315–17.

Kew, M.C., Dusheiko, G.M., Hadziyannis, S.J. and Paterson, A.C. (1984) Does delta infection play a part in the pathogenesis of hepatitis B virus related hepatocellular carcinoma? *British Medical Journal*, **288**, 1727.

Kew, M.C., Geddes, E.W., Macnab, G.M. and Bersohn, I. (1974) Hepatitis-B antigen and cirrhosis in bantu patients with primary liver cancer. *Cancer*, **34**, 539–41.

Kew, M.C., Hodkinson, J., Paterson, A.C. and Song, E. (1982) Hepatitis-B virus infection in black children with hepatocellular carcinoma. *Journal of Medical Virology*, **9**, 201–7.

Kew, M.C., McKnight, A., Hodkinson, J. *et al.* (1989) The role of membranous obstruction of the inferior vena cava in the etiology of hepatocellular carcinoma in southern African blacks. *Hepatology*, **9**, 121–5.

Kew, M.C., Yu, M.C., Kedda, M.A. *et al.* (1997) The relative roles of hepatitis B and C viruses in the etiology of hepatocellular carcinoma in southern African blacks. *Gastroenterology*, **112**, 184–7.

Kramvis, A., Bukofzer, S., Kew, M.C. and Song, E. (1997) Nucleic acid sequence analysis of the precore region of hepatitis B virus from sera of southern African black adult carriers of the virus. *Hepatology*, **25**, 235–40.

Lancaster, M.G., Jenkis, R.P. and Philip, J.M. (1971) Toxicity associated with certain samples of groundnuts. *Nature*, **192**, 1095–6.

MacSween, R.N.M. and Scott, A.R. (1973) Hepatic cirrhosis: a clinicopathological review of 520 cases. *Journal of Clinical Pathology*, **26**, 936–42.

Mandishona, E., MacPhail, A.P., Gordeuk, V.R. *et al.* (1998) Dietary iron overload as a risk factor for hepatocellular carcinoma in black Africans. *Hepatology*, **27**, 1563–6.

Maraj, R., Kew, M.C. and Hyslop, R.J. (1988) Resectability rate of hepatocellular carcinoma in rural southern Africans. *British Journal of Surgery*, **75**, 335–8.

Mets, T.F. (1993) The disease pattern of elderly medical patients in Rwanda, central Africa. *Journal of Tropical Medicine and Hygiene*, **96**, 291–300.

Mohamed, A.E., Kew, M.C. and Groeneveld, H.T. (1992) Alcohol consumption as a risk factor for hepatocellular carcinoma in urban southern African blacks. *International Journal of Cancer*, **51**, 537–41.

Okuda, K. (1986) Early recognition of hepatocellular carcinoma. *Hepatology*, **6**, 729–38.

Ozturk, M., Bressac, B., Puisieux, A. *et al.* (1991) p53 mutation in hepatocellular carcinoma after aflatoxin exposure. *Lancet*, **338**, 1356–9.

Paterson, A.C., Kew, M.C., Dusheiko, G.M. and Isaacson, C. (1989) Liver cell dysplasia accompanying hepatocellular carcinoma in southern Africa. *Journal of Hepatology*, **8**, 241–8.

Paterson, A.C., Kew, M.C., Herman, A.A.B. *et al.* (1985) Liver morphology in southern African blacks with hepatocellular cacinoma: a study in the urban environment. *Hepatology*, **5**, 72–78.

Peers, F.G., Gilman, G.A. and Linsell, C.A. (1976) Dietary aflatoxins and liver cancer. A study in Swaziland. *International Journal of Cancer*, **17**, 167–76.

Peers, F.G. and Linsell, C.A. (1973) Dietary aflatoxins and liver cancer – a population based study in Kenya. *British Journal of Cancer*, **27**, 473–84.

Powell, L.W., Fletcher, L.M. and Halliday, J.W. (1995) Distinction between haemochromatosis and alcoholic siderosis, in *Alcoholic Liver Disease: Pathology and Pathogenesis* (ed. P. Hall), Edward Arnold, London, pp. 199–216.

Prince, A.M., Szmuness, W., Michon, J. *et al.* (1975) A case/control study of the association between primary liver cancer and hepatitis B infection in Senegal. *International Journal of Cancer*, **16**, 376–83.

Ryder, R.W. (1992) Hepatitis B virus vaccine in The Gambia, west Africa: synergy between public health research and practice. *Mt Sinai Journal of Medicine*, **59**, 487–92.

Ryder, R.W., Whittle, H.C., Sanneh, A.B. *et al.* (1992) Persistent hepatitis B virus infection and hepatoma in The Gambia, west Africa. A case-control study of 140 adults and their 603 family contacts. *American Journal of Epidemiology*, **136**, 1122–31.

Simson, I.W. (1982) Membranous obstruction of the inferior vena cava and hepatocellular carcinoma in South Africa. *Gastroenterology*, **82**, 171–8.

Sitas, F., Blaauw, D., Terblanche, M. and Madhoo, J. (1992) Cancer in South Africa, 1992, in *National Cancer Registry of South Africa* South African Institute for Medical Research, Johannesburg, p. 17.

Soni, P.N., Tait, D.R., Gopaul, W. *et al.* (1996) Hepatitis C virus infection in chronic liver disease in Natal. *South African Journal of Medicine*, **86**, 80–3.

Tabor, E., Gerety, R.J., Vogel, C.L. *et al.* (1977) Hepatitis B virus infection and primary hepatocellular carcinoma. *Journal of the National Cancer Institutes*, **58**, 1197–1200.

Van Rensburg, H.J. (1989) Liver pathology in the Transvaal: a biopsy study, dissertation, University of the Witwatersrand, pp. 9–16.

Van Rensburg, S.J., van der Watt, J.J. and Purchase, I.F.H. (1974) Primary liver cancer rate and aflatoxin intake in a high cancer area. *South African Journal of Medicine*, **48**, 2508a–d.

Vogel, C.L., Anthony, P.P., Sadkali, F. *et al.* (1972) Hepatitis-associated antigen and antibody in hepatocellular carcinoma: results of a continuing study. *Journal of the National Cancer Institutes*, **48**, 1583–8.

Yap, E.P.H., Cooper, K., Maharaj, B. and McGee, J.O.'D. (1993) p53 codon 249ser hot-spot mutation in HBV-negative hepatocellular carcinoma. *Lancet*, **431**, 251.

Yoshida, Y., Kanematsu, T., Matsumata, T. *et al.* (1994) A comparative study on hepatocellular carcinoma between South Africans and Japanese from the viewpoint of nuclear DNA content. *British Journal of Cancer*, **69**, 362–6.

EUROPE

P.J. Johnson

13.1 INTRODUCTION

Europe includes some of the countries with the lowest incidence of hepatocellular carcinoma (HCC). In northern parts of Europe, HCC is uncommon and is seldom related to chronic viral hepatitis. In the southern, eastern and Mediterranean areas, chronic hepatitis C and hepatitis B-related HCC are more prevalent. HCC mostly arises as a complication of alcoholic cirrhosis, and cases arising in other, rarer, forms of cirrhosis such as hemochromatosis also comprise a significant percentage of the total number of HCC cases. Aflatoxin exposure does not appear to be an important risk factor in Europe.

'Europe', however defined, spans a huge geographic area and it is racially highly heterogeneous. This makes it difficult to generalize about HCC. Also, while it is possible to compare features of HCC in Europe with other areas of the world from the literature, direct and formal comparisons have seldom been attempted. For this reason some of what is written here is based on the author's experience in Europe and Asia. Not all the contentions can be backed up by references to the literature.

The major differences between Europe and high-incidence areas relate to the epidemiology of HCC. Treatment options remain similar.

13.2 EPIDEMIOLOGY

The incidence of HCC across Europe ranges from <2 to around 10 per 100000 per year (Table 13.1). The tumor arises in an older age group than that reported in high-incidence areas with a mean age of presentation of around 65 years. Figure 13.1 compares the age distribution in northern Europe, southern

Table 13.1 Age-adjusted HCC incidence rates for representative countries in Europe. For comparison, typical figures for high-incidence areas are usually in the range of 20–50/100000 and may rise to as high as >100/1000. Figures vary in different parts of the country and the above are only meant as rough guidelines.

Country	Incidence rate (per 100 000/year)	
	Male	*Female*
Romania	11.8	7.9
Poland	8.3	4.9
Spain	6.9	5.1
Italy	6.9	2.7
France	4.9	0.7
Germany	3.6	1.5
Sweden	3.4	1.8
Denmark	2.9	1.6
UK	1.5	0.4

From Waterhouse *et al.* (1982).

Hepatocellular Carcinoma: Diagnosis, investigation and management. Edited by Anthony S.-Y. Leong, Choong-Tsek Liew, Joseph W.Y. Lau and Philip J. Johnson. Published in 1999 by Arnold, London. ISBN 0 340 74096 5.

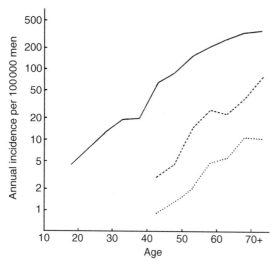

Fig. 13.1 Age distribution of HCC in populations at high (Zimbabwe, ———), intermediate (Spain, – – – –) and low (Norway, · · · · · ·) risk areas.

Europe and a high-incidence area outside the continent (i.e. Zimbabwe). It is noticeable that HCC <40 years of age is almost unheard of in Europe, whereas in Zimbabwe the annual incidence is already 50 per 100 000 by this age (Bosch and Munoz, 1987). As in most other areas of the world the incidence is several times greater in males than females and 70–90% of cases will have underlying cirrhosis (Johnson and Williams, 1987).

13.2.1 CHRONIC HEPATITIS B INFECTION AND HCC AMONG IMMIGRANTS FROM HIGH-INCIDENCE AREAS TO EUROPE

Subjects from high HCC incidence areas carry the increased risk of HCC with them when they emigrate to low-incidence areas such as Europe. The high risk of HCC among Chinese Americans has been recognized for >50 years. Studies from UK immigrants developing HCC show that most have been exposed to HBV infection and more than one-half will be HBsAg-seropositive. They usually acquire the infection in their country of birth, prior to residing in Europe. The risk is confined largely

to those who have evidence of underlying chronic liver disease (Zaman *et al.*, 1986).

13.2.2 COMMON ETIOLOGICAL FACTORS – CHRONIC ALCOHOL INTAKE AND HCV INFECTION ·

In Europe, most cases of HCC will arise in patients with alcoholic cirrhosis or chronic hepatitis C virus infection (Table 13.2). For patients with alcoholic cirrhosis the lifetime risk is about 15% in men and up to 5% in women. Meta-analysis has shown, however, that moderate alcohol consumption is associated with little or no increase in HCC. With higher consumption the relative risk is still only 1.5 (compared with >50 in HBsAg carriers) (Villa *et al.*, 1991). This is clearly at odds with the experience of Western hepatologists and presumably attests to the importance of cirrhosis, which develops in only a minority of heavy alcohol drinkers. It is likely that, while the association between HCC and alcohol is related to the underlying cirrhosis, there may be additional factors including chronic viral hepatitis.

With the development of serological tests for chronic hepatitis C virus infection it soon became apparent that the virus was responsible for a high percentage of cases of HCC, particularly in southern Europe where it has replaced hepatitis B as the most common cause of virus related HCC (Bruix *et al.*, 1989;

Table 13.2 Rate of positivity for anti-HCV in various European countries compared with a control population from the same country.

Country	Anti-HCV positivity (%)	Control population (%)
Italy	76	<1
France	58	<1
Spain	75	7.5
Greece	40	–
UK	10	<1

Colombo *et al.*, 1989; Table 13.2). The interactions between alcohol/cirrhosis/HBV infection and HCV infection are currently areas of intense research and considerable controversy (Walter *et al.*, 1988; Nappas *et al.*, 1990; Bode *et al.*, 1991).

13.2.3 THOROTRAST

No account of the epidemiology of HCC in a European context would be complete without the mention of the 'thorotrast tragedy.' Thorotrast, a radiological contrast medium containing a colloidal suspension of thorium dioxide (a powerful emitter of α-particles), was introduced into clinical practice in 1929 and was widely used throughout Europe until 1950. It contributed to many of the advances made in angiography, especially carotid angiography. Unfortunately, after a minimum period of 15 years following exposure, there was development of cirrhosis and primary liver tumors including, in 20% of cases, HCC, and other malignant neoplasms. The German Thorotrast study accumulated data on 1689 patients who received thorotrast and were known to have died. When these were matched with an appropriate control group the enormous increase in liver cancer deaths was readily apparent (Table 13.3). In the case of both liver cancer and cirrhosis a clear dose–effect relationship was established. The overall magnitude of the problem may never be known precisely but in Germany alone, 10–20 000 patients were treated and about one-third of these will have died from malignant liver tumors. Although grave doubts about its safety were raised as early as 1937, it was not withdrawn from use until 1950. Cases are still being encountered today (The German Thorotrast Study Group 1984).

13.2.4 ORAL CONTRACEPTIVE PREPARATIONS

Since the 1970s there has been considerable concern about the possibility that the birth control pill was associated with an increased risk of HCC. There now seems little doubt that there is a true association between such contraceptive preparations and *benign* hepatic adenomas (Jick and Herman, 1978), although the risk is extremely small. The risk that such lesions will lead to significant symptoms is even smaller. Epidemiological studies relating to the risk of HCC have been limited by the very small number of patients in individual studies, and the fact that the dose of estrogen in the various preparations has been usually decreasing over the years. This means that studies carried out in the 1970s may not be relevant to today's preparations. The current consensus, based on studies mainly in the UK, is that while there may possibly be a significantly increased risk of the development of HCC after prolonged (>8 years) usage, the absolute risk remains extremely small (Forman *et al.*, 1983, 1986; Neuberger *et al.*, 1986).

13.3 DIAGNOSIS, CLINICAL FEATURES AND PRESENTATION

Patients who develop HCC as the first presentation of cirrhosis, in a cirrhotic liver (as opposed to those who are already under medical care for 'known cirrhosis') will often have a delayed diagnosis because the physician will not be expecting a diagnosis of HCC. A liver mass in Europe is much more

Table 13.3 Causes of death in patients receiving thorotrast and a matched control group. Of the liver cancer patients, 75 also had cirrhosis.

Disease	Thorotrast (N=1689)	Control (N=1280)
Liver cancer	256	2
Myeloproliferative disease	27	2
Liver cirrhosis	132 (+75)	43
Bone marrow failure	16	1
Non-Hodgkin's lymphoma	12	5

likely to be a secondary deposit than a primary lesion. Furthermore, whereas in high-incidence areas the physician is likely to make the diagnosis on initial consultation, this seldom occurs in Europe. Apart from these points the investigative plan is similar to that described in Chapter 2.

In Europe the presentation is often with decompensation of already recognized cirrhosis. Asymptomatic detection following routine screening is also becoming a frequent occurrence. Patients with a wide variety of types of cirrhosis will also be seen including hemochromatosis, primary biliary cirrhosis and α-1-antitrypsin deficiency. Some presentations that are relatively common in the East are very rare in Europe, including hemoperitoneum from tumor rupture and membranous obstruction of the inferior vena cava.

13.4   TREATMENT

The same principles of treatment are applied in Europe as in other parts of the world. Surgical resection remains the only hope of long-term cure but it is only applicable in between 10 and 20% of patients. The recurrence rate is also high. Two points should, however, be noted. First, surgery in patients in whom the tumor complicates cirrhosis is a relatively late development in Europe; cirrhosis was often considered an absolute contraindication to resectional hepatic surgery. Second, because of the considerably greater availability of organs for transplantation, and the much lower numbers of HCC cases, the opportunity for transplantation as a treatment for HCC is much higher. If strict indications are laid down, then liver transplantation for all patients who would benefit is not an unrealistic aim in many European countries.

Palliative treatments have been attempted as in other countries. Indeed some of the only prospective controlled clinical trials in palliative treatments have been undertaken in Europe. Controlled clinical trials of transarterial chemoembolization from France have, in general, suggested that overall survival is unlikely to be improved (Trinchet *et al.*, 1995; Rougier *et al.*, 1997). Studies from Spain have shown that cutaneous alcohol injection, over a 3-year follow-up, gives survival figures similar to those obtained by surgical resection (Castells *et al.*, 1993). Other European studies have examined the efficacy of Tamoxifen and some have, remarkably, been quite positive (Farinati *et al.*, 1990; Martinez-Cerezo *et al.*, 1994; Castells *et al.*, 1995; Table 13.4). Larger randomized studies of hormonal manipulation are underway.

Table 13.4   European trials comparing the placebo and tamoxifen (TMX).

Author: Centre:		Farinati Padua, Italy	Martinez-Cerezo Barcelona, Spain	Castells Barcelona, Spain
Number of patients (deaths)	placebo	19 (18)	16 (3)	62 (36)
	TMX	19 (15)	20 (8)	58 (34)
	total	38	36	120
Median survival (months)	placebo	2	6	17
	TMX	9	9	20
Actuarial survival (1 year)	placebo	5%	9.1%	43%
	TMX	22%	48.5%	51%
	HR	0.48	0.66	0.79
	95%CI	0.21–1.09	0.28–1.55	0.49–1.26

HR = hazard ratio, CI = confidence interval

13.5 PROGNOSIS

There is the strong impression that the HCCs in a European population pursue a slightly less aggressive course and that median survival is better than in high-incidence areas. While this may be due, in part, to later presentation in high-incidence areas, the median survival in South Africa and many Asian countries is measured in terms of a few weeks *from first symptoms*. Such aggressive disease is seldom seen in Europe where survival is measured in months. This contention is supported by examination of the control groups in clinical trials where median survival in the untreated arm can be >1 year.

13.6 FIBROLAMELLAR HEPATOCELLULAR CARCINOMA

This tumor is almost unheard of in high-incidence areas whereas it will account for up to 5% of cases in Europe. It has several distinctive clinical features including a young age of presentation (median age 20–30 years), normal α-fetoprotein levels and lack of any association with cirrhosis. Patients are invariably HBV-negative (Craig *et al.*, 1980; Paradinas *et al.*, 1982). The histological picture is one of large polygonal malignant hepatocytes with abundant eosinophilic cytoplasm and lamella bands of dense connective tissue between groups of malignant cells. The tumor carries a better prognosis than the normal type of HCC. This relates partly to the fact that it is more often resectable and it has a less aggressive clinical course. Nonetheless, most patients will ultimately die from the tumor (Soreide *et al.*, 1986).

REFERENCES

Bode, J.C., Biermann, J., Kohse, K.P. *et al.* (1991) High incidence of antibodies to hepatitis C virus in alcoholic cirrhosis: fact or fiction? *Alcohol Alcoholism*, **11**, 26–30.

Bosch, F.X. and Munoz, N. (1987) Epidemiology of hepatocellular carcinoma, in *Neoplasms of the Liver* (eds K. Okuda and K.G. Ishak), Tokyo, Springer, pp. 3–20.

Bruix, J., Barrera, J.M., Calvet, X. *et al.* (1989) Prevalence of antibodies to hepatitis C virus in Spanish patients with hepatocellular carcinoma and hepatic cirrhosis. *Lancet*, **ii**, 1004–6.

Castells, A., Bruix, J., Bru, C. *et al.* (1993) Treatment of small hepatocellular carcinoma in cirrhotic patients: a cohort study comparing surgical resection and percutaneous ethanol injections. *Hepatology*, **18**, 1121–6.

Castells, A., Bruix, J., Bru, C. *et al.* (1995) Treatment of hepatocellular carcinoma with tamoxifen: a double-blind placebo controlled trial in 120 patients. *Gastroenterology*, **109**, 917–22.

Columbo, M., De Franchis, R., Del Ninno, E. *et al.* (1991) Hepatocellular carcinoma in Italian patients with cirrhosis. *New England Journal of Medicine*, **325**, 675–8.

Colombo, M., Kuo, G., Choo, Q.I. *et al.* (1989) Prevalence of antibodies to hepatitis C virus in Italian patients with hepatocellular carcinoma. *Lancet*, **ii**, 1006–8.

Craig, J.R., Peters, R.L. and Omata, M. (1980) Fibrolamellar carcinoma of the liver: a tumour of adolescents and young adults with distinctive clinicopathologic features. *Cancer*, **46**, 372–9.

Farinati, F., Salvagnini, M., de Maria, N. *et al.* (1990) Unresectable hepatocellular carcinoma: a prospective controlled trial with tamoxifen. *Journal of Hepatology*, **11**, 297–301.

Forman, D., Doll, R. and Peto, R. (1983) Trends in mortality from carcinoma of the liver and the use of oral contraceptives. *British Journal of Cancer*, **48**, 349–54.

Forman, D., Vincent, T.J. and Doll, R. (1986) Cancer of the liver and the use of oral contraceptives. *British Medical Journal*, **292**, 1357–61.

Jick, H. and Herman, R. (1978) Oral contraceptives induced benign liver tumors. The magnitude of the problem. *Journal of the American Medical Association*, **240**, 828–9.

Johnson, P.J. and Williams, R. (1987) Cirrhosis and the aetiology of hepatocellular carcinoma. *Journal of Hepatology*, **4**, 140–7.

Martinez-Cerezo, F.J., Tomas, A., Donoso, L. *et al.* (1994) Controlled trial of tamoxifen in patients with advanced hepatocellular carcinoma. *Journal of Hepatology*, **20**, 702–6.

Nappas, B., Diss, F., Pol, S. *et al.* (1990) Association between HCV and HBV infection in hepatocellular carcinoma and alcoholic liver disease. *Journal of Hepatology*, **12**, 70–4.

Neuberger, J., Forman, D., Doll, R. and Williams, R. (1986) Oral contraceptives and hepatocellular carcinoma. *British Medical Journal*, **292**, 1355–7.

Paradinas, F.J., Melia, W.M., Wilkinson, M.L. *et al.* (1982) High serum levels of vitamin B12 binding capacity as a marker of the fibrolamellar variant of hepatocellular carcinoma. *British Medical Journal*, **285**, 840–2.

Rougier, P., Pelletier, G., Ducreux, M. *et al.* (1997) Unresectable hepatocellular carcinoma: lack of efficacy of lipiodol chemoembolization. Final results of a multicenter randomized trial. *Proceedings of the American Society of Clinical Oncology*, **16**, A989.

Soreide, O., Czerniak, A., Bradpiece, H. *et al.* (1986) Characteristics of fibrolamellar hepatocellular carcinoma: a study of nine cases and a review of the literature. *American Journal of Surgery*, **151**, 518–23.

The German Thorotrast Study (1984) (eds G. van Kaick, H. Muth, and A. Kaul), Commission of the European Communities.

Trinchet, J.C. *et al.*, from the Group d'Etude et de Traitement du Carcinome Hepatocellulaire (1995) A comparison of lipiodol chemoembolization and conservative treatment for unresectable hepatocellular carcinoma. *New England Journal of Medicine*, **332**, 1256–61.

Villa, E., Melegari, M., Scaglioni, P.P. *et al.* (1991) Hepatocellular carcinoma: risk factors other than HBV. *Italian Journal of Gastroenterology*, **23**, 457.

Walter, E., Blum, H.E., Meier, P. *et al.* (1988) Hepatocellular carcinoma in alcoholic liver disease: no evidence for a pathogenic role of hepatitis B virus infection. *Hepatology*, **8**, 745–50.

Waterhouse, J.A.H., Muir, C., Shanmugaratnam, K. and Powell, J. (1982) Cancer incidence in five continents, in *International Agency for Research on Cancer* (IARC Scientific Publications no. 42), vol. 5, Lyon.

Zaman, S.N., Johnson, P.J. and Williams, R. (1986) Hepatocellular carcinoma in immigrants to the United Kingdom. *Quarterly Journal of Medicine*, **232**, 813–17.

JAPAN

M. Kage and M. Kojiro

13.7 INCIDENCE OF HEPATOCELLULAR CARCINOMA (HCC)

Hepatocellular carcinoma (HCC) is one of the most important neoplasms in Japan. The number of deaths due to HCC was 26 886 in 1994, accounting for 11% of all deaths due to malignant neoplasms in Japan. The incidence of HCC has been steeply increasing since about 1970, and it is the third commonest malignancy in the country following lung cancer and gastric cancer.

According to figures from the Liver Cancer Study Group of Japan of 13 991 cases of primary liver cancers occurring during a 2-year period from 1992 to 1993, 13 381 cases were HCC (95.6%), 432 were cholangiocellular carcinoma (3.1%) and 56 were mixed carcinoma (0.4%) (Liver Cancer Study Group of Japan, 1997).

13.8 ETIOLOGIC FACTORS IN HCC IN JAPAN

13.8.1 HBV AND HCV INFECTION

One of the characteristics of HCC patients in Japan is that the majority of cases are related to hepatitis virus infection (Shiratori *et al.*, 1995; Liver Cancer Study Group of Japan, 1997). Among 12 206 HCC patients examined from 1992 to 1993, HCV infection alone was demonstrated in 76.4%, whereas sustained HBV infection (HBsAg-positive) was found in 16.8%, and double infection, presenting both serum HCV Ab and HBsAg, was demon-

strated in 3.2% (Liver Study Group of Japan, 1997). The frequency of HBV-related HCC has decreased in recent years, while that of HCV-related HCC has increased in Japan. At present, the number of positive HBsAg cases is still lower compared with those in South-East Asia and Africa, but higher than those in the USA.

The average age of patients with HBsAg-positive HCC in Japan was 52 years and that of HCV Ab-positive patients was 62 years (Shiratori *et al.*, 1995).

13.8.2 OTHER ETIOLOGIC FACTORS

Viral hepatitis is an aggravating factor in various aspects of liver diseases including the development of HCC in Japan. A high prevalence of viral hepatitis, especially HCV infection, has been found in patients with HCC who have such underlying diseases as alcoholism and chronic *Schistosomiasis japonica*. Aflatoxin is quite unlikely to have a synergistic role in Japanese patients.

13.9 CLINICAL ASPECTS

A past history of acute or chronic hepatitis, blood transfusion and excessive alcohol intake was found in 70, 30 and 30% respectively in the patients with HCC (Liver Study Group of Japan, 1977). Abdominal pain is the most frequent of the presenting symptoms. Of the various objective signs, hepatomegaly is frequently found. However, large hepatomegaly is not common (Okuda *et al.*, 1984), indicating

Hepatocellular Carcinoma: Diagnosis, investigation and management. Edited by Anthony S.-Y. Leong, Choong-Tsek Liew, Joseph W.Y. Lau and Philip J. Johnson. Published in 1999 by Arnold, London. ISBN 0 340 74096 5.

that many of the HCCs in Japan arise from small viral cirrhosis unlike that in alcoholic cirrhosis.

13.10   PATHOMORPHOLOGIC FEATURES

13.10.1   GROSS CHARACTERISTICS

It is reported that the gross anatomic features as well as the incidence of HCC vary from one country to another (Okuda *et al.*, 1984; Kojiro *et al.*, 1990; Okuda 1992).

Of surgically resected HCCs in Japan, 80% were found to be of the nodular type or nodular type with varying degrees of perinodular tumor growth according to classification of the Liver Cancer Study Group of Japan (1977). The diffuse type is uncommon.

A high frequency of a capsule formation seems a characteristic of the Japanese cases compared with tumors in the USA and South Africa (Okuda *et al.*, 1984). A recent survey disclosed that 79% of 3443 surgically resected HCCs had capsule formation. Encapsulated expanding HCC develops almost always in cirrhotic or precirrhotic livers.

13.10.2   HISTOLOGICAL CHARACTERISTICS

Histologically, 75% of the carcinoma cells are arranged in a trabecular pattern, 14% in a solid pattern and 6% in a pseudoglandular pattern. A sclerosing pattern is rare. The fibrolamellar variant of HCC is extremely rare in all parts of Asia including Japan.

The grade of differentiation varies from case to case, largely depending on the tumor size. The smaller the tumor, the more differentiated it is. Almost all small HCCs <2 cm in diameter, usually sampled by liver biopsy or by hepatectomy, are well- or moderately differentiated, while 65% of autopsied HCCs demonstrate moderate differentiation, and 20% poor differentiation. The grade of differentiation is usually heterogenous within a tumor.

13.11   PATHOMORPHOLOGIC CHARACTERISTICS OF EARLY HCC

Along with the remarkable progress in various diagnostic imaging techniques, increasing numbers of small, early stage HCC have been detected and resected. Of all surgically resected HCCs, 18% are detected as small HCCs <2 cm in diameter (Liver Study Group of Japan, 1997). Accordingly, the pathomorphologic characteristics and the developmental process of early HCC have been clarified through histological examinations of resected HCC (Kojiro *et al.*, 1991; Okuda, 1992; Nakashima *et al.*, 1995).

13.11.1   GROSS FEATURES

Early HCCs <2 cm in diameter can be categorized into either the distinct or the indistinct nodular types. The latter is interpreted as the smallest HCC, which is currently clinically detectable. Many resected small HCCs are of the distinct nodular type and they frequently have a fibrous capsule. On the other hand, the indistinct nodular type is clearly detected as either a hypoechoic or hyperechoic nodular lesion in ultrasound examinations. However, the cancerous nodules are usually obscured and difficult to identify on gross examination (Figs 13.2a and b).

13.11.2   HISTOLOGICAL FEATURES

Early HCCs of the indistinct nodular type consist solely of well-differentiated cancerous tissues with little cellular and structural atypia, and they have portal tracts within the tumor. At the boundary between the tumor and the non-tumor, well-differentiated HCC cells proliferate along the adjacent hepatic cords by replacing normal hepatocytes. They are uncapsulated. When a small HCC grows to about 1.5 cm in diameter, it starts to show expansive growth with capsule formation and, importantly, de-differentiation of well-differentiated HCC cells also occurs. HCC at

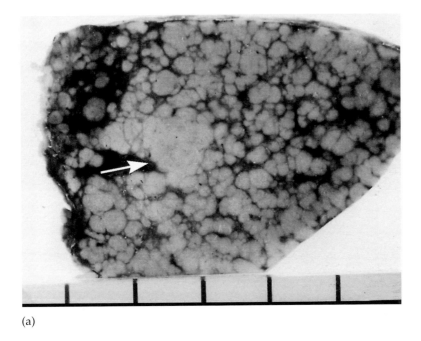

(a)

(b)

Fig. 13.2 A small HCC of indistinct nodular type in C cirrhosis. (a) The vaguely nodular subtype of HCC of 1 cm diameter is present (arrow). (b) Cancer cells with little atypia are arranged in an irregular thin trabecular pattern. Fatty change is also found in cancerous tissue. Arrows indicate the area of HCC.

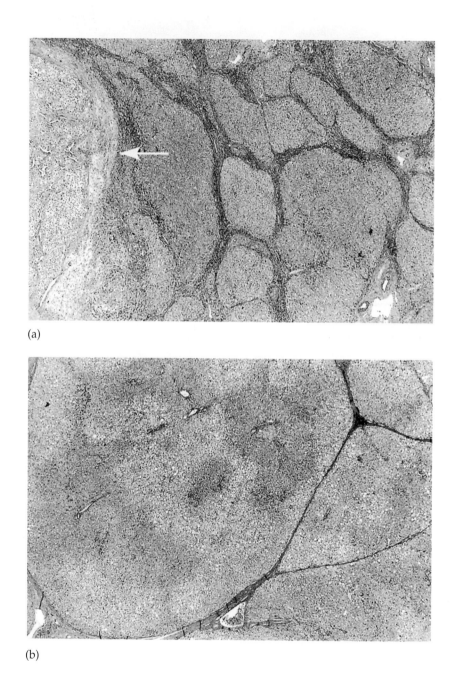

(a)

(b)

Fig. 13.3. Comparison of the pattern of fibrosis and regenerative nodules in C and B cirrhosis. (a) C cirrhosis: small nodules and relatively thick fibrous septa. Arrow indicates the presence of a HCC. (b) B cirrhosis: larger nodules and thin fibrous septa.

lower histological grades proliferates within the well-differentiated cancerous nodule; these moderately and/or poorly differentiated tumor cells replace the well-differentiated tissues (Kojiro *et al.*, 1991; Nakashima *et al.*, 1995). Thus, early HCCs develop into advanced HCCs.

13.12 HISTOLOGIC FEATURES OF THE NON-CANCEROUS LIVER TISSUE

Liver cirrhosis or fibrosis related to viral hepatitis is associated in >80% of autopsied cases of HCCs in Japan (Liver Study Group of Japan, 1997).

Our recent study on associated liver cirrhosis in HCCs has clarified significant histological differences between HCV-related cirrhosis (C cirrhosis) and HBV-related cirrhosis (B cirrhosis) (Shimamatu *et al.*, 1994). The histological characteristics can be summarized as follows:

- C cirrhosis: broadly expanded fibrous septa and small regenerative nodules (micro- or mixed-nodular type), relatively strong inflammatory reaction and frequent lymphoid aggregates in the fibrous septum (Fig. 13.3a).
- B cirrhosis: large regenerative nodules (macronodular type) with thin fibrous septa and quiescent inflammation (Fig. 13.3b).

Liver cell dysplasia is more frequently observed in B than in C cirrhosis. It is likely that such differences might be related to the severity and duration of active inflammation. In HCV hepatitis, active inflammation may continue through progression from chronic hepatitis to cirrhosis, while in HBV hepatitis inflammation subsides after the seroconversion. Subsequently, more vigorous regeneration is induced at the stage of cirrhosis.

REFERENCES

Kojiro, M., Nakashima, O., Kiyomatsu, K. *et al.* (1990) Comparative study of HCC between Japan and Spain, in *Viral Hepatitis and Hepatocellular Carcinoma* (eds I.L. Sung and D.S. Chen), Excerpta Medica, Amsterdam, pp. 545–8.

Kojiro, M., Sugihara, S. and Nakashima, O. (1991) Pathomorphologic characteristics of early hepatocellular carcinoma, in *Early Detection and Treatment of Liver Cancer* (eds K. Okuda, T. Tobe and T. Kitagawa), Japan Scientific Societies Press, Tokyo, pp. 29–33.

Liver Cancer Study Group of Japan (1997) *Primary Liver Cancer in Japan* (Report no. 12), Kyoto, Shinko (in Japanese).

Nakashima, O., Sugihara, S., Kage, M. *et al.* (1995) Pathomorphologic characteristics of small hepatocellular carcinoma: a special reference to small hepatocellular carcinoma with indistinct margins. *Hepatology,* **22**, 101–5.

Okuda, K. (1992) Hepatocellular carcinoma: recent progress. *Hepatology,* **15**, 948–63.

Okuda, K., Peters, R.L., Simson, I.W. *et al.* (1984) Gross anatomic features of hepatocellular carcinoma from three disparate geographic areas. *Cancer,* **54**, 2165–73.

Shimamatu, K., Kage, M., Nakashima, O. *et al.* (1994) Pathomorphological study of HCV antibody-positive liver cirrhosis. *Journal of Gastroeterology and Hepatology,* **9**, 624–30.

Shiratori, Y., Shiina, S., Imamura, M. *et al.* (1995) Characteristic difference of hepatocellular carcinoma between hepatitis B- and C- viral infection in Japan. *Hepatology,* **22**, 1027–33.

Korea

C. Park and Y.-N. Park

13.13 INTRODUCTION

Primary hepatocellular carcinoma (HCC) is one of the most common malignant tumors in man, but its incidence shows a marked geographic variability. The incidence of HCC among Koreans is relatively high at 30 and 7 per 100 000 population for males and females respectively. Notably, the incidence rates among Korean adults between 40 and 64 years of age is 74.8 for males and 15.6 for females per 100 000 population, which are the highest figures in the world (Ahn et al., 1989). Moreover, HCC is the second most common cause of cancer mortality in Korea.

As the majority of chronic liver diseases among Koreans are caused by hepatitis virus infection, hepatitis B virus (HBV) and hepatitis C virus (HCV) may be regarded as the primary causes of death due to liver diseases. Since approximately 65% of HCC patients are positive for serum HBsAg and about one-half of the remaining cases are positive for serum anti-HCV, it can be estimated that HBV or HCV infection has a role in the causation of approximately 80–85% of HCCs. Liver cirrhosis is found in about 79% of HCCs, including 68–78.5% of HBV-related HCCs and 81.5–84.3% of HCV-related HCCs.

In general, HBV-infected patients are younger than HCV-infected patients, and among patients with HCC, those testing positive for serum HBsAg are younger than those positive for anti-HCV. It has been postulated that this may be the result of vertical or perinatal transmission of HBV.

Among Koreans, approximately 7% of the total population and 5% of the female population are seropositive for HBsAg. Since about 20% of the HBsAg-positive females are positive for HBeAg, approximately 1% of pregnant women would be responsible for vertical transmission of the disease, if the HBsAg-negative cases with precore mutation are excluded. Moreover, among the HBsAg carriers who began their carrier state in infancy following vertical transmission of HBV, >90% develop chronic liver diseases by adulthood, which is tremendously greater than that exhibited by HBV carriers who contracted the virus in adulthood. Regenerative nodules in cirrhosis have been shown to be an important factor in the genesis of HCC and the development of HCC in HBV-infected patients has been estimated to take approximately 45 years on average (Chen, 1987). These observations imply far-reaching consequences of vertical transmission of HBV. Approximately 10–30% of patients with HBV-associated chronic hepatitis develop cirrhosis. According to a national report that investigated the natural course of HBV-associated chronic hepatitis, the annual incidence rate of HCC is 0.8%, and the cumulative incidences of HCC are 2.7–3, 11, 25 and 35% after 5, 10, 15 and 20 years, respectively, following the initial diagnosis (Lee et al., 1997).

More than 50% of HCV infection turn chronic, a figure much greater than that exhibited by HBV infection during adulthood. However, because only 1–1.4% of the Korean

Hepatocellular Carcinoma: Diagnosis, investigation and management. Edited by Anthony S.-Y. Leong, Choong-Tsek Liew, Joseph W.Y. Lau and Philip J. Johnson. Published in 1999 by Arnold, London. ISBN 0 340 74096 5.

population is infected with HCV, the incidence of HCC associated with HCV is far smaller than that associated with HBV. Among Korean patients with HCV-associated cirrhosis, the annual incidence of HCC is 9.0%, and the cumulative incidences of HCC at 3 and 6 years after diagnosis are 22.0 and 54.8% respectively, and they are 6.8, 18.3 and 34.7% in HBV-associated cirrhosis (Lee *et al.*, 1996). These figures are in agreement with those reported from Japan where HCV is more prevalent. The findings imply that, when only cirrhotic patients are considered, the development of HCC from HCV cirrhosis is greater than that from HBV cirrhosis, regardless of the regional variation of hepatitis viruses prevalence.

13.14   PATHOLOGY

Advances in diagnostic techniques and pathologic studies on the early stage of HCC indicate that many HCCs are multicentric in origin. Morphologically, there are combinations of HCC nodule and other nodules, such as a dysplastic nodule of high grade with or without HCC foci (early HCC), or a well-differentiated HCC nodule containing moderately or poorly differentiated HCC foci. These combinations indicate that multiple nodules can be produced within a liver by multicentric *in situ* tumor formation rather than by intrahepatic metastasis. In our materials obtained through surgical resection, 12.5% of patients with HCC have dysplastic nodules of high grade containing HCC foci. This percentage is much less than that of other studies using explanted liver or autopsy material (Soxena *et al.*, 1997). The frequency of such changes seen in explanted and autopsy cases may be a more accurate reflection of the true incidence of multicentric tumors, because microscopic examination is limited to only the immediate vicinity of the main tumor, and patients with multiple small tumors may not

undergo surgery. About 50% of the multicentric HCC cases that we examined occurred in the non-cirrhotic liver, suggesting that cirrhosis is not a requirement for multicentric HCCs.

Among advanced HCCs, approximately 45% of cases are encapsulated by continuous fibrous band. The presence of a capsule depends on the presence of cirrhosis in the remaining liver. Capsules are found in >90% of HCCs developing in cirrhotic livers with the expansive growth pattern, whereas capsules occur in only about 20% of the non-expanding type HCCs in the non-cirrhotic liver. Fibrous septum formation within the tumor is also a frequent finding. Fibrous septum formation occurs in about 75% of HCCs in the cirrhotic liver compared with about 40% of HCCs in the non-cirrhotic liver (Park *et al.*, 1991).

In our series of 377 surgically removed or biopsied HCCs from 1984 to 1997, most were of the usual histologic type and there were no cases of fibrolamellar type. There were two cases of combined HCC and cholangiocarcinoma and four cases of sclerosing hepatic carcinomas (Park and Park, 1994).

13.15   GENETIC ALTERATIONS

Although chronic hepatitis/cirrhosis is the major etiologic cause of HCC, malignant transformation of hepatocytes has much to do with genetic changes. Proto-oncogenes are rarely altered in primary HCC, suggesting that inactivation of tumor suppressor genes (TSGs) is critical for hepatocarcinogenesis. TSGs are usually inactivated by the combination of intragenic mutation in one allele with loss of the other corresponding allele, termed loss of heterozygosity (LOH). Many chromosomal arms have been reported as candidate sites of putative tumor suppressor genes for HCCs, including 1p, 4q, 5q, 8p, 8q, 10q, 13q, 14q, 16q and 17p (Boige *et al.*, 1997; Nagai *et al.*, 1997).

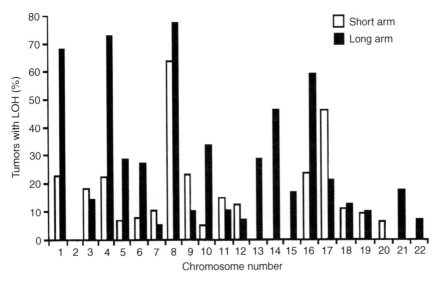

Fig. 13.4 Frequency of allelic imbalance in hepatocellular carcinoma.

Among our cases, chromosomes 1q(68.1%), 4q(72.7%), 8p(63.6%), 8q(77.3%) and 16q(59.1%) were found to have allelic imbalances at a high rate >50%, when using 68 microsatellite markers which covered all the non-acrocentric chromosomal arms (Piao *et al.*, 1997). The frequency of allelic imbalance on each chromosome arm is summarized in Fig. 13.4. LOH of the known TSGs are found in 86% of the Korean HCCs and frequent LOH is noted in *p53* (17p13.1) (50–66%), *Rb1* (13q14) (33%), *EXT1* (8q24) (33%) and *APC* (5q21) (20%) (Piao *et al.*, 1998).

Because *p53* mutation is not observed in tissues other than malignant tumors, and also because it has no correlation with tumor size, histology or the degree of differentiation, it must be a very important gene for the malignant transformation of cells. In our cases, the LOH of *p53* and/or the accumulation of LOHs are related to the poor differentiation of HCCs, suggesting that a progressively more aggressive malignant tumor is produced during the course of hepatocarcinogenesis as the result of continuous genetic alterations (Piao *et al.*, 1998). In the Korean HCCs, p53 mutation does not involve the

exon 7 codon 249 (TGC–TTC transition), which has been reported to be the hot point in the aflatoxin B1-associated HCCs.

REFERENCES

Ahn, Y.O., Park, B.J., Yoo, K.Y. *et al.* (1989) Incidence estimation of primary liver cancer among Koreans. *Journal of the Korean Cancer Association*, **21**, 241–7.

Boige, V., Laurent-Puig, P., Fouchet, P. *et al.* (1997) Concerted nonsyntenic allelic losses in hyperploid hepatocellular carcinoma as determined by a high-resolution allelotype. *Cancer Research*, **57**, 1986–90.

Chen, D.S. (1987) Hepatitis B virus infection, its sequela, and prevention in Taiwan, in *Neoplasms of the Liver*, 1st ed, (eds K. Okuda and K.G. Ishak), Springer, Tokyo, pp. 71–80.

Lee, K.J., Han, K.H., Chun, J.Y. *et al.* (1997) Natural history of chronic hepatitis type B throughout long-term follow-up. *Korean Journal of Gastroenterology*, **29**, 343–51.

Lee, H.S., Lee, J.H., Choi, M.S. *et al.* (1996) Comparison of the incidence of hepatocellular carcinoma in HBV- and HCV-associated liver cirrhosis: a prospective study. *Korean Journal of Hepatology*, **2**, 21–8.

Nagai, H., Pineau, P., Tiollais, P. *et al.* (1997) A comprehensive allelotyping of human hepatocellular carcinoma. *Oncogene*, **14**, 2927–33.

Park, C. and Park, Y.N. (1994) Immunohistochemial profile of sclerosing hepatic carcinoma. *Korean Journal of Pathology,* **28**, 636–42.

Park, Y.N., Han, E.K. and Park, C. (1991) Gross anatomical typing of hepatocellular carcinoma: classification of 49 lobectomized hepatocellular carcinoma. *Korean Journal of Pathology,* **25**, 83–92.

Piao, Z., Kim, H., Jeon, B.K. *et al.* (1997) Relationship between loss of heterozygosity of tumor suppressor genes and histologic differentiation in hepatocellular carcinoma. *Cancer,* **80**, 865–72.

Piao, Z., Park, C., Park, J.H. *et al.* (1998) Allelotype analysis of hepatocellular carcinoma. *International Journal of Cancer,* **75**, 29–33.

Soxena, R., Suriawinata, A., Schwatz, M. *et al.* (1997) An analysis of incidental multifocal and in-situ hepatocellular carcinoma in liver explant. *Hepatology,* **26**, 240A.

Taiwan: Progress in the past decade 1988–1997

J.-H. Kao and D.-S. Chen

13.16 INTRODUCTION

The annual incidence of HCC reaches as high as 10–25 cases per 100 000 population in Taiwan. Thus HCC is a major health problem in this country, and many basic and clinical research topics have been conducted in the past decade. In this chapter, the advances in our understanding of HCC with respect to etiological factors, genetic mechanisms responsible for hepatocarcinogenesis, diagnosis and therapy are reviewed.

13.17 ETIOLOGY

13.17.1 VIRUSES

In Taiwan, 80–90% of chronic liver diseases and HCC are caused by HBV (Chen, 1993) and HCV is the next most common etiologic agent (Chen et al 1990; Jeng and Tsai 1991; Lee *et al.*, 1992; Kao *et al.*, 1994). The prevalence of antibody to HCV (anti-HCV) in hepatitis B surface antigen (HBsAg)-negative patients is around 70–80%, and most of such patients are viremic. However, some HCV endemic townships have been recently identified in southern Taiwan, and most HCC cases from these townships are anti-HCV-positive instead of HBsAg (Lu *et al.*, 1997a).

The role of HBV and HCV in HCC in Taiwan differs in different age groups. HBsAg positivity is extremely high in the young people with HCC and the positivity rate declines gradually (Fig. 13.5). In the seventh decade the HBsAg-negative cases begin to

outnumber the HBsAg-positive HCCs. Because most HBsAg-negative HCCs are associated with chronic HCV infection, this age distribution indicates the relative importance of HBV in young patients and HCV in elder patients with HCC.

It has been reported that both anti-HCV as well as the carrier status of HBsAg and HBeAg were significantly associated with HCC, showing a multivariate-adjusted odds ratio of 24.8 for carriers of HBsAg alone, 33.5 for carriers of both HBsAg and HBeAg, and 23.7 for those who were positive for anti-HCV. In addition, the population-attributable risk percentage was estimated as 3% for anti-HCV alone, 69% for HBsAg carrier status alone, and 6% for both anti-HCV and HBsAg in Taiwan (Yu *et al.*, 1991).

The incidence of HCC has also been studied by prospective follow-up of patients with cirrhosis by regular hepatic ultrasound examinations and serum α-fetoprotein (AFP) surveillance in the following four groups: (1) 300 HBsAg-positive patients; (2) 151 anti-HCV positive patients; (3) 144 both positive patients; and (4) 62 both negative patients. Each year, 3–5% developed HCC, and the difference in incidence between the four groups was not statistically significant. The mean age when HCC was detected was 56 ± 10, 63 ± 9, 55 ± 11 and 60 ± 14 years in each group, respectively (Chen, 1995). These data indicate a high incidence of HCC in cirrhotic patients in Taiwan, whether the cirrhosis was related to HBV or HCV. Although most of our anti-HCV-positive patients with HCCs had

Hepatocellular Carcinoma: Diagnosis, investigation and management. Edited by Anthony S.-Y. Leong, Choong-Tsek Liew, Joseph W.Y. Lau and Philip J. Johnson. Published in 1999 by Arnold, London. ISBN 0 340 74096 5.

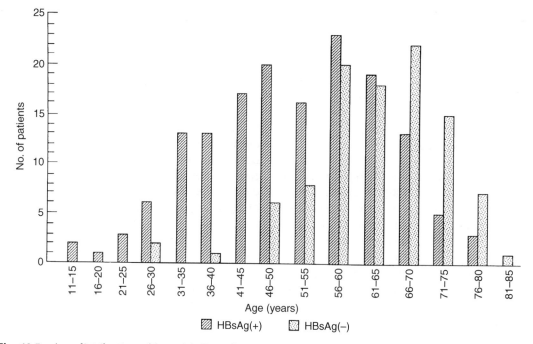

Fig. 13.5 Age distribution of hepatitis B surface antigen (HBsAg) positive and negative hepatocellular carcinoma in 254 cases. Data collected from National Taiwan University Hospital, 1987–92.

cirrhosis, HCC also occurred in some patients without cirrhosis. Further molecular studies showed that some of the non-cirrhotic HBsAg-negative and anti-HCV-positive HCC patients were actually positive for HBV DNA in the tumor tissue by PCR (Chen, 1995). However, the possible role of HBV in the etiology of HCC in such patients needs to be confirmed by a large-scale survey.

As to the interaction between HBV and HCV infection in hepatocellular carcinogenesis, some reports suggested both viruses have a synergistic effect to the pathogenesis of HCC but this is controversial (Chuang *et al.*, 1992; Sheu *et al.*, 1992a; Tsai *et al.*, 1994; Sun *et al.*, 1996). Hepatitis D virus (HDV) superinfection in HBV carriers can produce additional damage in an already injured liver; however, HDV superinfection may not accelerate the development of HCC (Huo *et al.*, 1996).

Although GB virus-C/hepatitis G virus (GBV-C/HGV) infection was found in 10% of

patients with HCC (Kao *et al.*, 1997), the effect of this newly identified flavivirus, alone or in combination with other hepatitis viruses, on the development of HCC seems unremarkable. However, a definite conclusion remains to be drawn.

13.17.2   CHEMICAL CARCINOGENS

Epidemiologic surveys have revealed a significant correlation between aflatoxin ingestion and incidence of HCC in Taiwan (Zhang *et al.*, 1991; Chen *et al.*, 1992; Hatch *et al.*, 1993; Chen *et al.*, 1996a; Wang *et al.*, 1996a; Yu *et al.*, 1996, 1997) but, aflatoxins are not generally regarded as an important causative agent in Taiwan today.

13.17.3   OTHER

Independent and interactive effects related to HCC risk have been assessed, and a significant association with HCC was observed for liver cirrhosis, low education level, low vegetable intake, low serum retinol level, elevated serum testosterone level, cigarette smoking, heavy alcohol consumption and a history of HCC among intimate family members (Chen *et al.*, 1991; Pan *et al.*, 1993; Yu and Chen, 1993; Yu *et al.*, 1994, 1995b; Hung *et al.*, 1996).

Several investigators have studied the genetic predisposition to the development of HCC in HBV carriers, and they found the HLA-B17 and L-myc genotype to be significantly associated with HCC risk (Yang *et al.*, 1989a; Hsieh *et al.*, 1996). In addition, polymorphisms of cytochrome P450 2E1 and null genotypes of glutathione *S*-transferase M1 and T1 polymorphisms may play a role in cigarette smoking-related and AFB-1-related hepatocarcinogenesis (Yu *et al.*, 1995a; Chen *et al.*, 1996b).

Because of the extreme complexities of host factors, these areas need to be investigated further. Further understanding of the etiologic factors will certainly help us to find effective measures to prevent hepatocarcinogenesis.

13.18 CARCINOGENESIS

13.18.1 VIRAL HEPATOCARCINOGENESIS

The mechanism of viral-related HCC is not yet clear. Integration of HBV sequences into the liver cell genome has been detected in most, but not all patients with HBsAg-positive chronic hepatitis or HCC (Chen *et al.*, 1982, 1988; Lai *et al.*, 1988, 1990). This evidence has identified HBV as a major etiological factor for HCC in Taiwan; however, this may not contribute directly to the hepatocarcinogenesis. In contrast, most of the woodchuck HCCs, like the human counterpart, contain integrated viral DNA with preferential integration site. Thus we need to re-evaluate HBV integration in human HCCs, using tissue specimens from a larger number of cases. Recently, an inverse polymerase chain reaction (PCR) that allows rapid cloning and sequence analysis of HBV

integration sites was developed. By this procedure, the junctional fragment can be rapidly amplified and the immediate cellular flanking sequences can then be analyzed (Tsuei *et al.*, 1994). Further studies are ongoing in our institute.

Unlike HBV, HCV is not a DNA virus and it does not integrate into the genome of liver cells. It is more likely that HCV occurs against a background of inflammation and regeneration, associated with liver injury due to chronic hepatitis. Most, if not all, cases of HCV-related HCC occur in the presence of cirrhosis, suggesting that it is the underlying liver disease *per se* that is the risk factor for HCC rather than HCV infection. We have reported that HCV genotype 1b infection and increasing viral loads are more likely to result in the progression of HCC (Kao *et al.*, 1995, 1996), larger studies are needed to confirm these preliminary findings.

13.18.2 MOLECULAR HEPATOCARCINOGENESIS

With the recent advent of molecular genetics, development of HCC also has been proposed to be a multistep evolution involving many important and stage-wise genetic changes. However, unlike the sequential genetic changes of colorectal cancers, most of those in hepatocarcinogenesis remain virtually unknown. Recent studies from Taiwan by using cytogenetic and subsequent molecular genetic characterization have shown interesting findings in many aspects. First, amplification and overexpression of known proto-oncogenes such as *cyclin D1* and *c-myc* in human HCC have been demonstrated (Peng *et al.*, 1993; Zhang *et al.*, 1993), and activation of *c-myc* occurs more frequently in young patients having elevated serum AFP levels or HBV infection (Peng *et al.*, 1993), and is perhaps related to the biologic behavior of HCC.

Second, because cytogenetic analysis of HCC cell lines and primary HCC tissues show chromosome 1p to be the region most commonly affected, genetic abnormalities of chromosome 1p in HCC by microsatellite polymorphism analysis were also explored (Chen *et al.*, 1993, 1996b). In half of the HCCs studied, chromosome 1p aberrations were found (Yeh *et al.*, 1994), and the abnormalities can be classified into three groups: typical loss of heterozygosity, 2–3-fold increase of allelic dosage, and novel microsatellite polymorphism. These abnormalities clustered at the distal part of chromosome 1p, with a common region mapped to 1p35–36, which is also the region with frequent loss of heterozygosity in neuroblastoma and colorectal and breast cancers. In addition, allelic loss on chromosomes 4q and 16q by using the same strategy was also studied (Yeh *et al.*, 1996). The frequency of allelic loss on chromosome 16q was 70%, and the common region was mapped to 16q22–23. An even higher frequency (77%) was found on chromosome 4q with the common region mapped to 4q12–23. Of interest, the allelic loss of chromosome 4q was associated with HCC of elevated serum AFP (Yeh *et al.*, 1996). Thus, further positional cloning to search for putative HCC-relevant tumor suppressor genes on chromosome 4q and 16q are mandatory, and the one on chromosome 4q may contribute to the AFP expression in HCC.

Third, it is known that tumor-suppressor gene *p53* can transactivate the transcription of genes that down-regulate cellular growth-related genes and become oncogenic as a result of the production of mutant proteins or the loss of its protein expression. In Taiwan, the association between *p53* gene mutation and hepatocarcinogenesis has been extensively studied (Sheu *et al.*, 1992b; Hsu *et al.*, 1993, 1994b; Diamantis *et al.*, 1994; Lunn *et al.*, 1997), showing mutant p53 protein, mutations in *p53*, and specific codon 249 mutations were detected in 37, 29 and 13%, respectively, of the HCC cases (Lunn *et al.*, 1997). The p53 protein was overexpressed more frequently in HCC with elevated serum AFP level, in large HCC, and in invasive HCC (Hsu *et al.*, 1993).

Meanwhile, the overexpression of p53 protein was closely correlated with p53 mRNA overexpression and *p53* mutation. Clinically, HCCs with p53 protein expression (group A) and those negative for both p53 protein and mRNA expression (group B) had an unfavorable outcome, while HCC with no p53 protein but with p53 mRNA overexpression (group C) had the best outcome; the 4-year survival rate was 26.1, 26.3 and 62.5% in the three groups, respectively (Hsu *et al.*, 1993). Thus, the p53 protein and mRNA expression patterns in HCC correlate with *p53* mutation and tumor behavior, and may serve as a molecular prognostic marker. Although a specific hot-spot mutation at codon 249 of *p53* has been frequently found in aflatoxin-related HCC, the specific mutation is much less related to hepatocarcinogenesis in Taiwan where contamination of food by aflatoxin is not heavy in recent decades (Sheu *et al.*, 1992b; Lunn *et al.*, 1997). The mutation of *p53* in the Taiwanese HCC is widely distributed throughout exons 5 to 8, and a new hot-spot for point mutations, T/A transversions with an amino acid change from serine to threonine was identified in codon 166 of *p53* (Diamantis *et al.*, 1994). On the other hand, alterations of the highly conserved consensus intervening sequences at the splice junctions may also lead to the inactivation of *p53* (Lai *et al.*, 1993; Hsu *et al.*, 1994a).

Recently, a gene that encodes the CD24 protein was cloned from the cDNA library of human HCC by using the differential display technique. In this study, CD24 mRNA was overexpressed in 66 and 68% of unicentric and multicentric HCC, respectively, and an increased frequency of CD24 mRNA overexpression in patients <50 years of age with HCC, in serum HBsAg-positives, in those with an elevated serum AFP level, and in HCC with AFP mRNA expression was observed. Besides, there was a strong correlation of CD24 mRNA overexpression with *p53* mutation in HCC and poorly differentiated HCC. However, the CD24 mRNA expression did not correlate with tumor size, tumor invasiveness or patient's prognosis. Thus, the *CD24* gene expression appears to be a common event in HCC and may serve as an early but not prognostic biomarker for HCC.

13.18.3 CLONALITY OF HCC

DNA clonal heterogeneity of HCC has been studied by integrated HBV DNA patterns and DNA fingerprinting, and multiple HCC and recurrent HCC usually have different clonalities (Chen *et al.*, 1989; Hsu *et al.*, 1991; Sheu *et al.*, 1993). These findings reinforce the importance of eliminating the underlying cause and the contributing factors of hepatocarcinogenesis.

13.18.4 OTHERS

Several studies have investigated the role of hormone and growth factor in the formation of HCC, and the presence of glucocorticoid receptors, insulin-like growth factor (IGF-II) and vascular endothelial growth factor (VEGF) in HCC suggest that these factors may be important in the growth of HCC (P'eng *et al.*, 1988; Wu *et al.*, 1988a; Lui *et al.*, 1993; Chow *et al.*, 1997). These data may help the design of future intervention for HCC.

13.19 DIAGNOSIS

13.19.1 TUMOR MARKERS

Among the markers for HCC, serum AFP is the most intensely studied and widely used. However, the sensitivity and specificity of AFP testing remains a problem. Although a serum AFP level of 400 ng/ml and above is generally thought to confer high specificity for HCC, the sensitivity of such high serum AFP levels for detecting HCC appears to be inadequate. Thus several attempts to improve the sensitivity and specificity of AFP testing have been carried out (Chen *et al.*, 1995; Wang *et al.*, 1996a). The diagnostic indices of lentil lectin

affinity of AFP in detecting HCC have been evaluated, and the proportion of AFP-L3 was significantly higher in patients with HCC. Using the proportion of AFP-L3 >35% as a parameter, the sensitivity, specificity, positive predictive value, negative predictive value and accuracy in detecting HCC was 57, 89, 83, 67 and 73%, respectively (Wang *et al.*, 1996b). Thus lentil lectin affinity of AFP may provide a moderately high sensitivity and a high specificity in the detection of HCC for persons with high AFP levels, and it may be a useful adjuvant of sonography and total serum AFP levels in a mass survey of HCC for a high-risk population.

Other proteins also have been reported to be potential markers for HCC (Ho *et al.*, 1989; Tsai *et al.*, 1990; Chan *et al.*, 1991). Elevated levels of des-γ-carboxy prothrombin (DCP), an abnormal form of prothrombin, have been reported to occur in the plasma of patients with HCC. Elevated DCP activities were documented in 48% of patients with HCC <3 cm, 67% with HCC 3–5 cm, and 68% with HCC >5 cm, as well as in 28% of those with chronic hepatitis or cirrhosis. Although the plasma DCP levels did not correlate with the tumor size or serum AFP levels, plasma DCP levels are complementary to serum AFP levels in the diagnosis of HCC because up to 77% of patients with HCC had an abnormal elevation in either marker (Tsai *et al.*, 1990).

Other potential tumor markers including complements, circulating immune complexes and urinary transforming growth factor-β 1 have also been reported (Chang and Chuang, 1988; Tsai *et al.*, 1995, 1997). However, further studies are needed to confirm these preliminary results.

13.19.2 IMAGING

A variety of methods including ultrasonography (US), computer-assisted tomography (CT), and CT with lipiodol have been used to image the liver. The clinical utility of these imaging modalities in the diagnosis of HCC depends on their ability to detect small lesions reliably. It appears that US in experienced hands is a practical and reasonable technique to detect HCC but CT may be more accurate in staging the extent of tumor involvement. CT-lipiodol is best reserved for patients in whom a high index of suspicion is present, but other imaging techniques are negative. Intraoperative US may be a useful adjunct to assist the surgeon in localizing all hepatic masses and in limiting the resection size in patients with underlying cirrhosis (Sheu *et al.*, 1985; Wu *et al.*, 1992).

Recently CO_2 gas-enhanced ultrasonography, color Doppler sonography and Duplex-pulsed Doppler ultrasonography were introduced to Taiwan, and several studies have shown their usefulness in detecting small liver tumors, in differentiating HCC from hemangioma, and in identifying arterioportal shunting as well as portal vein invasion by HCC (Wang *et al.*, 1991; Lin *et al.*, 1992, 1997; Chen *et al.*, 1994).

We evaluated ultrasound-guided cutting biopsy for the diagnosis of HCC in 420 patients from 1981 to 1990. We found the procedure to be important for the diagnosis of liver cancer but that it should be applied only when the image diagnosis and results of fine needle biopsy are equivocal, to minimize possible complications (Huang *et al.*, 1996).

13.19.3   MASS SCREENING FOR HCC

The utility of screening for HCC is determined by both the sensitivity and specificity of testing, and by the effectiveness of therapy once the disease is detected. In Taiwan, the cirrhotic patients, as they are at an unusually high risk of developing HCC, are advised to receive regular follow-up. By periodic examinations of serum AFP levels and abdominal US, small HCCs can be screened and the patients can thus be treated earlier (Wu *et al.*, 1988b; Chen *et al.*, 1995). However, it is still not satisfactory because most HCCs, no matter how large or small, are already well-estab-

lished cancers that actually represent a rather late stage in the genesis of the disease. Only when we understand the mechanism transforming dysplastic lesions or regeneration nodules into frank HCC can methods in detecting truly 'early HCC' be developed to divert or delay the outcome.

13.20   THERAPY

13.20.1   SURGERY

Surgery is generally considered the only curative therapy for HCC, although surgical resection often is not possible because of the extent of the tumor or the poor condition of the host. Furthermore, the majority of those who received curative resections still die of HCC. Several pertinent surgical questions have been addressed in recent years.

After curative hepatectomy for HCC, currently the perioperative mortality rate ranges from 3 to 4%, and the 5-year actuarial survival rate ranges from 42 to 50% (Chen *et al.*, 1989; Chou *et al.*, 1994; Lee *et al.*, 1996; Sheen *et al.*, 1996). The mortality rate, revealed after long-term follow-up, is mainly attributable to tumor recurrence, which in turn, is strongly correlated with the invasive and refractory nature of HCC (Hsu *et al.*, 1988a; Chen *et al.*, 1994). A postoperative intrahepatic recurrence rate of as high as 80% by 5 years in 205 patients with resectable HCC was reported, and 26% of those with recurrent HCC had recurrences near the resected stump, 54% had a single nodular recurrence in the remnant liver, and 20% had wide-spread multinodular recurrence (Chen *et al.*, 1994). The recurrent tumors usually had different clonalities (Chen *et al.*, 1989; Sheu *et al.*, 1993), indicating *de novo* occurrence of new HCCs.

The long-term prognostic factors in surgically resected HCC have been studied (Chou *et al.*, 1994; Hsu *et al.*, 1988a, 1989; Chen *et al.*, 1994; Wu *et al.*, 1996; Chiu *et al.*, 1992, 1993; Jwo *et al.*, 1992). It has been shown that in both small and large HCCs invasive tumors were accompanied by high patient mortality rate from tumor recurrence, and thus invasiveness and intraportal venous spread of an HCC seems to be most crucial in determining the long-term outcome for the patient (Hsu *et al.*, 1988b). Other favorable conditions associated with long-term outcome in resected HCC include absence of cirrhosis, good liver function reserve, surgery in the early stage, tumor size <5 cm, adequate resected margin, low preoperative serum AFP level, marked local immune response as indicated by marked lymphocytes infiltration, DNA ploidy and S-phase fraction of HCC, low proliferative capacity of cells in the liver remnant, and low hepatic perfusion index (HPI) (Chou *et al.*, 1994; Chen *et al.*, 1994; Wu *et al.*, 1996; Hsu *et al.*, 1988b, 1989; Chiu *et al.*, 1992, 1993; Jwo *et al.*, 1992).

Management of recurrent HCC in a cirrhotic liver remnant remains a challenging problem. The long-term benefits between aggressive re-resection or transarterial chemoembolization (TACE) for recurrent HCC have been reported, and the results showed that the survival rates at 6 months and at 1, 2 and 3 years after diagnosis of recurrence were 92, 72, 64 and 45% in group 1 (repeated resection) and 83, 75, 67 and 48% in group 2 (TACE). The survival of patients with unresectable recurrent HCC was much worse: 6-month and 1-, 2- and 3-year survival after recurrence was 46.5, 29.2, 12.5 and 7.8%, respectively (Lee *et al.*, 1995). Thus aggressive treatment with repeated hepatic resection or TACE can prolong survival time after recurrence of HCC in selected patients. The prognostic factors after resection for recurrent HCC include gender, age, multiplicity (tumor number >3), and tumor invasiveness (Hu *et al.*, 1996).

Although TACE improves the treatment of HCC by causing tumor necrosis and shrinkage, preoperative TACE for resectable large HCC should be avoided because it does not provide complete necrosis in large tumors and results in delayed surgery and difficulty in the treatment of recurrent lesions (Wu *et al.*, 1995).

The prognosis of surgical treatment for HCC with unusual clinical manifestation or location including icteric type HCC, ruptured HCC, centrally located large HCC, and HCC in the caudate lobe is generally poor and needs to be improved (Chen *et al.*, 1988, 1994, 1995, 1996; Mok *et al.*, 1996; Wu *et al.*, 1993; Yang *et al.*, 1996; Lu *et al.*, 1997b).

13.20.2 CHEMOEMBOLIZATION

Chemoembolization for HCC is carried out by giving intra-arterial substances then occluding the vessel in the hope of obtaining high tumor drug levels in a hypoxic environment. In Taiwan, earlier randomized controlled trial suggested that transcatheter arterial embolization (TAE) is an effective palliative treatment that prolongs survival of patients with unresectable HCC (Lin *et al.*, 1988). Later, a retrospective series of 329 patients with HCC treated by TACE was analyzed, and found the overall cumulative 1-, 2- and 3-year survivals of 50, 25 and 15%, respectively. The median duration of survival was 12.7 months (Yang and Ho, 1992). Other smaller series also showed similar results (Yang *et al.*, 1989a; Hsieh *et al.*, 1990, 1992). The prognostic factors predicting a better outcome in terms of the median survival period and the survival value include a single tumor <5 cm, an intact capsule, a patent portal vein, and a good clinical status (Yang *et al.*, 1989b, 1992; Hsieh *et al.*, 1990, 1992a; Yen *et al.*, 1995).

It is recommended that all patients undergoing TAE or TACE should receive periodic evaluation of US, CT and perhaps angiography to determine whether repeated embolization is necessary. In addition, it has been reported that serum AFP data with good linear decline in the first month after TAE indicated good therapeutic results, and the mean half-life of AFP in the non-recurrent group was 5.0 days (range 2.9–7.2) (Hsieh *et al.*, 1992b). Other methods including Duplex-pulsed Doppler sonography and HPI have also been used to monitor the treatment effects of TACE and the timing selection of repeated TACE (Lin *et al.*, 1992, 1995).

13.20.3   ABLATION INJECTION

Percutaneously administered intratumoral injections of ethanol to cause tumor necrosis is promising, and may even be curative in the treatment of small HCC. In the mid-1980s, intratumoral injection of absolute ethanol under ultrasound guidance to treat small HCC (1–3 cm) was first introduced to Taiwan (Sheu *et al.*, 1987), and complete tumor necrosis or small peripheral residual cancer nest were observed in the treated patients who finally received surgical resection. To achieve more satisfactory results, steel coil implantation in the tumor before treatment and a needle with multiple side holes were applied (Sheu *et al.*, 1987). For larger HCC, percutaneous intravascular ethanol injection of the supplying vessel of the tumor using color Doppler imaging was also applied, and a remarkable decrease in the tumor size or massive tumor necrosis was shown after treatment (Lin *et al.*, 1996). Other intratumor injected agents such as OK-432, a biological response modifier, have also been used to treat small HCC and total necrosis of HCC could be achieved after the treatment (Huang *et al.*, 1990).

13.20.4   CHEMOTHERAPY

Several chemotherapeutic agents including adriamycin and interferon have been studied for palliative therapy of HCC, but most of them are disappointing. In a small pilot study, systemic IL-2, even in the combination with chemotherapy, has been shown not effective for the treatment of advanced HCC (Chien *et al.*, 1991).

In general, HCC is a chemoresistant tumor that frequently expresses a high level of p 170 glycoprotein of the multidrug-resistance (MDR) gene, and VP-16 has shown modest activity against HCC. Accordingly, the ther-apeutic efficacy of chronic oral VP-16 plus tamoxifen, a potential MDR-reversing agent, has been tested in patients with far-advanced HCC. The results showed that median survivals of the responders and non-responders were 8.0 and 3.0 months, respectively ($p<0.05$), and the median Karnofsky performance status of the responders improved (Cheng *et al.*, 1996). Thus chronic oral VP-16 and tamoxifen may be used as a palliative treatment for far-advanced HCC.

13.20.5   RADIATION

Radiotherapy, delivered by external beam via the administration of radioactive substances, is an option for primary therapy for unresectable HCC. The effects of external radiation therapy (3000–5000 cGY) on primary HCC and portal vein invasion have been evaluated. Although clinical improvement was observed after initiation of the therapy, regrowth of the tumor or recurrence of symptoms occurred in most of the patients (Chen *et al.*, 1992, 1994). Therefore the role of external radiation in the therapy of HCC remains palliative only.

I-131-lipiodol treatment for HCC with minimal toxicity has been recently reported with encouraging results. A pilot study injecting I-131-lipiodol for the treatment of HCC has been conducted in Taiwan (Lo *et al.*, 1992). Although 70% of the treated patients had a reduction of AFP and decrease of tumor sizes with an overall median survival of 9 months (range 2–17 months), this preliminary result needs to be confirmed further.

13.20.6   LASER

Laserthermia by a novel interstitial probe adapted to low power Nd-YAG laser machine has been used to treat small HCC in early 1990s (Huang *et al.*, 1991). The set condition was 43–45°C in thermocouple with a power of 2–3 W and a duration of 20–30 min. The preliminary results seemed promising and histological examination showed cell degeneration and necrosis. Thus low-power laserthermia may be potentially useful in the treatment of small HCC. However, the machines used were complicated and were not easy to maintain.

13.20.7 HORMONE THERAPY

Although previous basic studies have shown that the levels of glucocorticoid receptor correlate well with the elevated serum AFP levels in patients with HCC, and progesterone, a female hormone, is found to inhibit the expression of AFP in hepatoma cells (Lui *et al.*, 1991), the clinical usefulness of steroid hormones and/or their antagonists such as megestrol acetate and flutamide in the treatment of HCC is far from satisfactory (Chao *et al.*, 1996, 1997).

13.21 CHILDHOOD HCC

As has been mentioned before, HBV plays a key role in HCC of the young people (Fig. 13.5). Virtually all Taiwanese children who have HCC are HBsAg-positive, and most of their mothers are HBV carriers (Wu *et al.*, 1987; Chang *et al.*, 1989, 1991). This indicates

the critical role of maternal–infant HBV transmission in these children with HCC, as was also shown in adults with HCC (Chen *et al.*, 1988). Childhood HCC has a peak at 5–9 years of age and it can be separated from hepatoblastoma that always occurs before 5 years of age (Chen *et al.*, 1988). Most of them are cirrhotic (Hsu *et al.*, 1987), and there is also a male predominance. Most have advanced HCC at the time of diagnosis, with a 1-year survival rate in 10% only (Ni *et al.*, 1991). Taken together, the advanced HCC in these young children suggests that HBV-induced HCC can develop early and rapidly in man.

13.22 PREVENTION

The most practical and cost-effective way to prevent HBV-related HCC is likely the vaccination against HBV. In Taiwan, we have already confirmed that a universal vaccination program is feasible and effective in reducing HBsAg carriers (Chen *et al.*, 1987), the carrier rate in children decreasing dramatically from 10 to 1.3% 10 years after immunization (Chen *et al.*, 1996a). Most importantly, a trend of the declining incidence of childhood HCC was observed in the

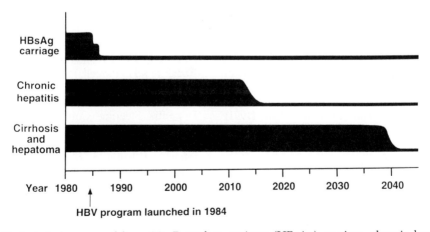

Fig. 13.6 Projected decrease of hepatitis B surface antigen (HBsAg) carriers, chronic hepatitis, and cirrhosis and hepatocellular carcinoma after national hepatitis B mass vaccination program in Taiwan. (Reproduced from Chen *et al.* (1997) with permission.)

later part of this period. The average annual incidence of HCC in children of 6–14 years of age declined from 0.70 per 100 000 children in 1981–86 to 0.57 in 1986–90, and further to 0.36 in 1990–94 ($p<0.01$) (Chang *et al.*, 1997). These data suggest the effect of the HBV mass vaccination program in controlling HBV-related HCC has begun to be seen in Taiwanese children, and it is very likely that it will be seen in young adults soon. We anticipate seeing a 80–85% decrease of HCC in all adults 3–4 decades later (Chen *et al.*, 1997) (Fig.13.6).

The decrease of HCC in children after the implementation of universal vaccination against HBV not only represents a practical prevention of a human cancer by vaccination first time in the history, but also it strengthens the etiologic role of HBV in causing HCC in man.

REFERENCES

Chan, C.Y., Lee, S.D., Wu, J.C. *et al.* (1991) The diagnostic value of the assay of des-gamma-carboxy prothrombin in the detection of small hepatocellular carcinoma. *Journal of Hepatology,* **13**, 21–4.

Chang, M.H., Chen, C.J., Lai, M.S. *et al.* (1997) Taiwan Childhood Hepatoma Study Group. Universal hepatitis B vaccination in Taiwan and the incidence of hepatocellular carcinoma in children. *New England Journal of Medicine,* **336**, 1855–9.

Chang, M.H., Chen, D.S., Hsu, H.C. *et al.* (1989) Maternal transmission of hepatitis B virus in childhood hepatocellular carcinoma. *Cancer,* **64**, 2377–80.

Chang, M.H., Chen, P.J., Chen, J.Y. *et al.* (1991) Hepatitis B virus integration in hepatitis B virus-related hepatocellular carcinoma in childhood. *Hepatology,* **13**, 316–20.

Chang, W.Y. and Chuang, W.L. (1988) Complements as new diagnostic tools of hepatocellular carcinoma in cirrhotic patients. *Cancer,* **62**, 227–32.

Chao, Y., Chan, W.K., Huang, Y.S. *et al.* (1996) Phase II study of flutamide in the treatment of hepatocellular carcinoma. *Cancer,* **77**, 635–9.

Chao, Y., Chan, W.K., Wang, S.S. *et al.* (1997) Phase II study of megestrol acetate in the treatment of hepatocellular carcinoma. *Journal of Gastroenterology and Hepatology,* **12**, 277–81.

Chen, C.J., Liang, K.Y., Chang, A.S. *et al.* (1991) Effects of hepatitis B virus, alcohol drinking, cigarette smoking and familial tendency on hepatocellular carcinoma. *Hepatology,* **13**, 398–406.

Chen, C.J., Lu, S.N., You, S.L. *et al.* (1995) Community-based hepatocellular carcinoma screening in seven townships in Taiwan (in Chinese). *Journal of the Formosan Medical Association,* **94** (Suppl. 2), S94–102.

Chen, C.J., Wang, L.Y., Lu, S.N. *et al.* (1996a) Elevated aflatoxin exposure and increased risk of hepatocellular carcinoma. *Hepatology,* **24**, 38–42.

Chen, C.J., Yu, M.W., Liaw, Y.F. *et al.* (1996b) Chronic hepatitis B carriers with null genotypes of glutathione S-transferase M1 and T1 polymorphisms who are exposed to aflatoxin are at increased risk of hepatocellular carcinoma. *American Journal of Human Genetics,* **59**, 128–34.

Chen, C.J., Zhang, Y.J., Lu, S.N. and Santella, R.M. (1992) Aflatoxin B1 DNA adducts in smeared tumor tissue from patients with hepatocellular carcinoma. *Hepatology,* **16**, 1150–5.

Chen, D.S. (1993) From hepatitis to hepatoma: lessons from type B viral hepatitis. *Science,* **262**, 369–70.

Chen, D.S. (1995) Hepatitis C virus in chronic liver disease and hepatocellular carcinoma in Taiwan. *Princess Takamatsu Symposium,* **25**, 27–32.

Chen, D.S., Hoyer, B.H., Nelson, J. *et al.* (1982) Detection and properties of hepatitis B viral DNA in liver tissue from patients with hepatocellular carcinoma. *Hepatology,* **2**, 42S–46S.

Chen, D.S., Hsu, H.M., Chang, M.H. *et al.* (1997) Hepatitis B vaccines: status report on long-term efficacy, in *Viral Hepatitis and Liver Disease* (eds M. Rizzetto, R.H., Purcell, J.L., Gerin and G. Verme), Minerva Medica, Turin, pp. 635–7.

Chen, D.S., Hsu, N.H.M., Sung, J.L. *et al.* (1987) The Hepatitis Steering Committee, The Hepatitis Control Committee. A mass vaccination program in Taiwan against hepatitis B virus infection in infants of hepatitis B surface antigen-carrier mothers. *Journal of the American Medical Association,* **257**, 2597–603.

Chen, D.S., Kuo, G., Sung, J.L. *et al.* (1990) Hepatitis C virus infection in an area hyperendemic for hepatitis B and chronic liver disease: the Taiwan experience. *Journal of Infectious Diseases,* **162**, 817–22.

Chen, H.L., Chang, M.H., Ni, Y.H. *et al.* (1996a) Seroepidemiology of hepatitis B virus infection in children: ten years of mass vaccination in Taiwan. *Journal of American Medical Association*, **276**, 906–8.

Chen, H.L., Chen, Y.C. and Chen, D.S. (1996b) Chromosome 1p aberrations are frequent in human primary hepatocellular carcinoma. *Cancer Genetics and Cytogenetics*, **86**, 102–6.

Chen, H.L., Chiu, T.S., Chen, P.J. and Chen, D.S. (1993) Cytogenetic studies on human liver cancer cell lines. *Cancer Genetics and Cytogenetics*, **65**, 161–6.

Chen, J.Y., Hsu, H.C., Lee, C.S. *et al.* (1988) Detection of hepatitis B virus DNA in hepatocellular carcinoma: methylation of integrated viral DNA. *Journal of Virological Methods*, **19**, 257–63.

Chen, M.F., Hwang, T.L., Jeng, L.B. *et al.* (1988) Surgical treatment for spontaneous rupture of hepatocellular carcinoma. *Surgery Gynecology and Obstetrics*, **167**, 99–102.

Chen, M.F., Hwang, T.L., Jeng, L.B. *et al.* (1989) Hepatic resection in 120 patients with hepatocellular carcinoma. *Archives of Surgery*, **124**, 1025–8.

Chen, M.F., Hwang, T.L., Jeng, L.B. *et al.* (1994) Postoperative recurrence of hepatocellular carcinoma. Two hundred and five consecutive patients who underwent hepatic resection in 15 years. *Archives of Surgery*, **129**, 738–42.

Chen, M.F., Hwang, T.L., Jeng, L.B. *et al.* (1995) Clinical experience with hepatic resection for ruptured hepatocellular carcinoma. *Hepatogastroenterology*, **42**, 166–8.

Chen, M.F., Jan, Y.Y., Jeng, L.B. *et al.* (1994) Obstructive jaundice secondary to ruptured hepatocellular carcinoma into the common bile duct. Surgical experiences of 20 cases. *Cancer*, **73**, 1335–40.

Chen, P.J., Chen, D.S., Lai, M.Y. *et al.* (1989) Clonal origin of recurrent hepatocellular carcinomas. *Gastroenterology*, **96**, 527–9.

Chen, R.C., Wang, C.S., Chen, P.H. *et al.* (1994) Carbon dioxide-enhanced ultrasonography of liver tumors. *Journal of Ultrasound Medicine*, **13**, 81–6.

Chen, R.J., Chen, C.K., Chang, D.Y. *et al.* (1995) Immunoelectrophoretic differentiation of alpha-fetoprotein in disorders with elevated serum alpha-fetoprotein levels or during pregnancy. *Acta Oncologica*, **34**, 931–5.

Chen, S.C., Lian, S.L. and Chang, W.Y. (1994) The effect of external radiotherapy in treatment of portal vein invasion in hepatocellular carcinoma. *Cancer Chemotherapy and Pharmacology*, **33** (Suppl.), S124–7.

Chen, S.C., Lian, S.L., Chuang, W.L. *et al.* (1992) Radiotherapy in the treatment of hepatocellular carcinoma and its metastases. *Cancer Chemotherapy and Pharmacology*, **31** (Suppl.), S103–5.

Chen, T.Z., Wu, J.C., Chan, C.Y. *et al.* (1996) Ruptured hepatocellular carcinoma: treatment strategy and prognostic factor analysis. *Chung Hua I Hsueh Tsa Chih (Taipei)*, **57**, 322–8.

Chen, W.J., Lee, J.C. and Hung, W.T. (1988) Primary malignant tumor of liver in infants and children in Taiwan. *Journal of Pediatric Surgery*, **23**, 457–61.

Cheng, A.L., Chen, Y.C., Yeh, K.H. *et al.* (1996) Chronic oral etoposide and tamoxifen in the treatment of far-advanced hepatocellular carcinoma. *Cancer*, **77**, 872–7.

Chien, C.H., Hsieh, K.H. and Yang, P.M. (1991) Immunochemotherapy with recombinant interleukin-2 and adriamycin in primary hepatocellular carcinoma. *Asian Pacific Journal of Allergy and Immunology*, **9**, 75–81.

Chiu, J.H., Kao, H.L., Wu, L.H. *et al.* (1992) Prediction of relapse or survival after resection in human hepatomas by DNA flow cytometry. *Journal of Clinical Investigation*, **89**, 539–45.

Chiu, J.H., Wu, L.H., Kao, H.L. *et al.* (1993) Can determination of the proliferative capacity of the nontumor portion predict the risk of tumor recurrence in the liver remnant after resection of human hepatocellular carcinoma? *Hepatology*, **18**, 96–102.

Chou, F.F., Sheen-Chen, S.M., Chen, C.L. *et al.* (1994) Prognostic factors after hepatectomy for hepatocellular carcinoma. *Hepatogastroenterology*, **41**, 419–23.

Chow, N.H., Hsu, P.I., Lin, X.Z. *et al.* (1997) Expression of vascular endothelial growth factor in normal liver and hepatocellular carcinoma: an immunohistochemical study. *Human Pathology*, **28**, 698–703.

Chuang, W.L., Chang, W.Y., Lu, S.N. *et al.* (1992) The role of hepatitis B and C viruses in hepatocellular carcinoma in a hepatitis B endemic area. A case-control study. *Cancer*, **69**, 2052–4.

Diamantis, I.D., McGandy, C., Chen, T.J. *et al.* (1994) A new mutational hot-spot in the p53 gene in human hepatocellular carcinoma. *Journal of Hepatology*, **20**, 553–6.

Hatch, M.C., Chen, C.J., Levin, B. *et al.* (1993) Urinary aflatoxin levels, hepatitis-B virus infection and hepatocellular carcinoma in Taiwan. *International Journal of Cancer*, **54**, 931–4.

Ho, C.H., Lee, S.D., Chang, H.T. *et al.* (1989) Application of des-gamma-carboxy prothrombin as a complementary tumor marker with alpha-fetoprotein in the diagnosis of hepatocellular carcinoma. *Scandinavian Journal of Gastroenterology*, **24**, 47–52.

Hsieh, L.L., Huang, R.C., Yu, M.W. *et al.* (1996) M1 genetic polymorphism and hepatocellular carcinoma risk among chronic hepatitis B carriers. *Cancer Letters*, **103**, 171–6.

Hsieh, M.Y., Chang, W.Y., Wang, L.Y. *et al.* (1992a) Treatment of hepatocellular carcinoma by transcatheter arterial chemoembolization and analysis of prognostic factors. *Cancer Chemotherapy and Pharmacology*, **31** (Suppl.), S82–5.

Hsieh, M.Y., Lu, S.N., Wang, L.Y. *et al.* (1992b) Alpha-fetoprotein in patients with hepatocellular carcinoma after transcatheter arterial embolization. *Journal of Gastroenterology and Hepatology*, **7**, 614–17.

Hsieh, M.Y., Wu, D.K., Lu, S.N. *et al.* (1990) The outcome of hepatocellular carcinoma treated with transcatheter arterial chemoembolization. *Kao Hsiung I Hsueh Ko Hsueh Tsa Chih*, **6**, 628–35.

Hsu, H.C., Chiou, T.J., Chen, J.Y. *et al.* (1991) Clonality and clonal evolution of hepatocellular carcinoma with multiple nodules. *Hepatology*, **13**, 923–8.

Hsu, H.C., Huang, A.M., Lai, P.L. *et al.* (1994a) Genetic alterations at the splice junction of p53 gene in human hepatocellular carcinoma. *Hepatology*, **19**, 122–8.

Hsu, H.C., Peng, S.Y., Lai, P.L. *et al.* (1994b) Allelotype and loss of heterozygosity of p53 in primary and recurrent hepatocellular carcinomas. A study of 150 patients. *Cancer*, **73**, 42–7.

Hsu, H.C., Tseng, H.J., Lai, P.L. *et al.* (1993) Expression of p53 gene in 184 unifocal hepatocellular carcinomas: association with tumor growth and invasiveness. *Cancer Research*, **53**, 4691–4.

Hsu, H.C., Wu, M.Z., Chang, M.H. *et al.* (1987) Childhood hepatocellular carcinoma develops exclusively in hepatitis B surface antigen carriers in three decades in Taiwan. Report of 51 cases strongly associated with rapid development of liver cirrhosis. *Journal of Hepatology*, **5**, 260–7.

Hsu, H.C., Wu, T.T., Sheu, J.C. *et al.* (1989) Biologic significance of the detection of HBsAg and HBcAg in liver and tumor from 204 HBsAg-positive patients with primary hepatocellular carcinoma. *Hepatology*, **9**, 747–50.

Hsu, H.C., Wu, T.T., Wu, M.Z. *et al.* (1988a) Evolution of expression of hepatitis B surface and core antigens (HBsAg, HBcAg) in resected primary and recurrent hepatocellular carcinoma in HBsAg carriers in Taiwan. Correlation with local host immune response. *Cancer*, **62**, 915–21.

Hsu, H.C., Wu, T.T., Wu, M.Z. *et al.* (1988b) Tumor invasiveness and prognosis in resected hepatocellular carcinoma. Clinical and pathogenetic implications. *Cancer*, **61**, 2095–9.

Hu, R.H., Lee, P.H., Yu, S.C. *et al.* (1996) Surgical resection for recurrent hepatocellular carcinoma: prognosis and analysis of risk factors. *Surgery*, **120**, 23–9.

Huang, G.T., Sheu, J.C., Yang, P.M. *et al.* (1996) Ultrasound-guided cutting biopsy for the diagnosis of hepatocellular carcinoma – a study based on 420 patients. *Journal of Hepatology*, **25**, 334–8.

Huang, G.T., Wang, T.H., Sheu, J.C. *et al.* (1991) Low-power laserthermia for the treatment of small hepatocellular carcinoma. *European Journal of Cancer*, **27**, 1622–7.

Huang, G.T., Yang, P.M., Sheu, J.C. *et al.* (1990) Intratumor injection of OK-432 for the treatment of small hepatocellular carcinoma. *Hepatogastroenterology*, **37**, 452–6.

Hung, Y.T., Lin, D.Y. and Chiu, C.T. (1996) Risk factors of hepatocellular carcinoma with familial tendency. *Chang Keng I Hsueh*, **18**, 8–13.

Huo, T.I., Wu, J.C., Lai, C.R. *et al.* (1996) Comparison of clinico-pathological features in hepatitis B virus-associated hepatocellular carcinoma with or without hepatitis D virus superinfection. *Journal of Hepatology*, **25**, 439–44.

Jeng, J.E. and Tsai, J.F. (1991) Hepatitis C virus antibody in hepatocellular carcinoma in Taiwan. *Journal of Medical Virology*, **34**, 74–7.

Jwo, S.C., Chiu, J.H., Chau, G.Y. *et al.* (1992) Risk factors linked to tumor recurrence of human hepatocellular carcinoma after hepatic resection. *Hepatology*, **16**, 1367–71.

Kao, J.H., Chen, P.J., Lai, M.Y. *et al.* (1995) Genotypes of hepatitis C virus in Taiwan and the progression of liver disease. *Journal of Clinical Gastroenterology*, **21**, 233–7.

Kao, J.H., Chen, P.J., Lai, M.Y. *et al.* (1997) GB virus-C/hepatitis G virus infection in an area endemic for viral hepatitis, chronic liver disease, and liver cancer. *Gastroenterology,* **112**, 1265–70.

Kao, J.H., Lai, M.Y., Chen, P.J. *et al.* (1996) Serum hepatitis C virus titers in the progression of type C chronic liver disease. With special emphasis on patients with type 1b infection. *Journal of Clinical Gastroenterology,* **23**, 280–3.

Kao, J.H., Tsai, S.L., Chen, P.J. *et al.* (1994) A clinicopathologic study of chronic non-A, non-B (type C) hepatitis in Taiwan: comparison between post-transfusion and sporadic patients. *Journal of Hepatology,* **21**, 244–9.

Lai, M.Y., Chang, H.C., Li, H.P. *et al.* (1993) Splicing mutations of the p53 gene in human hepatocellular carcinoma. *Cancer Research,* **53**, 1653–6.

Lai, M.Y., Chen, D.S., Chen, P.J. *et al.* (1988) Status of hepatitis B virus DNA in hepatocellular carcinoma: a study based on paired tumor and nontumor liver tissues. *Journal of Medical Virology,* **25**, 249–58.

Lai, M.Y., Chen, P.J., Yang, P.M. *et al.* (1990) Identification and characterization of intrahepatic hepatitis B virus DNA in HBsAg-seronegative patients with chronic liver disease and hepatocellular carcinomain Taiwan. *Hepatology,* **12**, 575–81.

Lee, C.S., Sheu, J.C., Wang, M. and Hsu, H.C. (1996) Long-term outcome after surgery for asymptomatic small hepatocellular carcinoma. *British Journal of Surgery,* **83**, 330–3.

Lee, P.H., Lin, W.J., Tsang, Y.M. *et al.* (1995) Clinical management of recurrent hepatocellular carcinoma. *Annals of Surgery,* **222**, 670–6.

Lee, S.D., Lee, F.Y., Wu, J.C. *et al.* (1992) The prevalence of anti-hepatitis C virus among Chinese patients with hepatocellular carcinoma. *Cancer,* **69**, 342–5.

Lin, D.Y., Liaw, Y.F., Lee, T.Y. and Lai, C.M. (1988) Hepatic arterial embolization in patients with unresectable hepatocellular carcinoma – a randomized controlled trial. *Gastroenterology,* **94**, 453–6.

Lin, W.Y., Wang, S.J. and Yeh, S.H. (1995) Hepatic perfusion index in evaluating treatment effect of transcatheter hepatic artery embolization in patients with hepatocellular carcinoma. *Neoplasia,* **42**, 89–92.

Lin, Z.Y., Chang, W.Y., Wang, L.Y. *et al.* (1992) Clinical utility of pulsed Doppler in the detection of arterioportal shunting in patients with hep-atocellular carcinoma. *Journal of Ultrasound Medicine,* **11**, 269–73.

Lin, Z.Y., Wang, J.H., Wang, L.Y. *et al.* (1996) Percutaneous intravascular ethanol injection of the supplying tumor vessel in the treatment of hepatocellular carcinoma larger than 3 cm. *Journal of Ultrasound Medicine,* **15**, 155–60.

Lin, Z.Y., Wang, L.Y., Wang, J.H. *et al.* (1997) Clinical utility of color Doppler sonography in the differentiation of hepatocellular carcinoma from metastases and hemangioma. *Journal of Ultrasound Medicine,* **16**, 51–8.

Lo, J.G., Wang, A.Y., Wei, Y.Y. *et al.* (1992) Preparation of (131I) lipiodol as a hepatoma therapeutic agent. *International Journal of Radium and Applied Instrumentation (A),* **43**, 1431–5.

Lu, C.L., Wu, J.C., Chiang, J.H. *et al.* (1997a) Hepatocellular carcinoma in the caudate lobe: early diagnosis and active treatment may result in long-term survival. *Journal of Gastroenterology and Hepatology,* **12**, 144–8.

Lu, S.N., Chue, P.Y., Chen, H.C. *et al.* (1997b) Different viral aetiology of hepatocellular carcinoma between two hepatitis B and C endemic townships in Taiwan. *Journal of Gastroenterology and Hepatology,* **12**, 547–50.

Lui, W.Y., P'eng, F.K., Liu, T.Y. and Chi, C.W. (1991) Hormonal therapy for hepatocellular carcinoma. *Medical Hypotheses,* **36**, 162–5.

Lui, W.Y., P'eng, F.K., Chang, Y.F. *et al.* (1993) Analysis of glucocorticoid receptors in human hepatocellular carcinoma and HepG2 cells. *Hepatology,* **18**, 1167–74.

Lunn, R.M., Zhang, Y.J., Wang, L.Y. *et al.* (1997) p53 mutations, chronic hepatitis B virus infection, and aflatoxin exposure in hepatocellular carcinoma in Taiwan. *Cancer Research,* **57**, 3471–7.

Mok, K.T., Chang, H.T., Liu, S.I. *et al.* (1996) Surgical treatment of hepatocellular carcinoma with biliary tumor thrombi. *International Surgery,* **81**, 284–8.

Ni, Y.H., Chang, M.H., Hsu, H.Y. *et al.* (1991) Hepatocellular carcinoma in childhood. Clinical manifestations and prognosis. *Cancer,* **68**, 1737–41.

Pan, W.H., Wang, C.Y., Huang, S.M. *et al.* (1993) Vitamin A, Vitamin E or beta-carotene status and hepatitis B-related hepatocellular carcinoma. *Annals of Epidemiology,* **3**, 217–24.

P'eng, F.K., Lui, W.Y., Chang, T.J. *et al.* (1988) Glucocorticoid receptors in hepatocellular carcinoma and adjacent liver tissue. *Cancer,* **62**, 2134–8.

Peng, S.Y., Lai, P.L. and Hsu, H.C. (1993) Amplification of the c-myc gene in human hepatocellular carcinoma: biologic significance. *Journal of the Formosan Medical Association*, **92**, 866–70.

Sheen, P.C., Lee, K.T., Chen, H.Y. *et al.* (1996) Conservative hepatic resection for hepatocellular carcinoma of cirrhotic patients. *International Surgery*, **81**, 280–3.

Sheu, J.C., Huang, G.T., Chou, H.C. *et al.* (1993) Multiple hepatocellular carcinomas at the early stage have different clonality. *Gastroenterology*, **105**, 1471–6.

Sheu, J.C., Huang, G.T., Lee, P.H. *et al.* (1992a) Mutation of p53 gene in hepatocellular carcinoma in Taiwan. *Cancer Research*, **52**, 6098–100.

Sheu, J.C., Huang, G.T., Shih, L.N. *et al.* (1992b) Hepatitis C and B viruses in hepatitis B surface antigen-negative hepatocellular carcinoma. *Gastroenterology*, **103**, 1322–7.

Sheu, J.C., Lee, C.S., Sung, J.L. *et al.* (1985) Intra-operative hepatic ultrasonography – an indispensable procedure in resection of small hepatocellular carcinomas. *Surgery*, **97**, 97–103.

Sheu, J.C., Sung, J.L., Huang, G.T. *et al.* (1987) Intratumor injection of absolute ethanol under ultrasound guidance for the treatment of small hepatocellular carcinoma. *Hepatogastroenterology*, **34**, 255–61.

Sun, C.A., Farzadegan, H., You, S.L. *et al.* (1996) Mutual confounding and interactive effects between hepatitis C and hepatitis B viral infections in hepatocellular carcinogenesis: a population-based case-control study in Taiwan. *Cancer Epidemiology, Biomarkers and Prevention*, **5**, 173–8.

Tsai, J.F., Chang, W.Y., Jeng, J.E. *et al.* (1994) Effects of hepatitis C and B viruses infection on the development of hepatocellular carcinoma. *Journal of Medical Virology*, **44**, 92–5.

Tsai, J.F., Chuang, L.Y., Jeng, J.E. *et al.* (1997) Clinical relevance of transforming growth factor-beta 1 in the urine of patients with hepatocellular carcinoma. *Medicine (Baltimore)*, **76**, 213–26.

Tsai, J.F., Jeng, J.E., Ho, M.S. *et al.* (1995) Clinical evaluation of serum alpha-fetoprotein and circulating immune complexes as tumour markers of hepatocellular carcinoma. *British Journal of Cancer*, **72**, 442–6.

Tsai, S.L., Huang, G.T., Yang, P.M. *et al.* (1990) Plasma des-gamma-carboxyprothrombin in the early stage of hepatocellular carcinoma. *Hepatology*, **11**, 481–8.

Tsuei, D.J., Chen, P.J., Lai, M.Y. *et al.* (1994) Inverse polymerase chain reaction for cloning cellular sequences adjacent to integrated hepatitis B virus DNA in hepatocellular carcinomas. *Journal of Virological Methods*, **49**, 269–84.

Wang, L.Y., Lin, Z.Y., Chang, W.Y. *et al.* (1991) Duplex pulsed Doppler sonography of portal vein thrombosis in hepatocellular carcinoma. *Journal of Ultrasound Medicine*, **10**, 265–9.

Wang, L.Y., Hatch, M., Chen, C.J. *et al.* (1996a) Aflatoxin exposure and risk of hepatocellular carcinoma in Taiwan. *International Journal of Cancer*, **67**, 620–5.

Wang, S.S., Lu, R.H., Lee, F.Y. *et al.* (1996b) Utility of lentil lectin affinity of alpha-fetoprotein in the diagnosis of hepatocellular carcinoma. *Journal of Hepatology*, **25**, 166–71.

Wu, C.C., Ho, Y.Z., Ho, W.L. *et al.* (1995) Pre-operative transcatheter arterial chemoembolization for resectable large hepatocellular carcinoma: a reappraisal. *British Journal of Surgery*, **82**, 122–6.

Wu, C.C., Ho, W.L., Yeh, D.C. *et al.* (1996) Hepatic resection of hepatocellular carcinoma in cirrhotic livers: is it unjustified in impaired liver function? *Surgery*, **120**, 34–9.

Wu, C.C., Yang, M.D. and Liu, T.J. (1992) Improvements in hepatocellular carcinoma resection by intraoperative ultrasonography and intermittent hepatic inflow blood occlusion. *Japanese Journal of Clinical Oncology*, **22**, 107–12.

Wu, C.C., Hwang, C.J., Yang, M.D. and Liu, T.J. (1993) Preliminary results of hepatic resection for centrally located large hepatocellular carcinoma. *Australia New Zealand Journal of Surgery*, **63**, 525–9.

Wu, J.C., Daughaday, W.H., Lee, S.D. *et al.* (1988a) Radioimmunoassay of serum IGF-I and IGF-II in patients with chronic liver diseases and hepatocellular carcinoma with or without hypoglycemia. *Journal of Laboratory and Clinical Medicine*, **112**, 589–94.

Wu, J.C., Lee, S.D., Hsiao, K.J. *et al.* (1988b) Mass screening of primary hepatocellular carcinoma by alpha-fetoprotein in a rural area of Taiwan – a dried blood spot method. *Liver*, **8**, 100–4.

Wu, T.C., Tong, M.J., Hwang, B. *et al.* (1987) Primary hepatocellular carcinoma and hepatitis B infection during childhood. *Hepatology*, **7**, 46–8.

Yang, C.F. and Ho, Y.J. (1992) Transcatheter arterial chemoembolization for hepatocellular carcinoma. *Cancer Chemotherapy and Pharmacology*, **31** (Suppl.), S86–8.

Yang, C.F., Ho, Y.Z., Chang, J.M. *et al.* (1989a) Transcatheter arterial chemoembolization for hepatocellular carcinoma. *Cancer Chemotherapy and Pharmacology,* **23** (Suppl.), S26–8.

Yang, M.C., Lee, P.O., Sheu, J.C. *et al.* (1996) Surgical treatment of hepatocellular carcinoma originating from the caudate lobe. *World Journal of Surgery,* **20**, 562–5.

Yang, P.M., Sung, J.L. and Chen, D.S. (1989b) HLA-A, B, C and DR antigens in chronic hepatitis B viral infection. *Hepatogastroenterology,* **36**, 363–6.

Yeh, S.H., Chen, P.J., Chen, H.L. *et al.* (1994) Frequent genetic alterations at the distal region of chromosome 1p in human hepatocellular carcinomas. *Cancer Research,* **54**, 4188–92.

Yeh, S.H., Chen, P.J., Lai, M.Y. and Chen, D.S. (1996) Allelic loss on chromosomes 4q and 16q in hepatocellular carcinoma: association with elevated alpha-fetoprotein production. *Gastroenterology,* **110**, 184–92.

Yen, F.S., Wu, J.C., Kuo, B.I. *et al.* (1995) Transcatheter arterial embolization for hepatocellular carcinoma with portal vein thrombosis. *Journal of Gastroenterology and Hepatology,* **10**, 237–40.

Yu, M.W. and Chen, C.J. (1993) Elevated serum testosterone levels and risk of hepatocellular carcinoma. *Cancer Research,* **53**, 790–4.

Yu, M.W., Chen, C.J., Luo, J.C. *et al.* (1994) Correlations of chronic hepatitis B virus infection and cigarette smoking with elevated expression of neu oncoprotein in the development of hepatocellular carcinoma. *Cancer Research,* **54**, 5106–10.

Yu, M.W., Gladek-Yarborough, A., Chiamprasert, S. *et al.* (1995a) Cytochrome P450 2E1 and glutathione S-transferase M1 polymorphisms and susceptibility to hepatocellular carcinoma. *Gastroenterology,* **109**, 1266–73.

Yu, M.W., Hsieh, H.H., Pan, W.H. *et al.* (1995b) Vegetable consumption, serum retinol level, and risk of hepatocellular carcinoma. *Cancer Research,* **55**, 1301–5.

Yu, M.W., Lien, J.P., Chiu, Y.H. *et al.* (1997) Effect of aflatoxin metabolism and DNA adduct formation on hepatocellular carcinoma among chronic hepatitis B carriers in Taiwan. *Journal of Hepatology,* **27**, 320–30.

Yu, M.W., Lien, J.P., Liaw, Y.F. and Chen, C.J. (1996) Effects of multiple risk factors for hepatocellular carcinoma on formation of aflatoxin B1–DNA adducts. *Cancer Epidemiology, Biomarkers and Prevention,* **5**, 613–19.

Yu, M.W., You, S.L., Chang, A.S. *et al.* (1991) Association between hepatitis C virus antibodies and hepatocellular carcinoma in Taiwan. *Cancer Research,* **51**, 5621–5.

Zhang, Y.J., Chen, C.J., Lee, C.S. *et al.* (1991) Aflatoxin B1–DNA adducts and hepatitis B virus antigens in hepatocellular carcinoma and nontumorous liver tissue. *Carcinogenesis,* **12**, 2247–52.

Zhang, Y.J., Jiang, W., Chen, C.J. *et al.* (1993) Amplification and overexpression of cyclin D1 in human hepatocellular carcinoma. *Biochemistry and Biophysiology Research Communications,* **196**, 1010–16.

USA: with emphasis on fibrolamellar carcinoma (FLHCC)

J.R. Craig

13.23 INCIDENCE

Hepatocellular carcinoma (HCC) exhibits a > 50-fold variation in incidence on a global basis and a similar variation in the various racial-ethnic groups within the USA. In general, the largest racial/ethnic group of the US population is of Western European extraction and this group has a low death risk from HCC. A low death rate may be defined as less than five deaths per 100 000 per year whereas in some Western European countries (France, Italy, Greece and Poland) a moderate death rate (of 5–20 deaths per 100 000 per year) is documented (Giovanni-Simonetti *et al.*, 1991). As a cancer-related cause of death within the USA, HCC is number 22, but selected racial groups have high rates (10 times the overall rate) which reflect the incidence in their native land (Tong *et al.*, 1989). In California, the most populous state in the USA, which has many ethnic groups, a recent increase in Asian women has been identified by the state cancer registry (R. Schlag, 1997, California State Cancer Registry, personal communication). Furthermore, racial differences have been recorded with the incidence in US black males double that of US white males (4.92 versus 2.33) (Bosch, 1997).

13.24 ETIOLOGY OF HCC

Several conditions associated with HCC in the USA include: (1) chronic hepatitis B, (2) chronic hepatitis C, (3) alcoholism, (4) cirrhosis (of various etiologies including categories 1, 2 and 3), and (5) other factors such as smoking. Chronic hepatitis B, well known to be associated with HCC in other regions of the world, affects many Asian born patients living within the USA (Tong *et al.*, 1989). Chronic hepatitis C virus (HCV) infection continues to rise in importance as an associated factor for HCC (Tong *et al.*, 1994). Tong *et al.* reported that in a large liver clinic group of 112 patients seen in 1982–92 in California, antibody to HCV was detected in 30% of 33 white patients and in 19% of 79 Asian patients. Up to 55% of HCC in Californian non-Asian patients may be attributed to HBV and/or HCV infection (Yu *et al.*, 1997).

Whereas the community blood supply has been effectively screened for HCV since 1990, there are patients with many post-transfusion chronic HCV infection within the general population that may evolve into HCC over the several decades usually required for such progression. In a study of 131 patients with post-transfusion HCV, 67% had cirrhosis at evaluation and the prior blood transfusion was an average of 35 years before the first liver clinic evaluation (range 1–76 years) (Tong *et al.*, 1995). HCC was detected at first evaluation in seven patients and was recognized in seven more during an average of an additional 36 months (range 7–121 months). Of this liver referral clinical group, eight died from liver failure and 11 succumbed to HCC. The average time from transfusion to HCC

Hepatocellular Carcinoma: Diagnosis, investigation and management. Edited by Anthony S.-Y. Leong, Choong-Tsek Liew, Joseph W.Y. Lau and Philip J. Johnson. Published in 1999 by Arnold, London. ISBN 0 340 74096 5.

was 28.3 years in the Tong study whereas cirrhosis was detected in an average of 20.6 years. These time intervals are similar to chronic hepatitis C progression in other countries. A third major causal factor of HCC is alcoholism and the associated cirrhosis (Craig *et al.*, 1989). Alcoholism was also identified as a common cause of cirrhosis and HCC in the large AFIP series of 804 North American patients (Nzeako *et al.*, 1996). Cigarette smoking is an additional factor identified by a careful epidemiologic study of HCC (Yu *et al.*, 1990).

13.25　FIBROLAMELLAR HCC – AN UNCOMMON BUT DISTINCTIVE HCC VARIANT IN THE USA

Fibrolamellar HCC (FLHCC) is a variant of HCC with distinctive histological and clinical features (Craig *et al.*, 1980, Craig, 1997). These distinctive histological features are: (1) large eosinophilic tumor cells with granular cytoplasm and prominent nucleoli, and (2) lamellar fibrous strands separating the liver cords (hence the name fibrolamellar). Occurrence in young persons, evolution in a non-cirrhotic liver and a prolonged survival compared with typical HCC are the typical clinical distinctive features. No etiologic factors such as specific viruses, toxins or drugs have been identified as possible causes of FLHCC.

13.25.1　CLINICAL

The incidence of FLHCC in the USA is variable according to the reference population but is approximately 1% of all HCC. Some selected series indicate up to 10% of HCC in non-cirrhotic patients may be FLHCC. Of the large 804 patient AFIP series, 4% was FLHCC type (Nzeako *et al.*, 1995). In a few selected cancer centers FLHCC may account for 40% of HCC in young persons. However, FLHCC is not common outside North America and there are case reports from Japan, Korea, Australia, Turkey and South Africa, and other countries.

This variant occurs with equal frequency in males and females and it has no association with cirrhosis. The average age in multiple series is in the 20s although there are a few cases identified >50 years of age. Because the clinical symptoms are mild, the patient has a prolonged prediagnostic course and a large tumor at diagnosis. Radiographic studies may be helpful in identifying a liver mass (or tumor) and plain films show minute microcalcifications in 50%. A central fibrous region (typical in most of the large tumors) produces a defect detected by CT scan or other studies and thus there may be confusion with focal nodular hyperplasia. Furthermore, the laboratory features are not diagnostic as the usual serum liver tests are not helpful and only slightly abnormal. The serum α-fetoprotein is normal in most patients (85%) and thus an elevated value is more typical of routine HCC. Selected serum tests that may be helpful include serum neurotensin, vitamin B12 binding globulin, and the abnormal prothrombin (des-γ-carboxyprothrombin) (Craig, 1997). In the recent large treatment evaluation group of 41 patients of FLHCC, the abnormal prothrombin was detected in all 10 patients tested (Pinna *et al.*, 1997).

13.25.2　PATHOLOGY

The key gross pathologic features of this tumor are: (1) origin in a non-cirrhotic liver and, (2) the common location in the left lobe. At the initial detection, a main mass is noted with several satellite nodules. At least 25% have a central fibrous nodule that is white, whereas the bulk of the tumor is dark brown, grey and even green (from bile) with focal red (hemorrhagic) areas. The resected tumor size is often large and has been documented as large as 3600 g. The microscopic pattern reveals large eosinophilic cells with granular cytoplasm that has prompted the term oncocytoma (Fig. 13.7). 'Pale bodies' are clear cytoplasmic areas and occur in about 50% of cases and are dispersed throughout the tumor usually as isolated cells (Fig. 13.8). In addition, a pelioid pattern occurs in at least 25% and is noted by large dilated sinusoidal spaces. The fibrous tissue surrounding the thin epithelial plates or cords forms thin multilamellar strands. In the central area, a large fibrous 'scar' includes scattered vessels and the margins demonstrate the flaying of the fibrous tissue into the lamellar strands. Sheets of the eosinophilic cells may account for more than one-half of the tumor and thus a selected small biopsy or needle biopsy may not reveal the diagnostic lamellar fibrous strands. The microcalcifications noted on radiographic study correspond to dystrophic calcification with foreign body reaction. The abundance of mitochondria within the granular cells is detected by electron microscopy.

The differential diagnosis of FLHCC includes focal nodular hyperplasia, ordinary HCC, metastatic adenosquamous carcinoma, sclerosing hepatic carcinoma and cholangiocarcinoma. The eosinophilic cells of the FLHCC variant have large nucleoli and often an acinar growth pattern whereas the sclerosing HCC lacks the large nucleoli and does not demonstrate the lamellar stranding of fibrous tissue. Some FLHCC have solid areas of the epithelial growth (without lamellar fibrosis), but the granular cytoplasm and pale bodies are diagnostic clues. Focal nodular hyperplasia does contain small pseudocholangiolar proliferation as well as benign small hepatocytes.

Cholangiocarcinoma is distinguished by glandular formation and often more diffuse

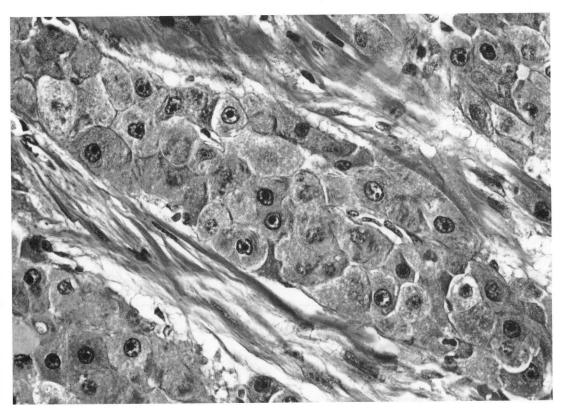

Fig. 13.7   FLHCC: fibrosis with a lamellar stranding and the trabeculae are 2–4 cells in thickness. Large nucleoli are present (H&E).

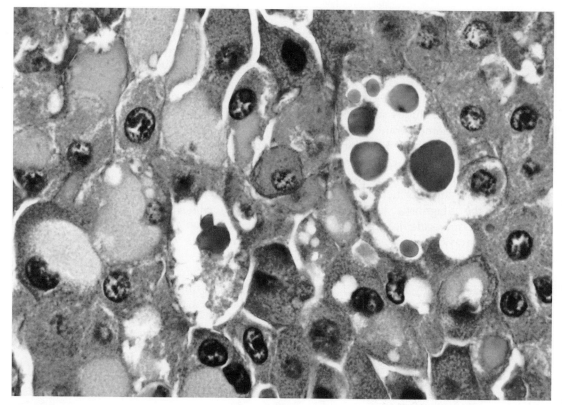

Fig. 13.8 High-power to show pale bodies (light grey cytoplasm) and the dense round cytoplasmic bodies that are PAS-positive (diastase resistant).

'hard' fibrosis. Adenosquamous carcinoma of the gall bladder with extension into the liver may produce a sclerosing carcinoma with large eosinophilic cells but the fibrosis is not lamellar and the cells do not have granular cytoplasm.

13.25.3   TREATMENT

The treatment and cure of FLHCC is best achieved with early diagnosis and surgical resection. Complete surgical resection and cure occur in 50–75% of cases. In the large series of 41 patients by Pinna *et al.* (1997), partial hepatectomy was completed in 28 patients and transplantation was completed in 13. Chemotherapy has been disappointing although others have reported neoadjuvant chemotherapy may allow tumor shrinkage and subsequent resection (Craig, 1997; Pinna *et al.*, 1997). The FLHCC variant had the most favorable long survival (of various subtypes of HCC) within the large series of 1063 North American patients from the AFIP group. Even after tumor recurrence, FLHCC had 1-, 3- and 5-year survival rates of 75, 48 and 21% (Craig, 1997). Resection of isolated metastatic tumors (in other organs) appears beneficial to longer survival.

REFERENCES

Bosch, F.X. (1997) Global epidemiology of hepatocellular carcinoma, in *Liver Cancer* (eds K. Okuda and E. Tabor) Churchill-Livingstone, New York, pp. 13–28.

Craig, J.R., Peters, R.L., Edmondson, H.A. *et al.* (1980) Fibrolamellar carcinoma of the liver: a tumor of adolescents and young adults with distinctive clinico-pathologic features. *Cancer,* **46**, 372–9.

Craig, J.R., Klatt, E.C. and Yu, M. (1989) Role of cirrhosis and the development of HCC: evidence from histologic studies and large population studies, in *Etiology, Pathology, and Treatment of Hepatocellular Carcinoma in North America* (eds E. Tabor and R.H. Purcell), Gulf, Houston, pp. 177–90.

Craig, J.R. (1997) Fibrolamellar carcinoma: clinical and pathologic features, in *Liver Cancer* (eds K. Okuda and E. Tabor) Churchill-Livingstone, New York, pp. 255–62.

Giovanni-Simonetti, R. Camma, C., Fiorello, F. *et al.* (1991) Hepatocellular carcinoma: a worldwide problem and the major risk factors. *Digestive Diseases Sciences,* **36**, 962–72.

Nzeako, U., Goodman, Z.D. and Ishak, K.G. (1995) Comparison of tumor pathology with duration of survival of North American patients with hepatocellular carcinoma. *Cancer,* **76**, 579–88.

Nzeako, U.C., Goodman, Z. and Ishak, K.G. (1996) Hepatocellular carcinoma in cirrhotic and non-cirrhotic livers. A clinico-histopathologic study of 804 North American patients. *American Journal of Clinical Pathology,* **105**, 65–75.

Pinna, A.D., Iwatsuki, S., Lee, R.G. *et al.* (1997) Treatment of fibrolamellar hepatoma with subtotal hepatectomy or transplantation. *Hepatology,* **26**, 877–83.

Tong, M.J., Schwindt, R.R., Lo, G. *et al.* (1989) Chronic hepatitis and hepatocellular carcinoma in Asian Americans, in *Etiology, Pathology, and Treatment of Hepatocellular Carcinoma in North America* (eds E. Tabor and R.H. Purcell), Gulf, Houston, pp. 15–23.

Tong, M.J., Lee, S., Hwang, S. *et al.* (1994) Evidence for hepatitis C viral infection in patients with primary hepatocellular carcinoma. *Western Journal of Medicine,* **160**, 133–8.

Tong, M.J., El-Farra, N.S., Reikes, A.R. *et al.* (1995) Clinical outcomes after transfusion-associated hepatitis C. *New England Journal of Medicine,* **332**, 1463–6.

Yu, M., Tong, M.J., Govindarajan, S. *et al.* (1990) Nonviral risk factors for hepatocellular carcinoma in a low-risk population, the non-Asians of Los Angeles County, California. *Journal of the National Cancer Institutes,* **83**, 1820–6.

Yu, M.,C., Yuan, J., Ross, R.K. *et al.* (1997) Presence of antibodies to the hepatitis B surface antigen is associated with an excess risk for hepatocellular carcinoma among non-Asians in Los Angeles County, California. *Hepatology,* **25**, 226–8.

FUTURE PROSPECTS 14

P.J. Johnson

14.1 INTRODUCTION

The aim of this book has been to survey the current status of diagnosis and management of hepatocellular carcinoma (HCC). In this final chapter some of the many problems that remain are examined and, in the light of these, the future prospects for treatment and prevention are reviewed. Much will depend on the general progress in the field of oncology but it will become apparent that progress in many non-cancer-related areas such as antiviral therapeutics, treatment of chronic liver disease, and public health initiatives will also be of central importance.

14.2 PROSPECTS FOR EFFECTIVE TREATMENT

Perusing this volume the author identifies eight major facets of the disease which impact on our ability to deliver effective treatment:

- The very high incidence rate.
- The frequent underlying liver disease.
- The late presentation.
- Lack of an effective systemic therapy.
- Limitation of regional treatments.
- Disease recurrence after surgical resection.
- Lack of research into palliative care.

Each of these will be considered separately and ways forward will be sought.

14.2.1 THE VERY HIGH INCIDENCE RATE

The simple observation that a hepatitis B seropositive male in a high-incidence area has almost a one in two chance of dying of liver cancer is enough to make the size of the problem apparent, especially when it is considered that in some areas of the world >10% of the population are carriers. The sheer magnitude of the problem has major implications for treatment. Any proposed treatment must, to have a public health impact, be cheap and simple to administer. This is particularly so in high-incidence areas, which are often in poorer, developing countries. For example, widespread use of liver transplantation which is an effective treatment for small tumors and used 'prophylactically' in patients with advanced liver disease would likely decrease the incidence of HCC, but it is not a practical option. If we consider the failure to deliver a simple, safe and effective vaccine against the hepatitis B virus to large parts of the world (including some wealthy countries), many years after it became readily and cheaply available, then the likelihood of delivering complex and expensive forms of therapy are put into perspective.

The implications for the future are plain. Therapy is becoming more complicated and, barring an unforeseen breakthrough, this trend will continue. The emphasis must

Hepatocellular Carcinoma: Diagnosis, investigation and management. Edited by Anthony S.-Y. Leong, Choong-Tsek Liew, Joseph W.Y. Lau and Philip J. Johnson. Published in 1999 by Arnold, London. ISBN 0 340 74096 5.

therefore rest on prevention. Perhaps if preventative measures are extensively applied over the next 20 years then, with the decreasing size of the problem, more complex and expensive therapies described below may become viable propositions in a public health setting.

14.2.2   THE UNDERLYING LIVER DISEASE

Of patients with HCC, 70–85% will have underlying liver disease, either chronic hepatitis or cirrhosis. Irrespective of the nature of the relationship between the two conditions, the presence of chronic liver disease has major implications for management of the disease. Diagnosis is more difficult because of the presence of cirrhotic nodules which may simulate tumor nodules; drug metabolism may be altered and, most importantly, the liver function may be so poor that patients cannot tolerate even minor resections or other therapeutic intervention that lead to some loss of functioning non-tumorous liver. The major implication from these observations is that in many cases the patient's prognosis would remain very poor even if the tumor could be completely treated by whatever means. Indeed, most of such patients who are in liver failure at presentation currently never even enter clinical trials. In the future therefore we must seek to:

- develop methods which delay or prevent the development of progressive chronic liver disease. Progress in this area may come from antiviral research, particularly that deriving from the AIDS research program. Already there are drugs that can effectively inhibit the replication of both the hepatitis B and C viruses. Whether this will have any effect on the development of HCC will be a fascinating observation. However, even if tumors continue to develop but do so in a less damaged liver, this may impact positively on the prognosis of HCC patients;

- and/or make the diagnosis of HCC earlier and, perhaps, thereby start treatment before the tumor has caused, or exacerbated, existing liver dysfunction. This possibility is discussed below.

14.2.3   LATE PRESENTATION

Diagnostic methods have certainly progressed rapidly over the last decade so that now a confident diagnosis can be arrived at within 1 week of presentation in most clinical units. The problem, however, remains that, by the time the tumor is detected after symptomatic presentation, up to 50% of patients will already be in liver failure so that no form of active treatment is indicated. Although there has been a general tendency to attribute late presentation to the failure of patients to report symptoms early in many cancers, this excuse seldom applies in the case of HCC. The duration of symptoms is usually less than a few weeks.

These observations inevitably lead to the question of early diagnosis. It is always taken as understood that early diagnosis would be beneficial, but before accepting this, it is as well to consider if, and why, this may be so. The most obvious reason is that at an early stage the tumor is more likely to be resectable. Further, less liver damage may have occurred, thereby increasing the chances of survival during the operation, or living longer thereafter. It is also clear that smaller tumors (or perhaps tumors with less vascular invasion) do not metastasize. A final, and perhaps, only theoretical reason, is that tumors may be more sensitive to chemotherapy when the burden of genetic changes is lower.

14.2.3.1   New approaches to early diagnosis

If delay in presentation is not due to the delay in seeking medical help, then screening becomes the only option. On the face of it HCC would appear to have some advantages here. The high-risk population is readily identifiable – namely patients with cirrhosis or those who are carriers of the hepatitis B or hepatitis C viruses. Second, screening techniques are available in the form of ultrasound scanning and α-fetoprotein (AFP) estimation. Nonetheless, the problems are enormous and have been described briefly in Chapter 2. Increasingly, wealthy people in high risk groups are having 3-monthly ultrasound and AFP estimations and all physicians involved in these programs have seen examples of early diagnosis and successful treatment. However, whether such programs can be translated into the public health domain is another matter.

We have recently proposed that it may be possible confidently to diagnose HCC at a preclinical stage, i.e. before it can be detected by conventional imaging techniques. The approach involves the use of 'hepatoma'-specific isoforms of AFP. We have shown that these isoforms may be detectable up to 18 months before the tumor manifests itself clinically (see Chapter 3). Two observations make us believe that this may offer an opportunity for novel therapeutic approaches. First is our experience with postoperative treatment. This is discussed in more detail below but in essence we have evidence to suggest that postoperative adjuvant therapy with lipiodol I[131] may prevent recurrence. The implication is that this form of therapy is effectively treating microscopic disease. Second, there is evidence, also discussed below, that interferon may be effective, if given while the disease is preclinical. These two evidences of effective treatment of microscopic disease have led us to consider starting treatment before there is any conventional evidence of tumor (i.e. imaging). This would be a very radical departure from conventional oncological principles, but with a disease so refractory to conventional approaches, such decisions may need to be taken (Fig. 14.1).

14.2.4 LACK OF EFFECTIVE SYSTEMIC TREATMENT

The observation that, in 1998, the overall median life-expectancy in high incidence areas is still only 3 months, it leaves one in no doubt about the efficacy of current treatment. Even allowing for the problem of late presentation, it must be admitted that systemic therapy has, to date, had no impact.

The failure of systemic therapy is important for two reasons. First, a systemic treatment is invariably much simpler and much cheaper to

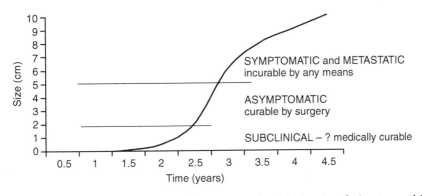

Fig. 14.1 Representation of the likely course of tumor growth with time in relation to curability. Tumors >5 cm in diameter are seldom curable by any currently available method of treatment as they have usually developed metastatic potential by this stage. Between 1 and 5 cm, both conventional surgical resection and transplantation have a high success rate. Is there a window of opportunity to treat tumors <1 cm in diameter by medical methods if they can be diagnosed at this stage?

260   *Future prospects*

administer (either orally or intravenously). Second, as local treatments get better, the problem of extrahepatic metastases increases. The prospects for conventional cytotoxic approaches look poor. The older agents have been extensively studied and none of these has achieved consistent response rates >20%. These have been known to be achievable with adriamycin for 20 years. The taxanes and topoisomerase inhibitors do not, in initial studies, appear effective and there are no other new promising agents on the horizon.

14.2.4.1 Hepatitis C and interferon therapy

There is no doubt that since assays for antibody to the hepatitis C virus were first developed in the late 1980s the importance of this virus in the pathogenesis of HCC has become increasingly apparent. In many areas of the world it is now recognized to be as important a cause of HCC as is the hepatitis B virus (Hadziyannis *et al.*, 1997). However, in the absence of any prospect of a vaccine the problem is, as HBV infection declines in importance, likely to become relatively greater. Further, there is increasing recognition that the rate at which HCV infection leads

to HCC is very high – perhaps 3–5% per annum (Zoli *et al.*, 1996; Vian, *et al.*, 1997). While the medical community has been remarkably comfortable in accepting that HCV is carcinogenic because it causes cirrhosis and chronic hepatitis, there is emerging evidence that the rate of HCC development is over and above that of other types of cirrhosis and that HCV may have a specific and direct role in carcinogenesis (Naumov *et al.*, 1997). Most encouragingly, there is emerging evidence that treatment with interferon, aimed primarily at combating the hepatitis C virus may, quite dramatically, coincidentally, decrease the incidence of HCC.

The role of interferons has been actively investigated in HCC and, in general, the response has been very limited once the disease is symptomatic. It is not the author's aim to review these further but merely to highlight very recent studies that may have major implications for the future. Nishiguchi *et al.* (1995) studied the role of interferon-α in patients with chronic hepatitis C virus infection in a prospective randomized controlled trial. They showed clearly that viral replication could be inhibited in many subjects. Most intriguingly, however, they also showed that

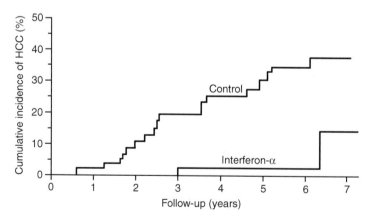

Fig. 14.2 Cumulative incidence of hepatocellular carcinoma in chronic carriers of the hepatitis C virus who receive interferon-α. Note that tumors start to be detected in the control group well within the first year, implying that they were already present on entry into the study although at a preclinical stage. Could the difference between the two curves represent those preclinical cases of HCC actually cured by interferon-α? (From Nishiguchi *et al.*, 1995.)

the group receiving the interferon-α had a significantly decreased incidence of HCC (Fig. 14.2). Several potential mechanisms were postulated including immune stimulation, direct inhibition of cell division preventing differentiation of precancerous cells, or slowing of hepatocyte degeneration and necrosis. However, inspection of Fig. 14.2 suggests an alternative explanation. We know that tumors must have a prolonged preclinical period before they become detectable by conventional imaging techniques – perhaps 3–5 years. It is very likely that both groups in Nishiguchi *et al's* series had similar numbers of tumors *already present* (but clinically undetectable) before the study started, since the time from entry to the first tumors becoming detectable was only 6 months. This may imply that the tumors were not prevented by the interferon but rather that microscopic disease was effectively treated. Similar data have recently been reported by Imai *et al.* (1997). This approach will no doubt become a major area for research over the next decade.

14.2.4.2 Gene therapy

The general despondency about therapy of HCC has, inevitably, led to consideration of gene therapy. This requires a gene to transfer and, in most cases, a vector to carry the gene, and a method of targeting the cell of interest – in this case the tumor cell. The procedure can be carried out *ex vivo*, after removal of some of the tumor cells and transduction of the therapeutic gene followed by reintroduction directly into the tumor mass. Alternatively the gene can be transduced *in situ* (i.e. *in vivo*) but while less cumbersome, this approach raises the additional problem of tumor cell targeting. A detailed discussion of the studies currently underway is beyond the scope of this chapter, but three examples will give a flavor of the direction in which research is likely to progress over the next few years.

The first, and perhaps most obvious, strategy is to replace a gene which is known to be defective and is likely to be responsible for the malignant phenotype. For example reintroduction of the 'wild-type p53' tumor suppressor gene (see Chapter 1) might possibly correct the genetic change responsible for the malignant phenotype. One idea is to use a replication-defective retrovirus containing wild-type p53 transcriptionally regulated by AFP transcriptional regulatory sequences (Xu *et al.*, 1994). It has already been shown that the new p53 gene is expressed specifically in AFP-positive HCC cells and that clonal growth of these cells is inhibited. Such approaches are now undergoing clinical trials.

A second approach is to introduce enzymes by gene therapy (Kanai *et al.*, 1997). Perhaps the most appealing approach is the 'suicide gene' paradigm. Here a gene, which codes for a specific enzyme, is introduced into the relevant tumor cell. The new enzymes activate a harmless 'prodrug' into a cytotoxic agent which can kill the cancer cell. In one example, the gene for thymidine kinase (TK, from herpes simplex type-1 virus) is transferred into hepatoma cells (Qian *et al.*, 1995). The drug gancyclovir is then administered. Those cells, hopefully the tumor cells which contain the functioning TK gene, will convert the harmless gancyclovir into its cytotoxic triphosphate form. Tumor cell specificity is again achieved by using a replication-deficient adenovirus, in which expression of the TK gene is under the control of the AFP promoter/enhancer, as the vector. As in the above-mentioned case, it has been shown that in animal models, tumor cell growth can be inhibited and that TK expression is confined to AFP expressing tumors (Wills *et al.* 1995).

Introduction of genes for various cytokines offers a third approach (Huang *et al.*, 1996). For example, it is possible to apply gene therapy to deliver high intratumoral concentrations of the cytokine TNF-α. This cytokine, originally known as 'tumor necrosis factor', does indeed cause tumor necrosis but is highly toxic to normal cells at the concentration required to kill tumor cells (Cao *et al.*,

1997). Thus, a considerable degree of selectivity is required if it is to be used as an anti-cancer agent. The approach has been to introduce the TNF-α gene into tumor cells and thereby increase local concentrations. Studies have aimed at *in vivo* transfer using, for example, the Moloney murine leukemia virus expressing the TNF-α gene under control of an albumin enhancer and promoter. It was shown, among many results, that the infected cells did, indeed, induce the expression of TNF-α in the culture medium of infected liver cells and that injection of the TNF-carrying retrovirus did lead to an inhibition of growth and prolongation of survival in an animal model.

The problems faced by gene therapy are still enormous. The retroviral vectors are rapidly inactivated *in vivo*. The requirement of dividing cells for retroviral transduction is also a problem. Not only are many cells in a tumor in 'G$_0$', i.e. not dividing, but normal cells around the tumor are often also replicating because of the associated hepatitis. Both AFP and albumin expression are extremely variable in malignant cells and normal hepatocytes. As Schuster and Wu (1997) have pointed out in comment on the TNF-α approach, these therapies are still essentially local therapies if the outcome is expression of cytokines by the infected cells rather than transduction of all tumor cells. Further, the number of genetic abnormalities in HCC is very large and targeting one of these, such as p53, the mutation of which may be quite a late event, is unlikely to reverse the malignant phenotype.

14.2.4.3 Immunotherapy and other novel approaches

In several areas of cancer research, stimulation of cell-mediated immunity by activation of cytotoxic T cells is entering clinical trials. Recent evidence suggests that one of the actions of interferon-γ (and other cytokines such as TNF) is to increase expression of MHC class I antigens on other molecules, such as ICAM, which may then become immunogenic. Such cells have now been shown to activate tumor-infiltrating and peripheral blood lymphocytes of HCC patients. These lymphocytes exhibit specific cytotoxicity against autologous tumor cells. In nude mice bearing human HCC, administration of such CTLs has led to significant tumor growth inhibition and an increase in survival time (Shi *et al.*, 1997).

Our own group's preference has been for internal radiotherapy, mainly with Yttrium-99 (see Chapter 10). Irrespective of any claims of improvement in survival, the treatment is remarkably non-toxic and the response, in terms of changes in AFP levels, looks identical to those following surgical resection. The implication of the observations that such tumor marker changes are not reflected by changes in the physical size of the tumor assessed by imaging is discussed below. Furthermore, both ourselves and others have noted that there is significant hepatic hypertrophy after radiation treatment which may actually improve, or at least stabilize, liver function (Robertson *et al.*, 1997; Lau *et al.*, 1998). Not only have several tumors become operable after such treatment, but the resected specimens have often had no, or only very few, viable tumor cells remaining.

The approaches described above do not rely on sensitivity to cytotoxic drugs and it may be that they, perhaps in combination with the new anti-angiogenesis agents, will prove to be the most appropriate therapeutic tools for the next few years.

14.2.5 LIMITATIONS OF REGIONAL TREATMENTS

Local treatment modalities that have been developed over the last 20 years are effective in their major aim of decreasing the tumor mass and yet convincing evidence of improved survival or improved quality of life remains elusive. It appears that there is little to choose between embolization, chemoembolization and alcohol injection. Indeed there is little evidence that any of these is better than no treatment. The most widely applied of these has been chemoembolization which has recently been subjected to prospective clinical trials and was found wanting (see Chapter 10). This may partly be due to damage to the non-tumorous liver caused by the embolization, which, in turn, precipitates liver failure. An alternative explanation is that prognosis is dependent on underlying liver function and not tumor progression. In any event this suggests that the important aims are to develop treatment which induces less damage, i.e. it is more tumor selective.

The story of local therapies also offers lessons for the future. All those in the field have seen numerous locoregional therapies come and go over the last 20 years. Each starts with enthusiasm only to crumble in the face of controlled trials or longer term follow-up. However, the huge number of patients treated before the approaches are subjected to controlled studies is unfortunate. In view of the difficulty in assessing the response to new approaches with currently available methods, the prospective randomized trial, using survival or quality of life as endpoints, and set-up early in the lifetime of any new treatment, becomes absolutely essential.

14.2.5.1 Surgical resection and liver transplantation

Although surgical resection has never been shown in a randomized trial to improve survival compared with either no treatment or any other specific therapy, the fact that in most surgical series the survival curve plateaus out at around 20–50% at 3 years implies that it does, indeed, improve survival. The same argument holds for liver transplantation where the long-term survival rates can be as high as 75% in selected cases (Schwartz, 1996). It would appear that the major technical problems associated with surgical resection of liver tumors and transplantation, and the

perioperative management, have reached their limit although artificial liver support in the postoperative period may decrease postoperative mortality further. The questions and problems that remain are therefore not surgical, but biological. They focus on the basic problem of local therapies in general, since both surgery and transplantation are, in effect, extreme local treatments. Autopsy studies show that once the tumor is >3 cm in diameter, or is multifocal, or has invaded vascular channels, there are virtually always systemic metastases (Ko *et al.*, 1996). Several questions therefore arise:

- Are these the source of postoperative recurrences, or does the surgeon seed tumor cells during surgery?
- Can systemic therapies deal with this extrahepatic disease?
- What is the effect of surgical resection on the hepatic secretion of hepatotrophic factors? Is it possible that these differentially stimulate micrometastases?
- What stimulates the cirrhotic liver to regenerate and hypertrophy – is this of any functional significance?

14.2.6 EFFECTIVE MONITORING OF TREATMENT

We cannot be sure that we would recognize a useful treatment if it became available. Conventional criteria for response are based on changes in the size of the tumor being treated. However, it is apparent that many liver tumors, or what is perceived of as the liver tumor, is in fact largely necrotic or, after treatment, fibrotic, non-malignant tissue. Furthermore, we have recently had the experience of treating liver tumors with internal radiation and observing the response, usually classified as 'partial' on radiological criteria, which have permitted surgical resection to be undertaken (see Chapter 11). The resected specimen has, in many cases, shown a complete pathological response in that no viable tumor cells were identified. The implication is clear; in some treatment modalities response defined on purely conventional radiological grounds is not satisfactory. What is needed is a physical method of addressing viable tissue. MRI may prove to be of great value in this role, as may a tumor marker which detects the viable tumor burden.

14.2.7   MANAGEMENT OF POSTOPERATIVE RECURRENCES

It is a depressing observation that most tumors 'recur' despite apparently successful resection. The actual recurrence rate will vary depending on the magnitude of the task the surgeon is comfortable to accept, but figures range between 40 and 80%. (In most cases these do represent genuine recurrences although occasionally, a 'new' tumor will develop. ('New' here implies a new clone. 'New' tumors and 'recurrences' can be distinguished by analysis of the integration site of HBV. If, following resection, the integration site in the resected specimen and any subsequent tumor that develops thereafter is the same, then a true 'recurrence' can be confidently diagnosed.) In the case of other tumors such as breast and colon cancer, postoperative adjuvant therapy has been proven to be successful in decreasing recurrence rates and prolonging survival. To date such an approach has not been successful in HCC although there have been some uncontrolled studies suggesting that adjuvant chemotherapy may prolong survival in patients undergoing liver transplantation for HCC (Olthoff *et al.*, 1995). It should be noted, however, that to demonstrate the efficacy of adjuvant therapy in terms of survival improvement in a prospective controlled trial setting, very large numbers of patients were required – well over 1000 in the case of colon cancer.

In our own randomized trial comparing postoperative lipiodol I^{131} to no adjuvant therapy there was a highly significant decrease in disease-free survival in the prelim-

inary analysis with only 20 patients in each arm – approximately 25 versus 75% (see Chapter 11). If these findings are confirmed, and the increase in disease-free survival translates into survival advantage, this will have major implications for future treatment. It will also imply that postoperative lipiodol I^{131} administration is an effective treatment for microscopic disease. This in itself gives credence to the possibility of treating HCC in the preclinical phase as suggested above. An alternative approach is the use of polyprenoic acid, an agent which inhibits experimental hepatocarcinogenesis and induces differentiation and apoptosis in cell lines. In a prospective randomized trial of patients treated with this agent after surgical resection or alcohol injection, the incidence of 'second primary' (i.e. 'new') tumors was very significantly reduced (Muto *et al.*, 1996). Similar approaches will no doubt be investigated in the future, as will the application of chemo-preventative agents to cirrhotic patients at high risk of HCC.

14.2.8   LACK OF RESEARCH INTO PALLIATIVE CARE

Considering that the great majority of patients with HCC will die within 6 months of first symptoms, the impact of this devastating cancer on the individual patient and family cannot be over-emphasized. Currently, the vast majority of clinical resources are concentrated on that small percentage of patients that may be suitable candidates for surgical resection or clinical trials. Palliative treatment which will relieve pain and keep patients out of hospital for a few months are therefore of the utmost importance to the patient, and yet research into this area of management is minimal. Similarly, the impact of current therapies, including local treatments, which are usually classified as 'palliative', is still judged almost entirely by survival analysis with no attempt to address quality-of-life issues.

This is partly due to lack of interest (and insight) among the medical profession and partly to a predilection of research fund-awarding bodies (and medical journals and conferences) for 'exciting' new approaches to treatment. All too often, 'novelty' comes before quality and value, so that in the age of 'patient-centered' medicine we find no area where patients' needs are, in practice, less considered. And yet, while widely perceived as a 'soft' area of research, the problems which need addressing in the assessment of quality-of-life issues, and the integration of these into clinical trials, are, in reality, extremely demanding and of a comparable intellectual challenge to anything being attempted in gene therapy.

14.3 PROSPECTS FOR PREVENTION

Prevention, like palliative care, is or at least has been, an area of research that has not been fashionable. Perhaps it is the lack of funding for projects which do not offer quick answers and which do not meet currently perceived conceptions of the correct direction. Others have suggested that the general public prefer to support research that targets the individual with whom they feel more sympathy rather than the general needs of their community. Nonetheless, any overall cost or utility analysis of 'basic' research, clinical therapeutics and epidemiology/public health approaches to HCC, would indeed leave the latter a long way ahead today and probably well into the next century. It is here that the brightest prospects for the future lie.

14.3.1 IMMUNIZATION AGAINST THE HEPATITIS B VIRUS

Universal immunization against the hepatitis B virus at birth is, today, the major hope for control of this tumor. There is now little doubt that this approach will be effective. In countries where vaccination has been utilized for >10 years the carrier rate falls from 12 to around 1%. Some authorities have even started to talk about eradication of the virus as a realistic prospect. It seems likely that universal vaccination or eradication would lead to a reduction in around 60–75% of all HCC. Already in areas such as Taiwan where a large scale-vaccination program was initiated in 1984 the adjusted mortality ratio for HCC (calculated from 1974 to 1993, relative to 1974) has significantly decreased over recent years. Two major factors may limit this potential success story. The first is lack of political will. Although the vaccine is effective and cheap, delivery to many countries where this tumor is prevalent is still limited. The second limiting factor will be the development of mutant viruses which have the capability to 'escape' the protection offered by the current immunization procedures.

14.3.2 AFLATOXIN

Epidemiological evidence was collected in the 1970s and 1980s by several excellent studies in Africa and the Far East (Van Rensburg *et al.*, 1985; Yeh *et al.*, 1989). They showed a clear correlation between exposure to aflatoxin and the development of HCC. It is sad that the authors of these painstaking studies have, in a time when viral carcinogenesis was fashionable, not received more credit for their work. In fact they showed that the correlation of HCC with aflatoxin exposure better explained the geographical variation than did the prevalence of hepatitis B virus carriage. More recently biomarkers have been established which allow the exposure to aflatoxin to be measured directly (Qian *et al.*, 1994) using a detection system for aflatoxin adducts in the urine. These data not only confirm that aflatoxin is a significant risk factor for HCC but also preliminary evidence suggests that simultaneous chronic carriage of the hepatitis B virus is multiplicative. Although it has been HBV that was identified as having a synergistic effect with aflatoxin exposure, albeit on a small number of patients, the author would predict that the result is not specific to HBV but would be found with any type of chronic liver disease. This latter observation is of crucial importance since while vaccination may eventually lead to eradication of hepatitis B, the problem will persist for several decades to come, and the prospect will be of little comfort to those who are currently HBV carriers. In contrast, control of aflatoxin exposure could theoretically decrease the risk of HCC in those who are current carriers. The first approach, to store grain in conditions which do not support the growth of the *Aspergillus* mould, is obvious and mainly a question of political and financial will. The second approach is chemoprevention.

14.3.3   PROSPECTS FOR CHEMOPREVENTION

Aflatoxin is activated in the liver to a carcinogenic metabolite (Fig. 14.3). The drug oltipraz can induce specific isoforms of glutathione transferase which enhance an alternative pathway leading to an inactive metabolite which is excreted through the biliary system. It has already been shown in animal studies that the administration of oltipraz can almost completely abolish the carcinogenic effects of

aflatoxin and it has been confirmed that the mechanism is as described above and in Fig. 14.3. Field trials of this agent are now underway in China and offer the most hopeful prospect of risk reduction for those who are currently chronic carriers of the hepatitis B virus.

As noted above, one of the strategies for gene therapy involves replacement of mutant p53 and this may have important implications for aflatoxin-related HCC since a direct link between aflatoxin exposure and a specific p53 mutation, namely a G>T transversion at the third base pair of codon 249 (Ozturk, 1994) has been proposed. If this is proven it may open another avenue for the treatment of aflatoxin-related HCC. However, the association between the p53 mutation and aflatoxin exposure has been accepted almost entirely on the basis of surrogate markers of aflatoxin exposure and much more critical appraisal is still needed (Lasky and Magder, 1997).

14.3.4   OTHER PROSPECTS FOR PREVENTION

Excessive alcohol consumption is one of the major factors contributing to HCC in the West and any advance in this area will be depend-

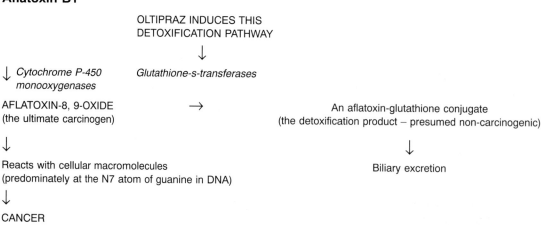

Fig. 14.3   Simplified representation of the activation of aflatoxin B1 and the mechanism by which oltipraz (4-methyl-5-[2-pyrazynyl]-1,2-dithiole-3-thione) may encourage the alternative detoxification pathway. The aflatoxin-glutathione conjugate is (8,9-dihydro-8-(*S*-glutathionyl)-9 hyroxy-aflatoxin B1).

ant on overall measures to control the alcohol problem, and for this the omens are not good. More hopeful is the large number of antiviral agents becoming available, largely as a result of the AIDS research program. If hepatitis C virus infection can be treated early, it is possible that there will be a concomitant impact on HCC development. Unfortunately, a vaccine against hepatitis C seems a long way off, although routine screening of all blood products for HCV will no doubt continue to limit the spread of this infection.

14.4   CONCLUSIONS AND PREDICTIONS

The author makes the following predictions for the next decade by way of a conclusion to this final chapter. He hopes to be in the field long enough to be able to review his personal predictive accuracy in 2008.

1. World-wide, there will be a steady decrease in the incidence of hepatitis B-related HCC; mutant escape viruses will become an increasing clinical problem but will not halt the effectiveness of hepatitis B immunization.
2. Hepatitis C will, at least in relative terms, become an increasing problem. The disparity in incidence between East and West will start to fall, and the West will focus more resources on HCC. No vaccination will become available for hepatitis C but curative antiviral agents, or combinations of agents, will be developed and, given early enough, will prevent HCC development.
3. New cytotoxic drugs and gene therapy will have no impact on the overall survival; rather any improvement in survival will be based on combinations of systemic therapies which are currently available (cytotoxic agents and interferons) and locoregional approaches.
4. Further controlled trials of purely local therapies will demonstrate little or no effect on overall survival although quality of life will be shown to be improved by some.
5. Results of resectional surgery will not change unless adjuvant therapy is proven to be effective. However, it is possible that, as local and systemic treatments improve, initially inoperable lesions will become operable. This approach, analogous to the management of hepatic tumors in childhood, may show significant progress over the next decade.
6. Transplantation will be used increasingly, and prophylaxis of HCC in high-risk cirrhotic patients will become an indication. With better antiviral agents both hepatitis C- and hepatitis B-related disease will become more common indications for HCC related to these viruses.
7. Attempts to justify screening high risk patients will fail to show cost or utility benefit but screening will, nonetheless, become a *de facto* management procedure.
8. Oltipraz will be shown to significantly decrease HCC development in areas of the world where aflatoxin exposure is widespread, but logistical problems, analogous to those encountered in screening, will impede any large-scale public health benefit.
9. MRI will become the definitive imaging procedure for HCC.
10. From the personal perspective of the authors of this volume, we believe that internal radiotherapy will be shown to be the best local approach for treatment of inoperable disease and will significantly improve survival after surgical resection. Preclinical treatment will, we anticipate, be an exciting novel approach to management.

REFERENCES

Cao, G., Kuriyama, S., Du, P. *et al.* (1997) Complete regression of established murine hepatocellular carcinoma by *in vivo* tumor necrosis factor alpha gene transfer. *Gastroenterology,* **112**, 501–10.

Hadziyannis, S., Rodes, J., Bruix, J. *et al.* (1997) Impact of HBV, HCV and HBV on hepatocellular carcinomas in Europe: results of an European Concerted Action. *Journal of Hepatology*, **26**, 139.

Huang, H., Chen, S.H., Kosai, K.I. *et al.* (1996) Gene therapy for hepatocellular carcinoma: long term remission of primary and metastatic tumors in mice by interleukin-2 gene therapy *in vivo*. *Cancer Gene Therapy*, **3**, 980–7.

Imai, Y., Kawata, S., Yabuuchi, I. *et al.* (1997) Incidence of hepatocellular carcinoma in chronic hepatitis C following interferon treatment. *Proceedings of the Annual Meeting of the American Association for Cancer Research*, **37**, A3305.

Kanai, F., Lan, K.H., Shiratori, Y. *et al.* (1997) *In vivo* gene therapy for alpha-fetoprotein producing hepatocellular carcinoma by adenovirus-mediated transfer of cytosine deaminase gene. *Cancer Research*, **57**, 461–5.

Ko, S., Nakajima, Y., Kanehiro, H. *et al.* (1996) Liver transplantation for hepatocellular carcinoma: consideration from the findings on autopsy. *Transplant Proceedings*, **28**, 1691–2.

Lau, W.Y., Ho, S., Leung, W.T *et al.* (1998) Selective internal radiation therapy for inoperable hepatocellular carcinoma with intraarterial infusion of yttrium^{90} microspheres. *International Journal of Radiation Oncology, Biology and Physics* (in press).

Lasky, T. and Magder, L. (1997) Hepatocellular carcinoma p53 G > T transversions at codon 249: the fingerprint of aflatoxin exposure? *Environmental Health Perspectives*, **105**, 392–7.

Muto, Y., Moriwaki, H., Adacho, S. *et al.* (1996) Reduction of second primary tumor in patients with hepatocellular carcinoma with acyclic retinoid: a double blind placebo-controlled study (Meeting abstract). *Proceedings of the Annual Meeting of the American Society of Clinical Oncology*, **15**, A339.

Naumov, N.V., Chokshi, S. Metivier, E. *et al.* (1997) Hepatitis C virus infection in the development of hepatocellular carcinoma in cirrhosis. *Journal of Hepatology*, **27**, 331–6.

Nishiguchi, S., Kuroki T., Nakatani, S. *et al.* (1995) Randomised trial of effects of interferon-alpha on incidence of hepatocellular carcinoma in chronic active hepatitis C with cirrhosis. *Lancet*, **346**, 1051–5.

Olthoff, K.M., Rosove, M.H., Shackleton, C.R. *et al.* (1995) Adjuvant chemotherapy improves survival after liver transplantation for hepatocellular carcinoma. *Annals of Surgery*, **221**, 734–41.

Ozturk, M. (1994) p53 mutation in hepatocellular carcinoma after aflatoxin exposure. *Lancet*, **338**, 1356–9.

Qian, C., Bilbao, R., Bruna, O. *et al.* (1995) Induction of sensitivity to gancyclovir in human hepatocellular carcinoma cells by adenovirus-mediated gene transfer of herpes simplex virus thymidine kinase. *Hepatology*, **22**, 118–23.

Qian, G.-S., Ross, R.K., Yu, M.C. *et al.* (1994) A follow-up study of urinary markers of alfatoxin exposure and liver cancer risk in Shanghai, People's Republic of China. *Cancer Epidemiology, Biomarkers and Prevention*, **3**, 3–10.

Robertson, J.M., Lawrence T.S., Andrews J.C. *et al.* (1997) Long-term results of hepatic artery fluorodeoxyuridine and conformal radiation therapy for primary hepatobiliary cancers. *International Journal of Radiation Oncology, Biology and Physics*, **37**, 325–30.

Schuster, M.J. and Wu, G.Y. (1997) Gene therapy for hepatocellular carcinoma: progress but many stones yet unturned! *Gastroenterology*, **112**, 656–9.

Schwartz, M.E. (1996) Liver transplantation for hepatocellular carcinoma: the best treatment, but for which patient? *Hepatology*, **24**, 1539–41.

Shi, L.H., Che, X.Y., Wu, M.C. *et al.* (1997) Adoptive immunotherapy for hepatocellular carcinoma with tumor specific CTLs generated *in vitro* by stimulating TILs or PBLs with the cytokine treated tumor cells and bispecific monoclonal antibody. *Proceedings of the Annual Meeting of the American Association for Cancer Research*, **37**, A3278.

Van Rensburg, A.J., Cook-Mozaffari, P., Van Schalkwyk, D.J. *et al.* (1985) Hepatocellular carcinoma and dietary aflatoxin in Mozambique and Transkei. *British Journal of Cancer*, **51**, 713–26.

Vian, A., Starzi, A., Lorenzoni, U. *et al.* (1997) Incidence of hepatocellular carcinoma (HCC) in HCV, HBV and both virus related cirrhosis: a 15 year prospective study. *Journal of Hepatology*, **26**, 139.

Wills, K.N., Huang, W.M., Harris, M.P. *et al.* (1995) Gene therapy for hepatocellular carcinoma: chemosensitivity conferred by adenovirus-mediated transfer of the HSV-1 thymidine kinase gene. *Cancer Gene Therapy*, **2**, 191–7.

Xu, G.W., Sun, Z.T. and Forrester, K. (1994) Growth inhibition of hepatocellular carcinoma *in vitro* by tissue-specific expression of the p53 tumor suppressor gene. *Proceedings of the Annual Meeting of the American Association for Cancer Research*, **35**, A3593.

Yeh, F.-S., Yu, M.C., Mo, C.-C. *et al.* (1989) Hepatitis B virus, aflatoxins, and hepatocellular carcinoma in Southern Guangzi, China. *Cancer Research*, **49**, 2506–9.

Zoli, M., Magalotti, D. and Bianchi, G. (1996) Efficacy of a surveillance program for early detection of hepatocellular carcinoma. *Cancer*, **78**, 977–85.

INDEX

Note: US spelling is used in the index. References to figures are in **bold** and references to tables are in *italics*. Abbreviations used are: AFP = α-fetoprotein; CT = computed tomography; HBV = hepatitis B virus; HCC = hepatocellular carcinoma; HCV = hepatitis C virus; MRI = magnetic resonance imaging.

Abdominal pain
  analgesia 209
  diagnosing HCC 19–20, *23*, 64, 193
Abdominal paracentesis 209
Adenocarcinomas 121, 124
Adenoma, hepatocellular
  etiology 115, 221
  focal nodular hyperplasia 118
  hepatocarcinogenesis 111
  identification 111
  macroscopic appearance 115, **116**
  microscopic appearance 115, **116**, 117
  presenting signs 115
  risk factors for HCC 11
Adenomatous hyperplasia *see* Dysplastic nodules
Adenomatous hyperplastic nodules *see* Dysplastic nodules
Adenosquamous carcinoma of gall bladder 253–4
Adenovirus vectors, gene therapy 142, 261
Adjuvant analgesic drugs 209
Adjuvant therapy 164–5, 167, 259, 264, 267
Adrenal tumors
  HCC mimics 44, **44**
  metastasis from HCC 51, **51**
Aflatoxins 265–6
  Africa 214
  chemoprevention 266, **266**, 267
  etiology of HCC 9, 131
  gene therapy 266
  hepatocarcinogenesis 12, 135–6, 139, 214, 233, 238, 265–6
  Hong Kong 89
  Japan 225
  Taiwan 236, 237, 238
AFP (α-fetoprotein) 26
  chemoembolization 241
  erythrocytosis 199
  fibrolamellar HCC 22, 252

gene therapy in HCC 142, 261
immunocytochemical staining 85
need for biopsy 107
non-cirrhotic HCC *23*
postoperative follow up 155
preoperative investigations 151
recurrent HCC 27, 28, 35, 67
as tumor marker 31–6, 39, 239
  aldolase A 38
  alkaline phosphatase 37
  α-1-antitrypsin 38
  benign liver disease 32–3
  des-γ-carboxy prothrombin 38
  cholangiocarcinoma 123
  clinico-pathological features of HCC 32
  detecting isoforms 33–5, **34**, **35**, 39
  γ-glutamyltranspeptidase 37
  internal radiotherapy 262
  isoelectric focusing 33–5, **34**, **35**, 39
  lectin-binding 33, 239
  metastatic tumors 123–4
  monitoring treatment responses 35–6, 185
  5'-nucleotide phosphodiesterase V 38
  prognostic significance 35–6, 38
  recurrent HCC 35
  screening programs 259
  serum ferritin 37
  time trends 33
Africa and HCC 213–15
  aflatoxins 214
  etiology 4, 6, 213–14
  incidence 1, **2**, 3, 213
  prevention 215
  risk factors 213, 214–15
  spontaneous rupture of tumor 193
  survival rates 215
  treatment 215
African iron overload (AIO) 215

Age factors 4
  AFP levels 32
  diagnosing HCC 23
  fibrolamellar HCC in USA 252
  HCC in Europe 219–20, *219*
  HCC in Japan 225
  HCC in Korea 231
  HCC in Taiwan 235, **236**, 243
Alanine aminotransferase (ALT) 153
Albumin
  diagnosing HCC 23, 123, 124
  preoperative risk assessment 154, *154*
Alcohol consumption
  carcinogenesis of HCC 12, **132**
  etiology of HCC 6–7, 214–15, 220, 225, 252
  future prospects 266–7
Alcohol (ethanol) injections 164, 185–6, 195, 222, 242, 263
Aldolase A, as tumor marker 38
Algae 9
Alkaline phosphatase (ALP, SAP) 23, 37
Allelotyping 138, 139, 232–3, **233**, 238
Alphafetoprotein *see* AFP
America *see* Mexico; South America; USA
[^{14}C] aminopyrine breath test 153
Amsacrine *174*
Analgesics 208–9
Anatomy of liver 147–9, **148**, **149**, **150**
Androgen
  etiology of HCC 5
  hormonal therapy 175
Angiography
  hepatic *see* Hepatic angiography
  thorotrast HCC 9, 221, *221*
Anticonvulsants 209
α_1-Antitrypsin (α_1AT, AAT)
  deficiency 6
  as tumor marker 38, 123–4
Antiviral drugs 167, 258, 267
Aorta, cross-clamping 158
Arterial portography, CT (CTAP) 52, 54–5, **68**, 69
Arteriography, CT (CTA) 52, 54, **55**
Ascites
  palliation 209–10
  postoperative complications 161
  preoperative risk assessment 154, **154**
Asia
  etiology of HCC 3–4, 6, 8–9
  incidence of HCC 1, **2**, 3, 4
  spontaneous rupture of tumor 193
  see also Hong Kong; Japan; Korea; Taiwan

Aspartate aminotransferase (AST) 23
Aspergillus spp 9, 135, 266
Aspirin 208, 209
Atypical regenerative nodules *see* Borderline (dysplastic) nodules
Australia, incidence of HCC **2**, 3

Benign nodular proliferations of hepatocytes 110–18
Bile duct 21, 43–4
  cholangiocarcinoma 102
  natural history 101
  obstructive jaundice 195–6, **196**, **197**
  postoperative complications 161
  ultrasonography 48, **49**
Bile duct epithelial cells 78, **78**
  combined HCC and cholangiocarcinoma 102, 121
  cytokeratin positivity 124, **125**
Bilirubin
  diagnosing HCC 23
  postoperative complications 162
  preoperative risk assessment 153, 154, *154*
Biopsy 26–7, 107
  complications 67, 76–7, 107, 151
  contraindications 66, 76, 107
  diagnostic algorithm **68**, 69
  differential diagnoses 108
    benign nodular proliferations of hepatocytes 110–18
    HCC 108–10, **109**
    malignant tumors 121–3, **122**, 124, **125**
    non-neoplastic tumor-like proliferations 118, 120–1
    special stains 123–4, **125**
  extrahepatic metastases 67
  fine-needle aspiration 67, 75–7, 151
  hemangiomas 25
  image-guided percutaneous 66–7, **68**, 76, 108, 240
  portal vein tumors 67
  preoperative investigation 151
  sample adequacy 107–8
Bismuth's nomenclature 45, **46**
Bleomycin *174*, 210
Blood transfusions, etiology of HCC 251–2
Bone metastases
  diagnostic imaging 44, **45**, 46, **46**, 65
  hypercalcemia 199
Borderline (dysplastic) nodules (DN) 10–11, 110–13, **112**, 115, **132**

Borderline nodules *see* Dysplastic nodules
Brain metastasis 44
BRCA2 gene 140
Budd–Chiari syndrome 6, 21

Carbamazepine 209
Carbon dioxide-enhanced ultrasonography 50–1, 240
Des-γ-carboxy prothrombin (DCP) 37–8, 239, 252
Carcinoembryonic antigen (CEA) stain 85, **85**, 123, 124
Carcinogenesis of HCC 12–13
    chemical carcinogens 135–6, 139, 214, 233, 236, 238, 265–6
    chromosomal alterations 12, 134, 137–41, **138**, **141**
        Korea 232–3, **233**
        Taiwan 238
    cirrhotic livers 5, 12, **132**, 136–7
    dysplastic nodules 111
    genomic instability 137–9
    growth-related genes 136–7
    hepadnaviruses infection 12–13, 131, 133–6, 236, 237, 260
    proposed sequence 131, **132**
    proto-oncogenes 136, 137, 232, 237
    Taiwan 237–9
    telomerase activity 141, **141**
    tumor suppressor genes 137, 138, 139–40, 232, 233, 238
Carcinoid syndrome 200
Carcinoid tumors 123
Carcinomas, metastatic 123, 124
Catheterization, hepatic angiography 62, 64–5
    see also Transcatheter treatment
CD24 gene 238–9
CD31, immunocytochemical staining 79, 86
CD34, immunocytochemical staining 79, **80**, 86
Celiac axis
    arteriogram 61, 62
    catheterization 62
Celiac plexus block 209
Chemical agents
    etiology of HCC 8–9, 131, **132**, 214, 236, 265–6
    molecular studies 135–6, 139, 237, 238
Chemoembolization 164–5, 178–9, *179*, 222, 241–2, 262–3
Chemotherapy 173–5
    adjuvant 164, 167, 259, 264
    before resection 159
    combination 173–4, *174*
    complications 176

    contraindications 175
    early diagnosis 258
    fibrolamellar HCC 254
    future prospects 259, 267
    hormonal 175, 179, 222, *222*, 243
    intra-arterial 176–8, *177*, *178*, *179*
    intraperitoneal 210
    liver transplantation 167, 267
    monitoring response to 36, 38
    survival rates 175, 176, *177*
    Taiwan 242
    transcatheter treatment 60, 61, 65, 69
Chest radiography
    diagnosing HCC **22**, 26, 46, **46**, **68**, 69
    preoperative investigations 151
Children
    etiology of HCC 4, 5, 6
    HCC in Taiwan 243–4
    hepatoblastoma 102–3, 103–4, 121, 123, 243
    incidence of HCC in 102, 243–4
    mesenchymal hamartoma 118
    pathology of HCC in 103–4, **104**
Child's hepatic functional reserve 154
China
    etiology of HCC 3–4, 8–9
    incidence of HCC 1, **2**, 3, 4
    see also Hong Kong
Cholangiocarcinomas 121
    with combined HCC 102, **102**, 121, **122**, 124
    fibrolamellar HCC 253
    or HCC variant 23
    immunochemical stains 123, 124, **125**
Cholesterol 199
Chromosomal alterations in HCC 12, 137–41, **138**, **141**
    by HBV DNA 134
    Korea 232–3, **233**
    Taiwan 238
Chronic liver disease
    carcinogenesis of HCC **132**, 136
    diagnosing HCC 20, 34–5, **35**, 258
    prospects for HCC treatment 258
    screening programs 24
    see also Cirrhosis
Cirrhosis
    carcinogenesis of HCC 5, 12, **132**, 136–7
    diagnosing HCC 19, 43, 258
        AFP levels 32–3
        biopsies 67, 108, **109**
        with CT 52, 54, **56**, 69
        decompensation 20, *23*, 222

Cirrhosis – *continued*
  diagnosing HCC – *continued*
    diagnostic algorithm 67, **68**
    erythrocytosis 21
    in Europe 221–2
    magnetic resonance imaging 60
    nuclear imaging 65, 66
    ultrasound scans 25, 47, 48, 49
  differentiation from HCC 108, **109**, 111, 113, **113**, **114**
  dysplasia 113, **113**, **114**
  etiology of HCC 5–6, 7, 213–14, 220–1, 231, 251, 252
  HCC in Africa 213–14, 214–15
  HCC in Europe 220–1, 221–2
  HCC in Korea 231
  HCC in Taiwan 235–6
  hepatectomy 155–9
    in Europe 222
    functional liver reserve 154
    postoperative complications 160, 161, 162
    postoperative prognosis 163
    preoperative investigations 152
    preoperative risk assessment 152–5
    resection margin 164, *164*
  histology of HCC in Japan **227**, **228**, 229
  histology of HCC in Korea 232
  incidence of HCC 89
  liver transplantation 165–6, 167, 222
  macroregenerative nodules 110, 111, 113
  metastatic HCC 101
  molecular studies 136–7
  morphine 209
  prospects for HCC treatment 258
  recurrent HCC 241
  rupture of tumor 193, 195
  screening programs 67–9, **68**, 240
  variceal hemorrhage 197, 210
Cisplatin *174*, 176, 177–9, *177*, *178*, *179*
Clotting function, preoperative 152, 154, *154*
Color Doppler ultrasonography 49, 50, 66, 240
Comparative genomic hybridization (CGH) analysis 139, 140
Computed tomography (CT) 25, 51–6
  advantages 51–2
  applications 51–2, 54, 55, 56
  arterial portography 52, 53–4, **68**, 69
  arteriography 52, 54, **55**
  contrast-enhanced 51, 52–4, **68**, 69
  delayed 55
  detection sensitivity 51, 52, 53–4, 56

hemangiomas 25, 54, 56
  limitations 51, 52
  lipiodol 52, 56, **56**, 62, **68**, 69, 152, 239–40
  monitoring therapy response 36
  MRI compared 53, 56
  preoperative investigations 151, 152, 153
  radiotherapy **182**, **184**
  single photon emission 65–6
  skull metastasis **45**
  spiral 51–2, 53–4, **54**, 55
  Taiwan 239–40
  tumor structures 53, **53**
  ultrasonography compared 47, 51, 53
Concanavalin A (Con A) 33
Congenital abnormalities 4, 5–6
Contrast-enhanced imaging
  CT 51, 52–4, **68**, 69
  MRI 59–60, 111
  ultrasonography 50–1
Cork sign 196, **196**
Couinaud, C.
  hepatectomy classification 149, 150, **150**, *150*
  liver division classification 147, 148, **148**
Cryosurgery 165
Cutaneous symptoms 200
Cycads 9
Cyclin-dependent protein kinases (CDKs) 140
Cytochrome P450 system 7, 135–6, 237
Cytokeratins 111, 123, 124, **125**
Cytokines
  gene therapy 261–2
  postoperative complications 162
  see also Interferon therapy
Cytology of HCC 67, 75–86
  bile duct epithelial cells 78, **78**
  biopsy technique 76
  clear cells 95, **96**
  complications of biopsy 76–7, 151
  contraindications to biopsy 76
  cytoplasmic inclusions 97
  hepatic (liver-like) cell variant 95, **95**
  history 75–6
  immunocytochemical staining 79, **80**, 85–6, **85**, 97
  Kupffer cells 78
  microhistology compared 151
  normal hepatocytes 77–8, **77**
  oncocyte-like cells 95
  pathologist–radiologist cooperation 76
  pleomorphic large cells 81–3, **82**, *85*, 95, **96**
  poorly differentiated cells 83, **83**, **84**, *85*, **96**
  spindle cells 95, 97

well-differentiated cells 79–81, **79**, **80**, **81**, *85*, **95**
WHO classification 95
Cytotoxic drugs 173–5, *174*, 176
  intra-arterial 176–9, *177*, *178*, *179*
  use in Taiwan 242

Decompensation, hepatic 20, *23*, 222
Delayed computed tomography 55
Des-γ-carboxy prothrombin (DCP) 37–8, 239, 252
Diagnostic algorithm 67–9, **68**
Diagnostic imaging 25–6
  algorithm 67–9, **68**
  Bismuth's nomenclature 45, **46**
  computed tomography *see* Computed
    tomography
  future prospects 267
  gross morphology of HCC 43–4, **44**, **45**, 53, **53**
  hepatic angiography 60–5
  magnetic resonance imaging 56–60, **57**, **58**, **68**,
    69, 111
  nuclear 62, 65–6, 69, 111, 183–4, 267
  plain radiography **22**, 26, 45–6, **46**, **68**, 69, 151
  preoperative investigations 151–2
  role 45
  Taiwan 239–40
  ultrasonography *see* Ultrasonography
Diaphragm
  invasion by HCC **22**, 44, 46, **46**
  resection 159, **160**
Direct intralesional treatment 185–6, 195, 222, 242
Diuretics, ascite palliation 209
DNA 12, 131, **132**
  chromosomal alterations 139, 238
  cirrhotic livers 5, 136
  clonality of HCC 239
  genomic instability in HCC 138, 139
  HBV and aflatoxins 135–6
  HBV and HCV genomes 12, 131, 133, **133**, 237
  HBV transactivation of cellular genes 134–5
  insertional mutagenesis by HBV 133–4
Doloxene Co 209
Doppler ultrasonography 49, 50, 66, 240
Doxorubicin 174–5, **174**, 176, 177–8, *177*
Drug treatments
  etiology of HCC 6
  HCC therapy *see* Chemotherapy
Duplex Doppler ultrasonography 49, 240
Dysplasia 10, 11, 113–15, **114**
  in Africa 213–14
  carcinogenesis of HCC **132**
Dysplastic nodules (DN) 10–11, 110–13, **112**, 115, **132**

E-cadherin gene 139
Early HCC *see* Small (early) HCC
Edmondson grading system 97–8, **99**
Elderly people, etiology of HCC 4
Embolization
  before resection 159
  future prospects 262–3
  hepatic arterial 186
  ruptured HCC 64–5, 194–5
  transarterial chemoembolization 164–5, 178–9,
    179, 222, 241–2, 262–3
  transcatheter arterial 241
Encephalopathy
  diagnosing HCC *23*
  preoperative risk assessment 154, **154**
Endocrine syndromes 21–22, 200
Epidemiology of HCC 1–3, *2*, 89, 131
  Africa 1, **2**, 3, 213
  Europe 1, **2**, 3, 4, 219–21
  incidence in children 102, 243–4
  incidence of metastatic HCC 101
  incidence trends 4
  Japan **2**, 3, 4, 225
  Korea 1, **2**, 3, 231
  prospects for treatment 257–8, 259
  Taiwan 1, **2**, 3, 235, 243–4
  USA 1, **2**, 3, 4, 251
4′-epidoxorubicin 174–5, **174**, 176, 178
Epithelioid hemangioendothelioma 23
Epstein–Barr virus 120
Erythrocytosis 21, 198–9
Erythropoietin (Epo) 199
Estrogen
  etiology of HCC 5, 221
  hormonal therapy 175, 179
Ethanol injection 164, 185–6, 195, 222, 242, 263
Ethiodol *see* Lipiodol; Lipiodolization
Etiology of HCC 3–9, 131, **132**
  Africa 4, 6, 213–15
  Europe 4, 8, 220–21
  Japan 6, 8, 9, 225
  Korea 231–2
  screening 259
  Taiwan 7–8, 235–7, 243–4
  USA 8, 251–2
Europe and HCC 219–23
  diagnosis 221–2
  epidemiology 1, **2**, 3, 4, 219–21
  fibrolamellar variant 223
  HCV 8, 220–1, *220*
  mortality rates 3

Europe and HCC – *continued*
  presenting signs 222
  prognosis 223
  spontaneous rupture of tumor 193
  treatment 222, *222*

Factor VIII 79, 86
Factor XIIIa 123, 124
Ferritin, as tumor marker 36–7
α-fetoprotein (AFP) *see* AFP (α-fetoprotein)
Fibrolamellar HCC
  chemotherapy 254
  clinical features 22–3, 26, 252
  differential diagnoses 253
  in Europe 223
  hepatectomy 254
  incidence 252
  liver transplantation 166, 254
  morphology 90, 93, 95, 252–4, **253**, **254**
  pleomorphic cells 83
  prognosis 254
  in USA 252–4
Fine-needle aspiration biopsy (FNAB) 67
  see also Fine-needle aspiration cytology
Fine-needle aspiration cytology 67, 75–86
  bile duct epithelial cells 78, **78**
  biopsy technique 76
  complications of biopsy 76–7, 151
  contraindications to biopsy 76
  history 75–6
  immunocytochemical staining 79, **80**, 85–6, **85**
  Kupffer cells 78
  normal hepatocytes 77–8, **77**
  pathologist–radiologist cooperation 76
  pleomorphic large cells 81–3, **82**, *85*
  poorly differentiated 83, **83**, **84**, *85*
  well-differentiated cells 79–81, **79**, **80**, **81**, *85*
Fluoropyrimidines *174*, 176, *177*
Focal necrotic nodule 120–1, **121**
Focal nodular hyperplasia (FNH) 117–18, **117**
Follicular dendritic cell tumor 120
Food storage, fungal infection 9, 135, 238, 266
Fouchet's stain 123
α-ʟ-fucosidase 39
Functional Life Index Cancer (FLIC) 206, **207**, 208
Functional liver reserve 154, **154**, 162
Fungi 9, 135
  see also Aflatoxins

Gadolinium-enhanced MRI 59, 60, 111
Gall bladder, adenosquamous carcinoma 253–4

Gallium-67 scintigraphy 65
Gastrointestinal bleeding
  causes 210
  diagnosing HCC 20, *23*, 43, 64
  palliation 210
  postoperative 160–1, **160**
  variceal 197, 210
Gelfoam, chemoembolization 178–9, *179*
Gendered differences in HCC
  AFP levels 32
  Africa 215
  diagnosis 19, *23*
  etiology 4–5, 5–6
  Europe 220
  Korea 231
  rare syndromes 200
  Taiwan 243
Gene therapy in HCC 142, 261–2, 266, 267
Gene transfer in HCC 142
Genetic factors in HCC 5–6, 215, 237
Genetic mutations 12–13, 131, **132**, 237–9
  aflatoxins 135–6, 139, 238, 266
  chromosomal alterations in HCC 12, 134,
    137–41, **138**, **141**, 232–3, 238
  cirrhotic livers 136–7
  gene therapy in HCC 142
  gene transfer in HCC 142
  genomic instability in HCC 137–9
  growth-related genes 136–7
  HCC in Africa 214
  HCC in Korea 232–3
  hepadnaviruses infection 12–13, 131, 133–6, 237
  proto-oncogenes 136, 137, 232, 237
  tumor suppressor genes 137, 138, 139–40, 232,
    233, 238
Genomic instability in HCC 137–9
  hepadnaviruses infection 12–13, 131, 133, 237
Geographic distribution of HCC 1–3, **2**
γ-Glutamyltranspeptidase isoenzyme 37
Glycogen storage disease 5
Goldsmith and Woodburne
  hepatectomy classification 149, *150*
  liver anatomy 147, 148
Growth factors
  carcinogenesis of HCC 136, 137, **137**, 140, 239
  gene therapy 261–2
  hypercalcemia 199
  hypoglycemia 198
  postoperative complications 162
  as tumor markers 239
Gynecomastia 22

Healey and Schroy
  hepatectomy classification 149, 150
  liver division classification 147–8, **148**
Helical (spiral) CT 51–2, 53–4, **54**, 55
Hemangiomas 25–6, 49, 50, 54, 56, 59
Hemobilia 21, 196
Hemochromatosis, genetic 5, 215
Hemodynamics
  color Doppler ultrasonography 49, 50
  postoperative complications 162
Hemoperitoneum
  diagnosing HCC 20, *23*, 43, 64
  management 193
Hemorrhage
  gastrointestinal 20, *23*, 43, 64, 160–1, **160**, 210
  intraoperative 157–9
  postoperative 160–1, **160**
  spontaneous tumor rupture 194, 195
  variceal 197, 210
Hep Par 1 (clone OCH 1E5) 124, **125**
Hepadnaviruses infection, carcinogenesis of HCC
    12–13, 131, 133–6, 236, 237, 260
  see also Hepatitis A; Hepatitis B; Hepatitis C;
    Hepatitis D
Hepatectomy
  adjuvant therapy 164–5, 267
  Africa 215
  anatomical vs non-anatomical 156–7
  classification 149–51, **150**, *150*
  early diagnosis 258
  Europe 222
  extending limits of 159, **160**
  fibrolamellar HCC 254
  future prospects 263, 267
  incisions 155
  intraoperative ultrasound 156
  liver insufficiency after 153–5, 162
  mobilization of liver 155–6
  palliative 165
  postoperative complications 160–2, *160*
  preoperative investigations 151–2
  preoperative preparations 160, 161, 162
  preoperative risk assessment 152–5
  prognosis 162–4, 240–1
  resection margin 156, 163–4
  retractors 155
  Taiwan 240–1
  transarterial chemoembolization 164–5
  vascular control 157–9
Hepatic angiography 60–5
  approaches 61–2

catheterization 62, 64
diagnostic algorithm **68**, 69
general appearances 63, *63*
hepatic arterial embolization 186
hepatic artery anomalies 60–1, **61**
hepatic vein invasion 63–4, **64**
preoperative 151, 152
spontaneous rupture of HCC 64–5, 195
transcatheter treatment 60, 61, 65, 69
Hepatic arterial embolization 186
Hepatic arterial perfusion scintigraphy 62,
    66, 69
Hepatic artery
  angiographic appearance 63, *63*
  anomalies 60–1, **61**
  catheterization 62
  intra-arterial chemotherapy 178
  portal vein invasion 63, *63*, **64**
  selective internal radiation 180–1
  selective Pringle maneuver 157–8
Hepatic decompensation 20, *23*, 222
Hepatic functional reserve 154, **154**, 162
Hepatic veins
  anatomical classifications 148–9
  intraoperative ultrasound 156
  invasion by HCC 21, 43
    computed tomography 51, **51**
    hepatic angiography 63–4, **64**
    natural history 101
Hepatitis A infection 8
Hepatitis B infection
  carcinogenesis of HCC 12–13
    see also Hepatitis B virus
  diagnosing HCC 19
    AFP levels 32–3, 35
    diagnostic algorithm 67, **68**
    Mallory bodies 97
  dysplastic nodules 11
  etiology of HCC 3, 5, 6–7
    Africa 213–14
    Europe 220–1
    Japan 225
    Korea 231–2
    Taiwan 7–8, 235–6, *236*, 237, 243
    USA 251
  histology of related cirrhosis **228**, 229
  immunization against 243–4, 265
  incidence of HCC 1–3, *2*, 89, 220, 257
  liver transplantation 167
  prospects for HCC therapy 257
  screening programs 24–5, 67–9, **68**, 259

Hepatitis B surface antigen (HBsAg)
  AFP levels 32
  HCC in Africa 213
  HCC in Japan 225
  HCC in Taiwan 235, **236**, 243
  immunocytochemical stains 85
  Mallory bodies 97
Hepatitis B virus 131, **132**
  aflatoxins 135–6, 265–6
  carrier rate 89, 265
  genome 12–13, 131, 133, **133**, 237
  HCC in Africa 213
  immunization 243–4, 265
  insertional mutagenesis of cellular genes
    133–4
  transactivation of cellular genes 134–5
Hepatitis C infection
  diagnosing HCC 19, 26
  etiology of HCC 8
    Europe 220–1, *220*
    Japan 8, 225
    Korea 231–2
    Taiwan 235–6
    USA 8, 251–2
  histology of related cirrhosis **228**, 229
  incidence of HCC 89, 133
  interferon therapy 260–1
  screening programs 24–5, 259
  see also Hepatitis C virus
Hepatitis C virus 131, **132**
  future prospects 267
  genome 131, 133, 237
  interferon therapy 260–1, **260**
Hepatitis D infection 8, 214, 236
Hepatitis E infection 8
Hepatitis G infection 236
Hepatoblastoma 102–3, 103–4, 121, 123, 243
Hepatocarcinogenesis *see* Carcinogenesis of HCC
Hepatocellular adenomas *see* Adenomas
Hepatocellular pseudotumors *see* Dysplastic
    nodules
Hepatocytes
  benign nodular proliferations 10–11, 110–18
  HCC 108–10, **109**
  immunochemical stains 124
  normal cytology 77–8, **77**
Hepatomegaly 20, 225–6
Heterozygosity, loss in HCC 138, **138**, 139–40,
    232–3, 238
Hilar structures, intraoperative bleeding 158–9
Histochemistry 123

Histology of HCC 26–7, 90–5, 107
  acinar cells 91, 93, **93**
  biopsy problems 107–8
  compact type 93, **94**
  differential diagnoses 108
    benign nodular proliferations 110–18
    HCC 108–10, **109**
    malignant tumors 121–3, **122**, 124, **125**
    non-neoplastic tumor-like proliferations 118,
      120–1
    special stains 123–4, **125**
  diffuse type 90, **91**
  encapsulation 90, **91**, 101, 226
  fibrolamellar 93, 95, 252–4, **253**, **254**
  Japan 226, **228**, 229
  Korea 232
  massive type 90, **91**
  multinodular type 90, **91**
  non-cancerous liver tissue **228**, 229
  pedunculated type 90, **91**
  pseudoglandular cells 91, 93, **93**
  scirrhous type 93, **94**
  smear cytology compared 151
  trabecular 90–1, **92**
Hong Kong
  chromosomal alterations in HCC 138, 139, 140
  etiology of HCC 4
  incidence of HCC 1, **2**, 3, 89
  mortality rates from HCC 3
  telomerase activity in HCC 141
Hormonal therapy 175, 179, 222, *222*, 242, 243
Hospice care 210
Hypercalcemia 22, 23, 199
Hypercholesterolemia 199
Hyperchromasia 97, **99**
Hyperthyroidism 22, 200
Hypoglycemia 22, 161–2, 198

Icteric type HCC 195–7, **196**, **197**, 241
Imaging in HCC diagnosis *see* Diagnostic
    imaging
Immunization, hepatitis 243–4, 265, 267
Immunochemical stains 79, **80**, 85–6, **85**, 97
  differential diagnoses 111, 113, 123–4, **125**
  see also Tumor markers
Immunotherapy *174*, 175–6, 242, 259, 260–1, 262
  radioimmunoglobulins 180
Incidence of HCC *see* Epidemiology of HCC
Incisions for hepatectomies 155
India **2**, 3, 6
Indocyanine green retention rate (ICG R) 153

Inferior vena cava
  anatomical classifications 148, 149, **149**
  etiology of HCC 6
  intraoperative cross-clamping 158
  invasion by HCC 21, **21**
    diagnostic imaging 43, **44**, 51, **51**
    natural history 101
  membranous obstruction 21, 214
Inflammatory pseudotumor 118, 120
Inhibin 124
Insulin-like growth factor II 198, 239
Interferon therapy *174*, 175–6, 242, 259, 260, 262
Internal radiotherapy
  with radioimmunoglobulins 180
  selective (SIR) 36, 180–5, 242, 262, 264, 267
Intra-arterial treatment 176–9, *177*, *178*, *179*
Intracranial metastasis 44, **45**
Intralesional treatment 185–6, 195, 222, 242
Intraoperative ultrasound (IUS) 50, 156, 240
Intraperitoneal chemotherapy 210
Iodine radionuclides
  nuclear imaging 65
  selective internal radiation 180–1, **181–2**, *182*,
    242, 264
Iron overload, African (AIO) 215
Isoelectric focusing (IEF), AFP isoforms 33–5, **34**,
  35, 39

Japan and HCC 225–9
  clinical aspects 225–6
  etiology 6, 8, 9, 225
  incidence **2**, 3, 4, 225
  pathomorphology 226–9, **228–9**
Jaundice 195–7
  diagnosing HCC 20, 21, *23*
  icteric type 195–7, **196**, **197**
  incidence 195
  natural history of HCC 101
  5'-nucleotide phosphodiesterase V 38

Korea and HCC 231–3
  genetic alterations 232–3, **233**
  incidence 1, **2**, 3, 231
  pathology 232–3, **233**
Kupffer cells 78, 162

Laminin 124
Laparoscopic ultrasonography 50
Large cell dysplasia (LCD) 10, 11, 113, **113**, 213–14
Laserthermia 242–3

Lectin-binding affinities of AFP 33, 239
Lentil lectin 33, 239
Leucovorin *177*
Levovist-enhanced color Doppler 50
Life expectancy
  early diagnosis 258–9
  palliative care 264
Lipiodol
  dysplastic nodules 111
  hepatic angiography 62
  selective internal radiation 180–1, **181**, **182**, *182*,
    242, 264
Lipiodol computed tomography 52, 56, **56**, 62, **68**,
  69
  preoperative investigations 152
  Taiwan 240
Lipiodolization 164, 177–8, *178*
Liver cell dysplasia (LCD) 10, 11, 113, **113**, 213–14
Liver function sufficiency 152–4, 162
Liver function tests 26
Liver transplantation 165–7
  Europe 222
  fibrolamellar HCC 254
  future prospects 263, 267
  monitoring response 35
Living standards 4, 6
Lobectomy, classification 149–50, **150**, *150*
Loss of heterozygosity (LOH) analysis 138, **138**,
  139–40, 232–3, 238
Lung metastasis **22**, 26, 44, **46**, 69, 101
Lung shunting, after SIR 184–5
Lymph node metastasis 101

Macroregenerative (dysplastic) nodules (DN)
  10–11, 110–13, **112**, 115, **132**
Magnetic resonance imaging (MRI) 56–60
  advantages 56
  applications 56–7, 57–8, 59
  contrast-enhanced 59–60
  conventional spin-echo 57–8, **57**
  CT compared 53, 56
  detection sensitivity 56, 59
  diagnostic algorithm **68**, 69
  dysplastic nodules 111
  fast (turbo) spin-echo 58–9, **58**
  limitations 56–7
  pseudocapsule **57**, 58
Mallory bodies 97
Malnutrition 6
Manganese-DPDP-enhanced MRI 60
Mechloethamine *177*

Membranous obstruction of inferior vena cava 21, 214
Men *see* Gendered differences in HCC
Mercedes–Benz incision 155
Mesenchymal hamartoma 118
Metabolic disorders 5, **132**
Metastases (non-HCC)
  adenocarcinoma 121
  carcinoid 123
  carcinoma 123, 124
  focal necrotic nodule 120
  hypercalcemia 199
  immunochemical staining 85–6, 123, 124
  spiral CT 54
Metastatic HCC 44
  computed tomography **44**, **45**, 51, **51**
  diagnostic algorithm 69
  early diagnosis 258
  image-guided biopsy 67
  natural history 101
  nuclear imaging 65
  plain radiography **22**, 26, 45–6, **46**
  preoperative investigations 151, 152
  rare presentations 21, **22**
  ultrasonography **44**, **45**, 49
Mexico, incidence of HCC 4
Microwave tissue coagulation 165
Middle East, HCC incidence 2, 3
Migrant populations
  etiology of HCC 4
  incidence of HCC 3, 220, 251
Mitomycin C *174*, *177*
Mitoxantrone 174–5, *174*
Molecular studies
  chemical carcinogens 135–6, 139, 237, 238
  chromosomal alterations in HCC 12, 134,
    137–41, **138**, **141**, 238
  cirrhotic livers 136–7
  gene therapy in HCC 142
  gene transfer in HCC 142
  genomic instability in HCC 137–9
  growth-related genes 136–7
  hepadnaviruses infection 12–13, 131, 133–6, 237
  Korea 232–3, **233**
  proto-oncogenes 136, 137, 232, 237
  Taiwan 237–9
  telomerase activity 141, **141**
  tumor suppressor genes 137, 138, 139–40, 142,
    232, 233, 238
Monoclonal antibodies 180
Morphine 209

Morphology of HCC 108–10, **109**
  biopsy problems 107–8, 151
  differential diagnoses 108
    benign nodular proliferations 110–18
    malignant tumors 121–3, **122**, 124, **125**
    non-neoplastic tumor-like proliferations 118,
      120–1
    special stains 123–4, **125**
  gross appearance 43–4, **44**, **45**, 89–90, **91**
    classification 43, 89–90
    contrast-enhanced CT 53, **53**
    Japan 226, **227**
    Korea 232
  microscopic appearance 90–101
    clear cells 95, **96**
    compact type 93, **94**
    cytological classification 95–7
    cytoplasmic inclusions 97
    fibrolamellar variant 93, 95, 252–4, **253**, **254**
    growth pattern 95, 97, **98**
    hepatic cells 95, **95**
    histologic classification 90–5
    hyperchromasia 97, **99**
    in Japan 226, **228**, 229
    Korea 232
    oncocyte-like cells 95
    pleomorphic cells 95, **96**, 97, 98, **99**
    prognostic significance 98–9
    pseudoglandular 91, 93, **93**, 97, **99**
    scirrhous type 93, **94**
    small (early) HCC 99–101
    spindle cells 95, 97
    trabecular pattern 90–1, **92**, 97, **99**
    tumor grading 97–9, **99**
    see also Cytology of HCC
Mortality rates
  from HCC 3
  postoperative 162–3, **163**
  spontaneous tumor rupture 195
mRNA expression **133**, 238

Naproxen 208
Narcotic analgesics 208, 209
Needle biopsy *see* Biopsy
Needle stick injuries 77
Neocarzinostatin *174*
Nodular regenerative hyperplasia (NRH) 11, 118,
  119
Nodules-in-nodules *see* Borderline (dysplastic)
  nodules
Non-cirrhotic HCC, diagnosis 23, *23*, 26

Non-cirrhotic nodulation (nodular regenerative hyperplasia) 11, 118, **119**
Non-neoplastic tumor-like proliferations 118, 120–1
Non-steroidal anti-inflammatory drugs (NSAIDS) 208–9
Nuclear imaging 65–6
  benign nodular proliferation of hepatocytes 111
  future prospects 267
  hepatic arterial perfusion scintigraphy 62, 66, 69
  radiotherapy 183–4
5'-Nucleotide phosphodiesterase V 38
Nutrition 6, 12

Obstructive jaundice 195–7
  diagnosing HCC 21
  icteric type classification 195–7, **196**, **197**
  incidence 195
  natural history of HCC 101
OK-432 242
Oltipraz 266, **266**, 267
Omentum, invasion by HCC 44, **45**
Oral contraceptives 5, 115, 221
Orthotopic liver transplantation 167

p53 12, 135, 139–40
  gene therapy in HCC 142, 261, 266
  HCC in Africa 214
  HCC in Korea 233
  HCC in Taiwan 238
Pain, diagnosing HCC 19–20, 23, 64, 193
Pain control 205, 208–9
Pain scales 205–6, **206**
Palliative care 205–10
  disease-orientated 205
    Europe 222
    hepatic arterial embolization 186
    see also Chemoembolization; Chemotherapy; Radiotherapy
  future prospects 264–5
  hepatectomy 165
  hospices 210
  pain control 205, 208–9
  pain scales 205–6, **206**
  palliation defined 205
  quality of life measures 206, **207**, 208
  role of 205
Paracentesis, abdominal 209
Paracetamol 208
Paraneoplastic syndromes 21–2, 197–200

Parasitic infections 6, **132**
Parathyroid hormone-related peptide 199
Partial nodular transformation (nodular regenerative hyperplasia) 11, 118, **119**
PAS stain 123
Pathology of HCC 89
  in children 102, 103–4, **103**
  with cholangiocarcinoma 102, **102**
  fibrolamellar 252–4, **253**, **254**
  gross appearance 43–4, **44**, **45**, 53, **53**, 89–90, **91**
  in Japan 226–9, **228–9**
  in Korea 232
  microscopic appearance 90–101
  natural history 101
  spread 101
  see also Cytology of HCC; Histology of HCC
Penicillium islandicum 9
Percutaneous ethanol injections (PEI) 185–6, 242
Percutaneous needle biopsy *see* Biopsies
Periodic acid-Schiff (PAS) stain 123
Peritoneal spread of HCC 44, **45**
Peritoneovenous shunting 209
Pesticides 8–9
Phenytoin 209
PiZ gene 6
Plain radiography **22**, 26, 45–6, **46**, **68**, 69, 151
Planar imaging 65
Plant carcinogens 9
Platelet-derived growth factor 140
Pleural effusion, postoperative 161
PML-RAR-α protein 137
Polyprenoic acid 164–5, 264
Porphyria, hepatic 5
Portal vein
  anatomical classifications 148, **149**
  extending resection limits 159
  intraoperative ultrasound 156
  invasion by HCC 43
    biopsy 67
    hepatic angiography 63, **63**, **64**
    natural history 101
    ultrasonographic scan **48**
  postoperative thrombosis 162
  selective Pringle maneuver 157–8
  variceal hemorrhage and thrombus 197
Positron emission tomography (PET) 66
Power Doppler ultrasonography 49
Precancerous changes 9–11
  dysplastic nodules 10–11, 110, 111
  nodular regenerative hyperplasia 11
  see also Carcinogenesis of HCC

Presenting modes of HCC 19–22, 258
Prevention of HCC 215, 243–4, 258–9, 265–7
Pringle maneuver 157–8
Prognosis
    AFP parameters 35–6, 38
    chemoembolization 178–9, 241
    chemotherapy 175, 176, *177*
    early diagnosis 258–9
    fibrolamellar HCC 254
    HCCs in Africa 215
    HCCs in Europe 223
    immunotherapy 175–6
    intralesional treatment 185
    late presentation 258
    pathologic parameters 98–9, 101
    postoperative survival 162–4, *163*, *164*, 166–7,
        166, 240–1
    radiotherapy 179–80, 185, 242, 264
    time course of tumor growth **259**
    tumor size 98–9
Protease inhibitor (Pi) genes 6
Prothrombin, des-γ-carboxy 37–8, 239, 252
Prothrombin time (PT)
    diagnosing HCC 23
    preoperative risk assessment 152, 154, *154*
Proto-oncogenes 136, 137, 232, 237
Public health, future of 257, 258–9
Pugh–Child hepatic functional reserve 154, **154**
Pyrexia of unknown origin 21
Pyrrolizidine alkaloids 9

Quality of life measures 206, **207**, 208

Radiation, etiology of HCC 9, 221, *221*
Radiography, plain *22*, 26, 45–6, *46*, **68**, 69, 151
Radioimmunoglobulins 180
Radionuclide scintigraphy *see* Nuclear imaging
Radiotherapy 179–85
    before resection 159
    external beam irradiation 179–80, 242
    internal irradiation with radioimmunoglobulins
        180
    monitoring response to 36, 185
    selective internal radiation 36, 180–5, 242, 262,
        264, 267
    side effects 180, 183, 185
    survival rates 179–80, 185
    Taiwan 242
Rb gene 140

Recurrent HCC
    adjuvant therapy 164–5, 167, 259, 264
    AFP 27, 28, 35, 67
    after tumor biopsy 67
    diagnosis 27–8
    fibrolamellar 254
    intralesional treatment 185
    management 241, 264
    postoperative prognosis 162–3, 240–1
    in transplanted livers 166–7
Redox tolerance index (RTI) 153
Regional nerve blocks 209
Retractors, hepatectomies 155
Retroperitoneal extension of HCC 44, **44**, 101
Retroviruses, gene therapy 142, 261, 262
Rex–Cantlie line 147, **149**
Risk factors for HCC 3–9, 19, 131, **132**
    Africa 4, 6, 213, 214–15
    Europe 4, 8, 220–1
    Japan 6, 8, 9, 225
    Korea 231–2
    screening 259
    Taiwan 7–8, 235–7
    USA 8, 251–2
RNA, HBV and HCV genomes 133
Rupture of tumor *see* Spontaneous rupture of
    HCC

Screening 23–5
    asymptomatic presentation of HCC 20–1
    for early diagnosis 258–9
    future prospects 267
    obstacles 24–5
    reasons for failure 24, *24*
    Taiwan 240
Segmentectomies 150–1, 156
Selective internal radiation (SIR) 36, 180–5, **181–4**,
        182, 242, 262, 267
Sepsis, postoperative 161
Sex hormones
    etiology of HCC 4–5
    hepatocellular adenoma 115
    hormonal therapy 175, 179, 222, 242, 243
    rare syndromes in HCC 200
Sex-related differences *see* Gendered differences in
    HCC
Sexual changes with HCC 200
Single photon emission CT (SPECT) 65–6
Skin problems 200
Skull metastasis 44, **45**
Small cell dysplasia (SCD) 11, **114**, 115

Small (early) HCC
  or borderline macroregenerative nodules 101, 111, 113
  criteria for 10
  early diagnosis 258
  early treatment 259
  intralesional treatment 185–6, 242
  intraoperative ultrasound 156
  Japan 226, **227**, 229
  laserthermia 242–3
  morphology 99–101, **100**
  time course of tumor growth **259**
Smoking 7, 215, 237, 252
Solitary necrotic nodule 120–1, **121**
South America, incidence of HCC 1, **2**, 3
Spiral CT 51–2, 53–4, **54**
  arterial portography 55
Spironolactone 209
Spontaneous rupture of HCC 20, *23*, 43, 193
  embolization 64–5, 194–5
  hepatic angiography 64–5, 195
  incidence 194
  management 193–5, **194**
  natural history 101
  presenting signs 193
  risk factors 193
Sterigmatocystin 9
Steroids
  adjuvant analgesia 209
  etiology of HCC 4–5
  hepatocellular adenoma 115
  hormonal therapy 175, 179, 243
  sex changes in HCC 200
Streptozotocin *174*, *177*
Styrene maleic acid neocarzinostatin (SMANCS) 177, *178*
Suicide gene paradigm 261
Sulfur colloid scintigraphy 65
Superior mesenteric vein 43
Superparamagnetic iron oxide-enhanced MRI 59–60
Surgical treatment
  adjuvant therapy 164–5, 167, 259, 264, 267
  Africa 215
  anatomical vs non-anatomical resection 156–7
  anatomy of liver 147–9, **148**, **149**, **150**
  assessing disease extent 151–2
  cryoablation 165
  early diagnosis 258
  Europe 222
  extending resection limits 159, **160**

fibrolamellar HCC 254
  future prospects 263, 267
  hepatectomy classification 149–51, **150**, *150*
  incisions for hepatectomy 155
  intraoperative ultrasonography 50, 156, 240
  mobilization of liver 155–6
  monitoring response to 35, 38, 67, **68**, 263–4
  palliative hepatectomies 165
  postoperative complications 160–2, *160*
  postoperative follow up 155
  postoperative survival rates 162–4, *163*, *164*, 167
    future prospects 263
    liver transplantation 166, *166*, 167
  preoperative investigations 151–2
  preoperative preparations 160, 161, 162
  preoperative risk assessment 152–5
  prognosis after resection 162–4, 240–1
  recurrences 27, 28, 162–3, 240–1, 264
  resection margin 156, 163–4
  retractors for hepatectomies 155
  spontaneous rupture of HCC 194, 195
  Taiwan 240–1
  transarterial chemoembolization 164–5
  transplantation 35, 165–7, 254, 263, 267
  tumor biopsy 27, 67, 151
  vascular control 157–9
Systemic chemotherapy *see* Chemotherapy

Taiwan and HCC 235–44
  carcinogenesis 237–9
  children 243–4
  diagnosis 239–40
  etiology 7–8, 235–7, 243
  incidence 1, **2**, 3, 235, 243–4
  prevention 243–4, 265
  treatment 240–3
Tamoxifen 175, 178–9, 222, *222*, 242
Technetium-99m nuclear imaging 62, 65, 66, 69, 183–4
Telomerase activity in HCC 141, **141**
Thallium-201 SPECT 66
Thorotrast 9, 221, *221*
Thrombi 159, 197
Thrombosis, postoperative 162
Thymidine kinase (TK) 261
Time course of tumor growth **259**
Tissue polypeptide antigen (TPA) 38–9
Tobacco smoking 7, 215, 237, 252
Transabdominal ultrasonography 47–8, **48**, **49**
Transarterial chemoembolization 164–5, 178–9, *179*, 222, 242–3, 262–3

Transcatheter arterial embolization (TAE) 241
Transcatheter treatment
    hepatic angiography 60, 61, 65, 69
    hepatic artery anomalies 61
Tumor markers 31–9, 239
    AFP 31–6, 37, 38, 39, 123–4, 185, 239, 259, 262
    aldolase A 38
    alkaline phosphatase 37
    α-1-antitrypsin 38, 123–4
    des-γ-carboxy prothrombin 37–8, 239, 252
    cholangiocarcinoma 123
    CT images compared 36
    differential diagnoses 123–4, **125**
    essential characteristics 31
    α-L-fucosidase 39
    γ-glutamyltranspeptidase 37
    inhibin 124
    internal radiotherapy 262
    laminin 124
    lectin-binding 33, 239
    metastatic tumors 123–4
    monitoring treatment responses 35–6, 185
    5'-nucleotide phosphodiesterase V 38
    screening programs 259
    serum ferritin 36–7
    Taiwan 239
    tissue polypeptide antigen 38–9
    uses 31
Tumor necrosis factor-α (TNF-α) 162, 261–2
Tumor suppressor genes 137, 138, 139–40, 232, 233, 238
    gene therapy in HCC 142, 261, 266
Tyrosinemia 5

Ultrasonography (US, USS) 25, 46–50
    advantages 46–7
    applications 46–7
    carbon dioxide-enhanced 50–1, 240
    CT compared 47, 51, 53

detection sensitivity 47, 49
diagnostic algorithm 67–9, **68**
Doppler 49, 50, 66, 240
hemangiomas 25, 49, 50
image-guided biopsy 66–7, 76, 108, 240
inferior vena cava invasion **44**
intraoperative 50, 156, 240
laparoscopic 50
limitations 47
metastases **44**, **45**, 49
mosaic pattern 47, **48**
preoperative 151
screening programs 259
Taiwan 239–40
transabdominal 47–8, **48**, **49**
USA and HCC 251–4
    etiology 8, 251–2
    fibrolamellar variant 252–4
    incidence 1, **2**, 3, 4, 251
    mortality rates 3

Vaccines, hepatitis 243–4, 260, 265, 267
Variceal hemorrhage 197, 210
Vinblastine *174*
Viral serology 26
Volume-acquisition (spiral) CT 51–2, 53–4, **54**, 55
VP-16 *174*, 242

Weight loss, diagnosing HCC 19, *23*
Wilson's disease 5–6
Women *see* Gendered differences in HCC
World distribution of HCC 1–3, **2**
World Health Organization (WHO)
    HCC classification 90–5
    pain control 208

Yttrium-90, internal radiotherapy 180, 181–5, *182*, **183**, **184**, 262